HEALING
IN A
CHANGING
AMERICA

Doctoring in a Nation of
Needless Suffering

GEORGE RUST, MD, MPH

JOHNS HOPKINS UNIVERSITY PRESS | BALTIMORE

© 2025 Johns Hopkins University Press
All rights reserved. Published 2025
Printed in the United States of America on acid- free paper
9 8 7 6 5 4 3 2 1

Johns Hopkins University Press
2715 North Charles Street
Baltimore, Maryland 21218
www.press.jhu.edu

Library of Congress Cataloging-in-Publication Data is available.

A catalog record for this book is available from the British Library.

ISBN 978-1-4214-5304-0 (hardcover)
ISBN 978-1-4214-5305-7 (ebook)

Special discounts are available for bulk purchases of this book. For more information, please contact Special Sales at specialsales@jh.edu.

EU GPSR Authorized Representative
LOGOS EUROPE, 9 rue Nicolas Poussin,
17000, La Rochelle, France
E-mail: Contact@logoseurope.eu

To Cindy,
The love of my life
Who taught me how to love
And to be loved.

CONTENTS

HEALING AND HOPE

HEALING IN A CHANGING AMERICA

FACTS

1.

Leaving White-World
A White Guy's Journey in a Non-White America

(Toto, I've got a feeling we're not in Kansas anymore)

I grew up in one world, but I've spent most of my life working in another. I grew up in white-world, where everyone looked like me and we all spoke English. From birth to high school and medical school, I lived in a world where white Anglo norms were society's norms. Other people's perspectives were "ethnic" or "cultural." Our sense of "normal" set the boundaries between us and others. And then the boundaries moved. Or I moved.

There came a moment when I decided that I needed to make a difference in the world. My own insecurities, my family dysfunction, and my college roommate's suicide all left me questioning my choices and my value as a person. All I had was this vague, poorly defined sense that I wanted to help people, especially the people who needed help most. I needed to be needed. So, I moved.

I switched first from being an English major at Harvard to being a premed chemistry major at the University of Miami. I learned about yogurt and Boston accents and arrogance at Harvard and Cuban coffee and Jesus at the U.

I was trying to find my place in the world. In one sense, I had grown up not only in white-world but in privileged white-world. Boca Raton. Palm Beach County. Bastion of wealth and privilege. I went to high school at an elite college prep school, with sons of real wealth and privilege. Children of the Dodge auto family and Musselman's applesauce. Son of a world-famous golf course designer. Sons of (ho-hum) doctors, lawyers, and airline pilots. But only the sons.

I didn't entirely fit in, and maybe that was good. I was a local kid, not a rich kid sent to boarding school. My dad was in real estate, and then he was a banker. Even so, he struggled to make ends meet for two boys and our stay-at-home artist mom. He had to push past crippling depression, working to pay for private school for his sons. I was one of the smarter kids, even in this elite prep school, which is how I ended up doing time at Harvard. I was also a school janitor on a work-study program. I studied with, hung out with, and cleaned the toilets of the kids I saw as the privileged ones.

Growing up white means never having to say race matters. My life was built on a rock-solid foundation of white norms and racial denial. For example, I grew up near the ocean. Only in my teen years did I begin to be vaguely aware that going to the beach was a white thing. After desegregation, African American families would come to the beach in groups and stay together. *"Why do they do that?"* white people would say, as they moved their towels farther up the beach. White fears were tied to white ignorance. We had no idea that Black families were scared of us. It still felt unsafe for them coming to beaches that used to be legally segregated. Ironically, white people were frightened by Black families who were keeping their distance to avoid frightening white people.

In the 1930s and 1940s, there was violence against African Americans seeking to use public pools in Pittsburgh, St. Louis, and Youngstown and in communities all across America.[1] A white woman in Marion, Indiana, said this—white people *"didn't want to be polluted by their Blackness."* And yet white people still look shocked when an African American adult says, *"I can't swim."*

I went to a public elementary school. I skipped second grade, ensuring that I would be the smallest kid in every class I ever attended. But in 1967, my parents decided that both I and my brother would now attend a college prep school. It was presented as an opportunity. *"You need to be with other kids who are smart,"* they said. *"We're afraid you'll be bored in public school."* What they didn't say was that school desegregation was now court-ordered. The high school would soon be admitting Black students from Boca's Black neighborhood, Pearl City. White fears took over, and a very expensive decision was made. *"We want you to reach your potential,"* they said.

Sure. In fact, the rapid expansion of private schools in the South was built on enabling white flight from public schools. How many other white families made similar choices at exactly this moment in history? Only about 25,000 students went to private schools in the South in 1966; within six years, by 1972, the number was 20 times higher, over half a million.[2] When I was in my junior year of high school, Hillary Clinton was a young law school student going undercover to show that too many of these southern schools were little more than "segregation academies."

In the dictionary next to white privilege would be St. Andrews, an elite Episcopal college prep school in Boca Raton. A private plane with wealthy parents once landed on the soccer field to attend the homecoming football game and galas. One kid got his parents to put *his* ski boat in the tiny pond near the dorms. My brother and I attended on scholarships and a work-study plan. Cleaning up rich kids' bathrooms left me with strong feelings about children of wealth and privilege.

My supervisor was the head janitor. White students at the school knew him only as "Joe the Janitor," never bothering to learn his last name. Mr. Newsome taught me dignity in work. He taught me to do a job with excellence not because someone was watching but because you could choose to be a *person* of excellence. He took pride in using a mop and wax to make a floor really shine. He had dropped out of school to support his mom and siblings. By example, he taught me about sacrifice and responsibility.

Students who were my friends also saw me after school cleaning toilets and mopping floors. I saw some of them with no earthly need to work, perhaps for the rest of their privileged lives. It gave me a unique perspective. I was part of this world, but I could still see it as an outsider.

I hung out with other scholarship kids from our town. I was also friends with the only two African American students in my class. We hung out together. We got drunk together. My father, in all of his racial insensitivity, called us "the Oreo kids." I couldn't convince him that this was an offensive racist term. *"But it's funny,"* he would say. *"You're white and walking around with a Black layer on either side."* No, Dad. It's not funny. Please stop.

Why do I have such a hard time thinking of myself as having privilege? I think of privilege as rich kids who drop cigarettes on the carpet and put bubble gum under their desks. I was the kid who turned into a janitor when the school bell rang and sometimes cursed these privileged rich kids under my breath. *Me, privileged?*

Here in North Florida, we have beautiful springs that emerge from underground aquifers. They pump out millions of gallons of beautiful, crystal-clear water at a constant temperature of 70 degrees. Floating down a spring-fed river in an inner tube is blissfully relaxing. Buses bring people to the starting point and let them float down the river to the pickup area. No one wants to paddle those floaty things back upstream against the current.

The tidal flow of privilege has carried me along all of my life. My parents both had a college education. My father had a white-collar job. Not an option for parents of color. My mom and dad sacrificed tremendously to give me a higher education, but I never experienced any of the racial stresses that my Black friends experienced. I was oblivious. Spending our privilege to deconstruct it is like trying to paddle an awkward floaty-thing upstream against the current.

But consider it from the perspective of those who lack privilege. I am a cisgender, straight, European American, Anglo, deeply spiritual but not-very-religious Protestant Christian white guy. I don't walk into a room thinking about my racial privilege or male privilege. But my advantage is just the flip side of another's disadvantage. People of color and gender-minoritized people are at a disadvantage in society. They have less economic opportunity. They experience tremendous discrimination and violence. They are disadvantaged in interactions with our justice system. But disadvantaged relative to what or to whom? Of course, it's disadvantage relative to white, male, cisgender guys like me. Which makes me "advantaged" relative to them. I have structural and societal advantage. I have privilege. *Damn.*

My first year of college was in Boston in 1973. White folks were rioting over the court-ordered busing of African American students to predominantly white schools. White adults threw stones at buses filled with frightened Black children. Still, many students at Harvard who had attended elite prep schools in the North looked down on Southerners as racist and ignorant. It was regional bias, dressed up in intellectual verbiage. It was arrogant.

I had a tough year. I had graduated high school at age 16. I was not at all ready to be on my own. But I had desperately wanted to get away from my dysfunctional family. I was cocky and insecure all at the same time. I made the dean's list but didn't feel very smart. I was drinking too much and often alone, wanting only to drown out the noise of inner doubts and inadequacies.

I was an English major. I wrote short stories and essays. The more I wrote, the more it felt like an exercise in self-absorption. After my roommate's Christmas suicide and my grandmother's spring funeral, I became more unsure every day of who I was. My confidence was nearly gone. I began to hunger desperately to do something meaningful, something important. I began to want to make a difference in the world and in people's lives. I needed to be needed. I wanted to be enough.

In the spring semester, I took my one required science class, *Human Physiology for Non-Science Majors*. Might as well call it *Science for Dummies*. But what an elegant world it opened up for me! The human body and its marvelously self-regulating systems. I loved the harmonies of homeostasis, the way our body systems stay in balance. For the first time, I thought about what it might be like to be a doctor. I imagined caring for people, like my gentle maternal grandfather had done.

So I moved. I moved from liberal arts to hard science. I moved from Harvard to the University of Miami. I was closer to home but still on my own. In that first year at the U, I found Jesus and I found my future wife. Both gave me unconditional love.

I applied to 12 medical schools. I was rejected by 10, put on a waiting list for another, and got accepted by one. Loyola University School of Medicine accepted me, largely on the basis of one interview in which I spoke honestly about wanting to help people in need. The basic science researcher who interviewed me believed that compassion and altruism would be a good thing in a doctor. Go figure.

After I completed medical school and an internship at the suburban ivory tower, I moved again. This time, I moved to the real-world blood and pus, grit and reality, of Chicago's urban public hospital. Making ward rounds at Cook County Hospital, I saw mostly people of color whose commonality was to be poor and un-insured. I saw people with all the end-stage diseases and bad complications that my colleagues at the university medical centers might never see. Money and insurance and education protect you from a lot of bad stuff. Poverty doesn't.

I treated infections that most doctors only see on Two-Thirds World mission trips. The patients were Black and Latine, or occasionally poor and white, sometimes with alcohol or drug addictions. The nurses, aides, and clerks were mostly Black or Filipino. The doctors were an international variety pack, but mostly from India, Pakistan, Viet Nam, Africa, and Latin America. Dozens of languages, hundreds of cultures, thousands of individuals. Most of them were non-white, non-Anglo, and delightfully diverse. At Cook County Hospital, I learned to practice medicine in a non-white world.

The emergency department (ED) at Cook County Hospital inspired the TV show *ER*, which didn't capture the half of it. The Cook County ED was more like a busy subway station during an earthquake, 24 hours a day. Walking through the ED jarred all your senses at once. It was a noisy cacophony of chaos that also smelled funky. Sometimes patients had fist-fights in the waiting area. Sometimes police brought people handcuffed to a stretcher. The Chicago Police Department had a substation at the back entrance. Mostly there were way too many people in a small space. Our patients were good and decent people who couldn't get health care anywhere else. They often had serious complications. Most of them were Black or brown. All of them were poor.

When we were interviewing students for internships, we would walk them through the emergency department. Some were idealistic and naive, like little Cub Scouts with a wide-eyed look in their eyes. They jerked their head around whenever a patient hollered. I was like that once, but an intense year of internship had toughened me up a little. We wanted interns who had idealism and compassion but with some grit. Maybe they had worked over-seas, or maybe they just had street-smarts. Maybe they grew up poor. Maybe they were just naturally cool. They strode confidently through the ED. Interested, but unafraid. Those were the ones we wanted.

Underneath the chaos, the ED was a finely tuned machine of triage and patient flow. The sickest or most injured were cared for first. Those with minor problems waited. Sometimes a long time. I saw a man once who couldn't even remember why he had come to the emergency department. When I saw him, he had de-veloped a temporary paralysis of his arm because he had fallen asleep with that arm draped over the back of a chair. We called it honeymoon paralysis or Saturday night palsy. It sometimes happened when lovers fell asleep, one's head nestled in the oth-er's arm. This man fell asleep just waiting for care.

We worked in different sections of the ED on different rota-tions. Some months it was the GYN area, treating vaginal infec-tions or caring for women with partial miscarriages. We would do D&Cs (scraping the inner lining of the womb) with just IV sedation. See one, do one, teach one. Except at Cook County, it was *"see one, do a hundred, teach a bunch, and then do some more."* Until one of our new residents perforated a woman's uterus. We got a little more supervision after that. At least for a little while.

We also worked in the surgical dispensary. If you got shot or mortally stabbed in a vital organ, you went straight upstairs to the trauma unit. But if you got stabbed just a little or got your arms slashed defending yourself, then you came to the dispensary for us to sew you up. We also drained a lot of pus. Often yellow-green, sometimes liquid, sometimes like *queso*—one friend said he had dreams about pus. It was during another wave of Chicago's ongo-ing heroin epidemic. Some shot up into their veins. Skin-poppers just injected their drugs under the skin. When they used a dirty needle, they got infections, which formed abscesses. We'd stab these pockets of pus with a sharp-pointed #11 scalpel and then irrigate with saline and dig around with forceps to break up all the pus pockets. Then we would stuff it with iodine-infused gauze to help the cavity to heal from the bottom up. Painful as hell because you can't numb pus.

As family practice residents, we mostly worked in the medical section of the ED. Patient after patient, waiting room full, all day and all night. They came with common conditions that were wildly out of control—diabetes and high blood pressure playing havoc with the kidneys, the heart, or the brain. I once blew the top off an old-fashioned blood pressure gauge trying to go high enough to measure a man's BP. I blew mercury out the top and onto the floor, creating my own little hazmat emergency.

We saw old diseases like syphilis and tuberculosis. I could spot a TB x-ray from across the room. I still can. Pneumonias were often severe, with patients turning septic with bacteria in their bloodstream. Liver damage was too often end-stage. Yellow-jaundiced patients, bellies stretched with peritoneal fluid, would drift in and out of consciousness. Heart attacks. Cardiac arrests. Code blue.

The sheer volume of it was unending. One time in three years, we came up for breath in the adult medical unit and said, *"Where's our next patient?"* Usually there were at least a few in the hallway on stretchers. In fact, we had learned to do hallway rounds. We had to make sure nobody died on a stretcher outside our small evaluation bays. But at 3 a.m. on one rainy night in October, there was no one left to be seen. The waiting room was empty. The old nurses who had been there for decades said they had never seen it before. We looked at each other and smiled in disbelief. We had cleared out the Cook County ER! It lasted about 10 minutes, and then it started filling up again. Back to work. But we had done it. No one could ever take that away from us.

We also saw a fair number of drug overdoses. Heroin OD patients came in not breathing and blue, until we gave the magic Narcan. It revived them almost instantly, turning them into angry shouting addicts whose blessed high we had just taken away. Angel dust (PCP) overdoses were the worst. Wild men, screaming and thrashing, hallucinating and strapped with leather cuffs to the stretchers. Sometimes they fought so hard they tipped the top-heavy old metal stretchers sideways onto the floor with a loud crash and a pathetic moan. *"Oowww. . . ."* We could recognize the sequence of sounds from the other room. The only thing good about PCP was that it would wear off, and the patient would become themselves again. Released from the stretcher, they would shake my hand and say, *"Thank you, doctor. I don't know how that happened. Someone must have put something in my drink."* Must have.

But it was all an organized chaos. GYN patients went to GYN. Kids went to the pediatric ED. Serious knife and gunshot wounds went straight up to the trauma unit. Medical problems came to the adult medicine section. Organized. Civilized. Most of the time. One time I was in medical bay #4 and picked up a chart to see my next patient on the stretcher. I pulled back the curtain only to see what looked like a small hole in his forehead. I glanced down at the chart. GSW. Gunshot wound. I reached for the phone before I even examined the patient. I called triage—*"What's this guy doing down here? I've got a 42-year-old male with a single gunshot wound to the forehead. We need to get him up to the trauma unit stat!"*

I was interrupted by someone tugging on the sleeve of my white coat. It was the patient. He looked at me quite sincerely and held up three fingers. It wasn't a single gunshot wound. He had been shot three times. *"Get him out of here now!"* I growled into the phone and hung up. I vowed that if I ever got shot three times, I would just lay down and die. Not this guy. County patients were tough.

Every now and then, a patient came through who didn't belong. I would see a white guy on a stretcher with vomit stains on a tailored suit. His hair would be a little mussed but neatly styled, expensive shoes freshly shined. The nurse handed me a clipboard with his vitals.

"Who's this guy?" I asked.

"DUI. Crashed his Mercedes into the rear end of a Chicago police cruiser."

"Ouch. He's having a bad day."

"Just watch him for DT's, okay?" she said from experience. *"His labs say he's an everyday drinker."*

And then our white male investment banker-lawyer-executive would start to wake up. The alcohol and the head injury would slowly clear until he realized that he was tied down to a stretcher somewhere he had never been before. His eyes would grow wide as he began to fully experience the noise and the chaos and the smell and the humanity of the Cook County ED. In an uncertain voice, he would ask the inevitable question. *"Where the hell am I?"*

Across America, lots of white guys, not just the rich ones, are also waking up to the humanity around them. They are asking the same question. *"Where the hell am I?"*

America is in transition. A white-majority population accustomed to setting the norms is moving into a new minority-majority reality. Dorothy and Toto really aren't in Kansas anymore. If you look at our kids' and grandkids' generation, brown and Black outnumber white. Diversity is now and forever the norm. Racially, America is no longer white. Ancestrally, America is no longer European. Religiously, America is no longer Christian. Gender is no longer binary. Sexuality sees a strong and increasingly "out" LGBTQ presence.

The Census Bureau says that the US population will comprise more minority persons than whites by the year 2045.[3] For those who imagine America as a mostly white Euro-American country, there will be tremendous cognitive dissonance between this new reality and their core identity. The real America doesn't look like the America they see in their heads. Already four states have white non-Hispanic populations of less than half, with more states to come.[4]

One reason for the "anti-woke" educational backlash in Florida is that public schools are already majority-minority institutions. White parents feel their sense of control and privilege slipping away. We are becoming more ethnically and linguistically diverse, only to trigger from some people a "speak English, dammit!" response.

I've lived and practiced amidst this transition in urban Chicago and in the small-town Deep South. In Chicago, I worked with immigrant doctors at Cook County Hospital and immigrant patients at our South Lawndale/La Villita clinic. Later in Central Florida, I served six years as medical director of the West Orange Farmworkers Health Association. I practiced in our smallest migrant clinic, on Highway 50 in Groveland, Florida. I did home visits on dirt roads on the Black side of town. Latine farmworkers were invisible. Just pick the citrus and disappear.

Groveland was also a town with an unspoken history of violent racial oppression, a divided family as sick as its secrets. And to maintain stability, these racial horrors were to me unspoken.

My patients in Groveland were a diverse mix of Latine and Anglo, Black and white, Haitian and Mexican, and US-born people. They all shared the one common denominator of being low-income and/or uninsured. I would rush from exam room to exam room, quickly shifting between my clumsy Spanish and American English. My accent would become more southern as I cared for low-income southern white patients. They lived in a suspended purgatory between poverty and racial privilege. My speech slowed to match the cadence of my African American patients who lived for generations in the shadow of Jim Crow.

In Groveland, at least in the Black and Latine and poor-white communities, I was Dr. Rust. Six miles away, in the less deeply southern town of Clermont, my wife was Dr. Rust, the area's only pediatrician. We were both on call 24/7. I was working 12-hour days. It worked for a while, but then we had two kids in the space of two years. Someone was going to have to raise them. We knew it was time to move again. I wrote an open letter to my patients in the local paper, saying that *"the only job for which I am truly indispensable carries the title, Daddy."*

My need to move was to find balance in my roles as husband, father, and physician and perhaps to teach others to do this work. I moved from Groveland to Atlanta, to the relatively new Morehouse School of Medicine. There it took a quarter-century of working in a historically Black medical school to help me find my soul, to make peace with myself, and in some ways to become comfortable in my own skin.

I often sat in meetings with dozens of people, where I was the only white person. I remember sitting in a historic church, surrounded by African American congregants. When the music started, the church came alive. First, just the choir, then voices in a call-and-response. Then a tapping of the feet on a wooden floor in a church with wooden pews and wooden walls until the tapping became a deep rhythmic beating. The church itself (pews and floor and people) became the instrument rising up in a glorious rhythm of breath and heartbeat and life.

My wife and I raised our children in Atlanta, the heart of the progressive New South. Even so, if you looked at Dekalb County where we lived, wealth and income levels were distributed unevenly from north to south. Racial segregation followed exactly the same pattern. It affected everything from property values to community resources to the quality of public schools.

Race affected health care as well. Grady Hospital is the large urban public hospital in Atlanta. It was founded in 1890 on the progressive premise that all people should receive care. It also reflected southern norms of segregation. In the African American community, Grady Health System is still called "the Grady's" because historically, it had functioned as two separate and not necessarily equal hospitals. A white nurse from my church described working different shifts in the white operating room and in the "colored" operating room. The blood bank separated colored blood from white blood. The hospital itself was built in the shape of an H, with separate wings designated for white and non-white patients. Still, African American patients born there often said proudly that they were a Grady baby. They trusted the Grady's because it had always been there for them.

Over the decades, I went to funerals and weddings. I learned Latine traditions and Catholic rituals. I grieved and celebrated with African American friends and colleagues. I drove across the heartland of Georgia to be with my chosen brother at his father's funeral, and he flew to Florida to be with me at my father's funeral. At each funeral, we hugged and exchanged whispers. *"Love you, my brother,"* we each said, words I had never spoken to any other man in my life except my biological brother. In those moments, I was still a white guy, but one who was loved and blessed to be included in a non-white community.

Unfortunately, many of us do not have such robust multiracial experiences. In 1965, the Moynihan Report said, "Our nation is moving toward two societies, one Black, one white—separate and unequal." Some want to embrace an aspirational postracial future as if we're already there. *"I don't see Black or white, I just see people,"* they say innocently. That's a luxury only white folks have in America, because it damn sure isn't true for everyone else.

Most white folks like me walk on eggshells, as many of us learned to do in our own dysfunctional families. If there's been abuse, we don't talk about it. The abusive ones will blow up the conversation with their sense of grievance and victimhood. Don't talk about race, because you might say the wrong thing. Stay quiet, because somebody's going to get hurt.

In 1955, James Baldwin said, "This world is white no longer, and it will never be white again."[5] For folks who have grown up in a world of invisible white culture, the world seems to be shifting beneath our feet. We can feel anxious and not even know why. We say things like *"Why does it always have to be about race?"* We can choose to pretend that it's not, while our brothers and sisters of color never can.

"Why are all the Black kids sitting together in the cafeteria?"[6] some ask, not noticing that all the white kids have been sitting together for a lot longer. Nobody called that a racial thing. It's hard to see our own whiteness, until we see it through others' eyes.

That is now my gift and perhaps my burden. At least sometimes, as through a mirror dimly, I can see through others' eyes. Colleagues of color more often have the gift of what W. E. B. Dubois called "double consciousness." They can see their own reality but can also see the world through white eyes. They have navigated their entire lives through institutions and culture defined by white male norms.

E pluribus unum. Out of many, one. It was the unofficial motto of the United States for our first 180 years. Five days after I was born in 1956, the US Congress made "In God We Trust" our nation's official motto. They did so in the moment of the Montgomery bus boycott, out of fear that their white Christian America was slipping away. Race and religion were melded together. Brace the fortress walls. *In God We Trust.*

The question is how we get from the *pluribus* to the *unum*, from a diversity of people to one nation. There is nothing special about forming a nation out of one people. The magic is in the *pluribus*, the making one out of many! Isn't that the highest, most beautiful and patriotic vision, one great America uniting each of us in all of our different colors and flavors and languages and genders?

It's not easy. White folks love to talk about America as a melting pot, so long as it's the minorities who do all the melting. Jimmy Carter spoke instead of the beautiful American tapestry with thousands of unique individual threads. No metaphor is perfect. Some talk of a salad instead of a melting pot. I prefer the metaphor of a Snickers bar. I can still taste specific ingredients, but in my mouth, the chocolate and the caramel and the peanuts all are one. It's a blissful experience of gooey goodness. Oh, what a wondrous and beloved community that would be!

And yet . . . . those thoughts are sadly naive. They fail to recognize just how scary or threatening these demographic changes can be. Roland Martin gave his book the subtitle, *How the Browning of America Is Making White Folks Lose Their Minds*.[7] A subset of white America is gripped with the fear that power and opportunity are slipping away. Maybe our norms are no longer America's norms. Maybe our culture is no longer America's culture.

Diversity does not automatically produce a beloved community. A loss of dominant culture status can lead to a sense of grievance and victimization, to anger and backlash. Polls show that a majority of white Americans now believe that white people face race-based discrimination.[8] *Really?*

At the end of 2023, Donald Trump began again using the anti-immigrant language that had fueled his 2016 emergence as a presidential candidate. This time, he chose words that evoked the writings of Adolf Hitler, saying that immigrants were "poisoning the blood of America." He didn't mention Eastern European immigrants like his wife. Instead, he focused on those coming north from Mexico, Central America, Africa, and Asia. All immigrants of color. He then equated them to dangerous people from prisons and mental institutions. Terrorists.

A week later, a poll showed that 42 percent of Republicans were *more likely* to support Trump for his "poisoning the blood" statement. That's Trump-ism. It's a feature, not a bug. And it's setting the stage for justifying violence against those he sees as "other."

Over the past four decades, I have been blessed to experience the wondrous and messy community of diversity. I have lived and worked in a non-white world. I was not always the only white person, but non-white persons made enough of a super-majority to define the culture and to have the power. And then I came home to Florida.

I moved back to teach at another mission-driven medical school, this one at Florida State University. We say that we train the doctors Florida really needs. And as good a job as this school does in achieving diversity, the organizational culture is still very white and a bit southern. I am also very white and a bit southern, but it struck me here how much my worldview and cultural norms had shifted. I realized that I had spent my entire career working in institutions where the culture and power were majority-minority. *Where did I belong?*

America is facing a similar crisis of identity. Those who grew up in white-world see the world through white (and often straight male) eyes. *Where do we belong? Or do we still belong at all?*

Some of us welcome the opportunity to grow and to learn new ways of seeing each other. We have found new relationships and new insights. We have embraced the rainbow. We're like the kids in *Pleasantville*, a movie in which two teens open the eyes of a 1950s black-and-white TV world, until more and more people embrace the joys of art and fun and books and sex in a marvelous world bursting with color and life.

Predictably, some of the townspeople of Pleasantville resisted the change, just as people in America are doing. Those who have power, or whose sense of self is defined by rigid gender roles, prefer their simpler black-and-white world. The rigid folks feel threatened in their identity and their narrow norms. They take to courtrooms and violence and book banning to make things go back to the way they once were.

Here in America, we are playing out our own version of Pleasantville. We are becoming more racially, ethnically, and gender diverse, but a lot of us straight white guys don't know how to deal with it. Some resist and explicitly call for America to return to some nostalgic time past. They won't acknowledge that those were terrible times for people of color living in segregation and the era of Jim Crow. Those were times when women had constrained career options and no reproductive choices. For LGBTQ people, their sexuality and even personhood were illegal.

The Trump/MAGA slogan *Make America Great Again* would seem to co-opt the first two lines of Langston Hughes's poem. "Let America be America again. Let it be the dream it used to be." But read on a few lines. To a Black poet writing this in the 1930s, "America never was America to me."

Beyond race, LGBTQ identities have always been present in America but often oppressed and hidden. More than 7 percent of all Americans identify as LGBTQ. Among the younger generation, it is more like one in five.[9] Given that many still do not feel safe coming out, what is the real number in America? What is the real number in your family or in mine?

Gender diversity now goes way beyond the binary male and female dichotomy that I grew up with. It challenges me, but I can begin setting down new tracks in my brain. I can see three-dimensional matrices of sexuality and gender identity. I can question the gender roles and identities I have learned as mental shortcuts. How much more robust and gloriously colorful is my world when I see an infinite range of possibilities for people's gender and sexuality and personhood?

But, wow, this stuff sure is threatening to folks whose gender identity is tied to their religion or their culture or their power. People who are insecure about their manhood will have a hard time ever embracing their inner feminine. They will forever lack balance. For many of us, these gender identities and sexual identities are at the very core of our own sense of self. For some, the very thought of nonbinary genders or gay sex is so intrusive and threatening that it must be attacked, oppressed, or stamped out.

Senator Ted Cruz recently drew raucous applause at a conservative convention with the declaration that "my pronouns are 'Kiss my ass'!" Is this something to be proud of? Are we so fragile, so insecure, and so incapable of showing grace that we can't adjust our language to help everyone feel included? In my state, drag shows are seen as a dangerous menace to society, even more so than legalizing no-permit, concealed-carry guns.

At our governor's urging, the Florida legislature has passed various acts of white denialism and male homophobia. For example, new laws prohibit classroom teaching about sexual and gender identity in the Don't Say Gay bill. They prohibit discussions of our racial history or structural inequalities in the Stop Woke Act. Governor DeSantis has bragged on his accomplishments, calling it "The Year of the Parent" and celebrating "parental rights."

What if I'm a gay parent—do I celebrate that my child is made to fear mentioning their two daddies? What if I'm a third-generation African American whose grandparents were killed in one of Florida's race massacres? Whose version of that history will I be taught? What if I'm a child, beginning to sense that my gender identity is not the sex I was assigned at birth?

In my current faculty position, I have several roles. I am a teacher, a researcher, and a tenured professor. I am a public health physician who serves as medical director for six county health departments. I also chair the Council on Diversity and Inclusion (now the Council on Engagement) at our College of Medicine. In all of these roles, my job is threatened by the grievance-driven political backlash.

It is now a third-degree felony for me to teach anything that would make [white heterosexual] students uncomfortable. DeSantis's attorneys argued before the Supreme Court that a professor's speech is government speech that can be compelled or restricted by the governor. I am outlawed from teaching that systemic racism and institutionalized inequities are root causes of health disparities. As a public health physician, I am not supposed to promote vaccinations that could save lives. By order of the state surgeon general, no one in the Florida Department of Health is *ever* supposed to use the phrase *health equity*. To say it would require us to acknowledge that we still have systemic *inequities*.

My colleagues and I are also handcuffed in the care we may provide to trans individuals or even to adult women making reproductive choices. Get out of my exam room! Is this what the governor calls *the Freedom State*? Limiting kids' freedom to read? Taking away women's control over their own bodies? *Freedom State?* What kind of Orwellian talk is that?

I can only understand it in a framing of conservatism offered by Frank Wilhoit, who said, "Conservatism consists of exactly one proposition. . . . There must be in-groups whom the law protects but does not bind, alongside out-groups whom the law binds but does not protect."[10]

This explains every anti-Black, anti-immigrant, anti-trans, anti-gay, anti-woman pro–gun law various governors and state legislatures have passed. Protect but do not bind the straight Christian white guys. Bind (but do not protect) everyone the white guys see as *others*.

Here's our challenge. White guys still think we live in a white-guy world. It frames all our perceptions and expectations. I still can be surprised by those whom I find "different." Forty years after I first started being intentional about expanding my cultural horizons, I can still be surprised. I need more learning. More diverse experiences. More openness. I need to be freed of my assumptions and biases, so deeply ingrained that I am constantly peeling back layers of my own onion. I need *healing*.

For some, our faith also is being threatened. Religious identity that conflated Christian evangelicalism with American patriotism is on the defensive. More than a third of Americans already did not identify as Christian, even before COVID-19 accelerated the decline.[11] Instead, we are becoming a nation not only of diverse religious backgrounds but of ecumenical religious collaboration, non-institutionalized spirituality, or no faith at all.

Fears of America becoming a post-Christian nation have further driven a backlash of Christian nationalism. This is painfully sad to me, because the Jesus I know embraces the poor and the oppressed. He takes the side of women and minorities, as well as immigrants and the incarcerated. He gets angry at those who stand in the way of grace. He teaches me both to receive and to give unconditional love.

Senator Cory Booker says, "Before you speak to me about your religion, first show it to me in how you treat other people; before you tell me how much you love your God, show me in how much you love all God's children; before you preach to me of your passion for your faith, teach me about it through your compassion for your neighbors."[12]

Southern Baptist comedian Grady Nutt used to weave gentle lessons into his church-humor storytelling. In one story about our spiritual future, he painted a verbal picture of a traffic jam at the pearly gates of heaven. He said there was a large holding pen just to the right of the entrance. It held people who just needed time to get over who else got into heaven. "Lutherans, Methodists, and good-golly even Presbyterians!" he would intone. These were the deepest layers of diversity the Baptist crowd's good humor would allow. He didn't mention Catholics or Mormons and certainly not Muslims. Gay or trans people? We weren't even using that language yet.

If you have an image of the great beyond, what does it entail? How do you imagine the people of heaven? They won't be mostly white people. Race and culture will be all over the map. Language too. There will be a lot of people speaking English and Mandarin, but Hindi and Spanish will be next, then French and Arabic. Swahili will be common, as will all the indigenous and tribal languages.

People freed to be their true spiritual selves will be male and female, queer and gender-fluid, and everything in between and different. And we'll need a holding pen by the entrance for lots of folks to get over it. But imagine walking through the gate like a child seeing a vivid, three-dimensional rainbow for the first time. Eyes open in wonder, *"Wow! So cool! I have so much more to learn and an eternity to learn it!"*

Here's the dilemma for white people who want to do the right thing and be on the right side of history. How do we come to grips with our own whiteness? For many of us, the opposite of being a white nationalist has meant denying race or pretending that we live in a postracial world. We have good intentions. But to deny our own racial identity or pretend that we don't see race is to gaslight the real everyday lived experience of people of color. It also denies our own lived experience of privilege.

How can I be a white guy who is a force for good in this nonwhite, multigendered world? George Will says that we have become "a nation of the woke and the wary, walking on eggshells."[13] But I wonder—is there a third path, one that boldly rejects white nationalism or white identity politics but also avoids the colorblind racism of claiming that race doesn't matter? Over the past few decades, I have paid attention to my own journey on this "third path." I have tried to encourage others to see their own true selves, including their own whiteness, through non-white eyes.

I see the dysfunction, and I wonder how and when the healing can begin.

FAMILY MEMBERS WHO APPEAR IN THE BOOK

Family member	Family history
Maternal grandfather	Son of German immigrants; Army Medical Corps doctor in World War I; orthopedic surgeon in Springfield, Illinois
Maternal grandmother	Daughter of Swedish immigrants; saw herself as a doctor's wife and mother of 3 daughters
Paternal grandfather	Son of German immigrants; US Marine Corps stretcher-bearer in horrific battles of World War I; disabled by poison gas in the war; struggled with undiagnosed posttraumatic stress disorder, alcohol, and violence
Paternal grandmother	Daughter of German immigrants; cancer survivor, domestic abuse survivor; working single mom
Father	Pilot, businessman, and Navy Reserve Officer; adult child of an alcoholic, abusive father raised by a single mom (after age 12) in Chicago
Mother	Artist and mom; grew up as oldest of surgeon's 3 daughters in Springfield, Illinois; attended Chicago Art Institute

TIMELINE AND LIFE JOURNEY

1956	Born in Lake Forest, Illinois (Chicago suburb)
1959–1973	Raised from age three in Boca Raton, Florida; attended public elementary school and then went to prep school (St Andrew's) for grades 7–12 as scholarship student and part-time janitor
1973–1974	Harvard University—Freshman year of college as an English major; Cambridge, MA
1974–1977	University of Miami—Remainder of college as pre-med chemistry major Came away with a BS degree and lifelong love relationship with future wife Cindy
1977–1981	Loyola University School of Medicine in the Chicago suburb of Maywood, IL *(married Cindy after first year of medical school)*

TIMELINE AND LIFE JOURNEY (CONTINUED)

1981–1982   Internal Medicine/Pediatrics residency at Loyola; left after first year to focus on primary care in underserved settings

1982–1985   Family Medicine residency (and fourth-year Chief Resident) at Cook County Hospital, Chicago

1985–1991   Medical Director, West Orange Farmworkers Health Association based in Apopka, FL
Clinic sites in Apopka, Winter Garden, and Groveland, where I practiced
Cared for our hospital patients at South Lake Memorial Hospital in Clermont, FL
Cindy was the only pediatrician in South Lake County
Dan and Christina were born (1989 and 1991)

1991–2016   Faculty at Morehouse School of Medicine (MSM) in Atlanta, GA; various roles, including Professor (teaching, patient care, and health equity research), interim Department Chair, Founder of MSM Faculty Development Program, and Founding Director of National Center for Primary Care

2016   Detailed from Morehouse half-time to US Department of Health & Human Services Agency for Healthcare Research and Quality (DHHS/AHRQ) as Senior Scientist

2016–present   Tenured Professor, Florida State University College of Medicine in Tallahassee, FL; Co-Director of the Center for Medicine & Public Health; Medical Director of the Leon County Health Department and Florida Department of Health units in five surrounding rural counties
Grandpa

FOR FURTHER READING

Allen S. *Real Queer America: LGBT Stories from Red States.*

Ansell DA (introduction by Quentin Young). *County: Life, Death, and Politics at Chicago's Public Hospital.*

Barber WJ II. *White Poverty: How Exposing Myths About Race and Class Can Reconstruct American Democracy.*

Booker C. *United: Thoughts on Finding Common Ground and Advancing the Common Good.*

Boykin K. *Race Against Time: The Politics of a Darkening America.*

Frank T. *What's the Matter With Kansas?.*

Gest J. *The New Minority: White Working Class Politics in an Age of Immigration and Inequality.*

Hawley G. *Demography, Culture, and the Decline of America's Christian Denominations.*

Karels C. *Cooked: An Inner City Nursing Memoir.*

2.

Unnecessary Suffering
The Human Face of Inequality

"Statistics are just tragedies with the tears wiped dry." My whole career, I've seen those tragedies over and over again. Preventable suffering. Countless tragedies. I've treated a bunch, comforted some, and wept with a few.

I flash back to being on-call, covering our Morehouse residents. We were admitting patients at Southwest Hospital, one of the last five historically Black hospitals in the nation at that time. Our patient was the 38-year-old father of a toddler. He worked a warehouse job all day and played jazz piano gigs at night to support his family. Simple hypertension. High blood pressure. He knew he had it. Knew he needed treatment. But he didn't have insurance. He didn't want to spend the family's food and rent money on a doctor visit. And then he had a stroke.

Not a little mini-stroke, with slurred speech and a little weakness that might go away in a few days. This was a full-blown hemiparesis, almost complete loss of muscle strength on the entire right side of his body. We got his blood pressure under control and started physical therapy right away. But he would never be the same. He could barely lift his right hand. I felt awful for him and his family. Could he lift his toddler to give him a hug or throw a ball with him? Would he ever be able to play jazz piano again?

We did the best we could and arranged follow-up care. On the day he was to be discharged, I brought him an old electronic piano keyboard. He seemed grateful and began moving his hands on it right away to find the right keys. It was clumsy, but he seemed sadly hopeful. I slipped out of the room.

Why did that patient hit me so hard? Because it was so unnecessary. Hypertension is so easily preventable, treatable with medicines that almost anyone can afford. I can get almost anyone's blood pressure under control with four-dollar-a-month meds from the Walmart formulary. But this patient brought back memories of my years in Chicago. I would ride the L to Cook County Hospital and see 30-year-old men limping along with one-sided weakness. Their hands and wrists were curled up by years of post-stroke contractures. Untreated high blood pressure. Unnecessary strokes. Preventable suffering.

Over the decades, I've seen hundreds of such patients. One in five people with high blood pressure in America don't even know that they have it.[1] Among the uninsured, three out of four with hypertension have out-of-control blood pressure.[2] Persons of color are twice as likely to have a first stroke and four times more likely to end up on dialysis for kidney failure. Preventable strokes. Heart attacks. Dialysis. Death.

After med school, I had started my residency training at Loyola. After only a few months, I knew that I was not being trained for the mission I wanted to do. The University Medical Center was in a Black township, but once you stepped inside, you were in white-world. Cultural diversity among our senior faculty meant Irish Catholic and Polish Catholic. Or Italian. How could I learn to deliver compassionate care for the poor in a place that cared mostly for the well-off and well-insured?

So, I moved. I made a conscious choice and switched to the Family Medicine residency program at Cook County Hospital. My teachers were passionate about community health and social justice. They were led by our chairman, Dr. Jorge Prieto, who at one time had worked alongside Cesar Chavez in the United Farmworkers movement. In Chicago, he founded clinics in low-income Black and Latine neighborhoods. Our program director had himself been a resident at Cook County when he and other residents went on strike. A few even went to jail. Their demands were simple—a blood pressure cuff on every ward and a curtain around every bed. An end to 32-hour shifts in the ER. Quality of care and just a little dignity.

Cook County was the first place I ever worked where being white and US-born was to be in the minority. Not just the patients, but staff, nurses, physicians, and even leaders were people of color. I was living and working in a non-white world. A global community of multilingual, multicultural diversity. Diversity in gender and sexuality. I was so eager to learn and yet so woefully unprepared.

It was a place of tough-minded idealism. Engraved in the granite walls of that great hospital building was this quote from Louis Pasteur: "One doesn't ask of one who suffers: What is your country and what is your religion? One merely says, 'You suffer. That is enough for me. You belong to me, and I shall help you.'"

We worked together ridiculous hours, day and night, with on-call shifts of 32 hours or more every third to fourth night. Our colleagues saw us in all of our imperfect humanity, tired and cynical and irritable. We saw tragedies born of social and medical and behavioral complexities. We tried to be excellent and caring physicians in a space where sometimes surviving was the best we could do. We cared for the poor, and in the US health care system, we *were* the poor.

At Cook County, I got to train with some of the best US-trained physicians. I also worked side-by-side with excellent physicians-in-training from countries and cultures all over the world. We were all shades of beige and brown. It helped me notice my own white bias and my own need to press on in my journey of cultural learning and healing.

Cook County Hospital was my lifeboat. It was okay to be idealistic, to care about things that mattered. I was surrounded by physicians who cared, not just about their patients or about practicing good medicine but about *health justice*. Many still do. They cared about all the social complexities of their patients. They cared about the health of marginalized communities. They taught me about seeing patients in context, as "free-range humans" living in impoverished but resilient neighborhoods.

My mentors taught me that true health equity and social justice would ultimately require structural change. They even taught me to quote Rudolf Virchow, a 19th-century physician-anatomist. He said, "The physician is the natural attorney for the poor. . . . Medicine is a social science, and politics is nothing more than medicine on a grander scale."[3]

Years later, I would join former US Surgeon General Dr. David Satcher in his push for health justice. We published a paper titled "What If We Were Equal?"[4] We showed that America could have prevented over 83,500 deaths each year from 1960 to 2000 if we had eliminated the Black–white mortality gap. Sadly, we also found that the overall Black–white disparity did not change over all those decades. Quality improvement guru W. Edwards Deming once said, "Every system is perfectly designed to get the results it gets." That's scary because it means that our system is *designed* to produce racially unequal outcomes.

A seminal paper described the variation in US death rates by race and region as the *Eight Americas*, as if we were living in different nations.[5] Fifteen years earlier, researchers had shown that "Black men in Harlem were less likely to reach the age of 65 than men in Bangladesh."[6] Poverty and racism are bad for your health.[7]

HIV death rates are six times higher in Black populations. Rates of end-stage diabetic renal disease are more than double in Hispanic communities.[8] In 2023, *JAMA* reported that nationwide, there were over 80 million excess years of potential life lost due to health disparities.[9] How many person-years of life can one community afford to lose? How many grandfather years or grandmother years can one community afford to lose? How many wisdom-years can our nation afford to lose?

Poor people get worse care than rich people.[10] People on Medicaid get worse care than those with private insurance. Having no insurance is worst of all. Meanwhile, over a million people across the nation were dumped from the Medicaid rolls in 2024. A quarter of those were in Florida.[11] It's not that they're all ineligible. States are purposely making the complex process of re-enrolling more difficult to navigate.

In the 1990s, our team at Morehouse documented myriad racial-ethnic disparities. We wanted to break through the denial. Every rock we turned over, out would come the cockroaches of racial inequalities. Infant mortality. Pain medicine during labor and delivery. Childhood asthma emergency department visits. HIV treatment. Cardiovascular disease. Depression treatment.

We also learned of a troubling trend. The very conditions for which we were making the greatest health gains in America were the conditions for which Black–white disparities were worsening.[12] In short, *advantaged* segments of the population were *taking advantage* of new lifesaving technologies at a greater pace than the disadvantaged. When HIV treatments finally became effective around 1996, rising mortality rates suddenly reversed and declined rapidly. But the Black and white trend lines diverged even more.

Certainly, African American patients were less eager to jump into the new treatments. But physicians were also withholding lifesaving therapy from patients whom they thought could not manage the complex regimens. They worried about the virus developing resistance to the drugs. This is when implicit bias kicked in. Is a Black or Latine patient less able to handle the complexity? How about a poor person or a homeless person? Even with the same Medicaid coverage, African American patients were less likely to receive lifesaving HIV treatment.[13]

During this time, many researchers started asking the "why" questions. There were so many other factors associated with racial disparities. Poverty. Education. Social determinants. Except that race is a driver of all those things, just as it is for adverse health outcomes. Do patients sometimes get treated badly in hospital emergency departments because they are uninsured, along with being Black or Latine? Absolutely. But what's the point of this research if it just leads to minimizing race as a factor? Race and social determinants are profoundly intertwined. Unintentionally, the emphasis on social determinants of health just plays into white denialism. *It's not racism, it's just poverty—whew!*

This can be particularly problematic when research teams lack the African American or Latine or Native voices that could bring nuanced understanding to their work. At Cook County, the residents had a saying that *"just because you know the lab result doesn't mean you know what it means."* In too many research articles, the technical methods are impeccable, but I can tell that the article was written by a non-diverse team. I can see their blinders. The same results might have been understood very differently by authentic community voices with lived experience.

One of the earliest reports documenting racial inequalities in health came in the US Department of Health Education and

Welfare's (DHEW's) 1985 Heckler report.[14] The report said that the Black population in 1983 had "barely reached a life expectancy already reached by Whites in the early 1950s, a lag of about 30 years."[15] Even today, an African American with a college degree has a shorter life expectancy than a white American who only graduated from high school.[16] In the words of Michael Eric Dyson, "The statistics of [health] disparities, and our ongoing impotence in eliminating these disparities, send a very clear message—'White lives matter more.'"[17]

Disproportionately bad health outcomes cause an excess of preventable suffering for marginalized groups of all types, including LGBTQ people. More than a quarter of trans patients have had to educate a medical provider about trans health issues. One in five trans individuals has actually been refused health care by a medical provider.[18]

Such discrimination is now being institutionalized in states like Texas. Parents who seek professional help with their child's gender identity are being investigated by child protective services. In Florida, the state Medicaid agency will no longer pay doctors to provide gender-affirming care. Physicians may even be subject to disciplinary action from the Medical Board for providing evidence-based treatment.

Imagine, then, the intersecting inequities experienced by those with more than one minoritizing identity. To be a Black man who has sex with men is different from being a white gay man or a Black straight woman. According to the National Transgender Discrimination Survey, a third of Black transgender people live in extreme poverty. Forty-one percent have experienced homelessness, and nearly half report having attempted suicide.[19]

Another area of disparity is for people with mental health or substance use issues. Nearly a third of Americans reported symptoms of anxiety or depression in 2023. A person with schizophrenia may have a shorter life span by 25 years. My wife's sister died in her 50s. Was it the alcohol? The smoking? Or was it the underlying mental illness, in her case schizoaffective disorder? Mental health is health.

Not long ago, I had a patient who was overcoming addiction and severe anxiety and depression. He attributed his progress to a rescue dog that was his constant companion. He had heart problems and failing kidneys, but we couldn't address any of those conditions until I first wrote a letter to his landlord. I had to advocate for him to be able to keep his dog. He loved that dog. Mental health is not just about antidepressants.

Individuals in mental health crisis too often end up in hospital emergency departments. It's worse in rural areas, where there are not enough mental health professionals. Here in my county in North Florida, *suicide is the third leading cause of death among children aged 5 to 14.* Homicide ranks fourth. Is this not a public health crisis?

Over the past several years, there has been a stunning rise in opioid overdose deaths. It takes me back to my days treating heroin addicts in Chicago in the 1980s. Now we see even stronger and more deadly opioids like OxyContin and fentanyl. In just the first year of the COVID pandemic, the United States saw a 31 percent increase in drug overdose deaths. Almost a million people have died since 1999 from drug overdose.[20] More preventable suffering.

There are also significant regional health disparities. The South is where bad health outcomes prevail. For decades, Georgia has consistently ranked near the bottom in rankings of states with the worst health outcomes in the nation. Public health folks in Georgia consoled ourselves with foxhole humor: *"At least we're not Mississippi."*

When I was co-chairing the Georgia Minority Health Advisory Council, I proposed conducting a Georgia Health Disparities Report. With a lot of late-night data-sifting, our team at the National Center for Primary Care got it done. We identified racial disparities in nine different domains across every county in Georgia.

We held a press conference to release the report and town hall meetings across the entire state. We had given each county two letter grades in each domain for how optimal and equitable the outcomes were. The *Atlanta Journal Constitution* published a front-page story reporting that Fulton County got an F in minority health. I got a lot of phone calls that week from angry county commissioners. But the most meaningful phone calls I got were from local leaders calling to ask, *"Okay, what do we do about it?"*

When we gave the statistics in town hall meetings, people's eyes glazed over. We had to translate our statistics into personal terms. We showed an image of a Black premature baby on a ventilator in the neonatal ICU. *"A baby dies every day in Georgia,"* I would say, *"who wouldn't have died if we could eliminate the Black–white infant mortality gap."* I could see the emotional hit on the faces of the audience. We had moved from the head to the heart. The crowd would become quiet and sad. Some would give a little *"ain't-it-awful"* shake of their heads. But in that same moment, the energy was sucked out of the room. Powerlessness and despair settled in. We had to follow that slide immediately with one that showed a cute, healthy toddler. *"We could save a baby's life every day in Georgia if we eliminated this gap."*

Florida is now the state in which a Black baby could be saved almost every day if we could eliminate this gap (324 excess infant deaths in 2021). Recently, our FSU research team projected when each of our 50 states would eliminate the Black–white infant mortality gap. A few states are on track to accomplish this in the next few decades. Sadly, Florida will achieve equality somewhere between 2066 and 2213.[21] Not in my lifetime.

Dr. Martin Luther King Jr. said, "Of all the forms of inequality, injustice in health care is the most shocking and inhumane."[22] But health disparities do not only happen to low-income Black women or the uninsured. Ask Serena Williams, who recently retired from tennis to focus on her daughter. The day after Olympia was born by cesarean section, Serena Williams became extremely short of breath. She knew the feeling. She had had a history of blood clots in her lungs several years before. Pulmonary embolism. Ms. Williams asked for a CT scan and blood thinners, but the medical team discounted her insights. Finally, under pressure, they did the CT scan. They found life-threatening blood clots in her lungs.

People of color, especially those of non-male genders, feel that too often they are being dismissed or ignored. They are not being listened to.[23] Black women are three times more likely than white women to have serious complications or even death related to childbirth.[24] Meanwhile, the Centers for Disease Control and Prevention (CDC) reports that four out of five maternal deaths are preventable.[25] It isn't just about education or income inequities. According to the New York Department of Health, "Black mothers who are college-educated fare worse than women of all other races who never finished high school."[26] Preventable suffering.

Just west of my home in Tallahassee is Liberty County. It's a small rural community with the lowest population of any county in Florida. There are more possums than people. The lumber-driven economy was crushed when Hurricane Michael barreled through, splintering half of the pine tree forests like toothpicks. Cotton is still a major cash crop. Liberty County has one small, 25-bed, critical access rural hospital.

Ms. Barbara Dawson was a 57-year-old African American woman being evaluated in the emergency department for shortness of breath. She was seen and quickly discharged, even though she insisted she still couldn't breathe. She refused to leave, so they called the police. Ultimately, she was handcuffed and forcibly removed. She collapsed while being put into the police car. She remained unconscious in the parking lot for 18 minutes. When they brought her back into the hospital, resuscitation efforts failed. She was pronounced dead.

Why did the hospital staff not take her complaints seriously? Was it because she was Black? A Black woman? An overweight Black woman? Was it because she was a so-called "frequent flier" who had had frequent visits to the emergency department? Had she been labeled by the insurance companies as an expensive "super-utilizer"? Was it overt prejudice or implicit bias? *Does it matter?*

It's not just people of color. I remember caring for a pregnant uninsured white woman at our little clinic in Groveland, Florida. She was three weeks past her due date. All of her previous labors had required medical induction. Her asthma was getting worse, and her blood pressure was rising to dangerous levels. The obvious treatment was for her to go to the hospital and have the labor induced.

I called the nearest hospital with an OB unit, 30 miles away. I could hear the private practice obstetrician on-call say to the nurse, *"I don't have to take care of those patients unless they're in labor. She's not in labor. And don't you dare give my phone number to Dr. Rust."* I slammed the phone down and tried to blur the curse that came out of my mouth in front of my patient. A piece of the phone broke off and flew up in the air.

I rarely show anger, but something in me had snapped. A colleague once told me that to do this work would be to personally share the powerlessness of the poor. I never felt more powerless than I did in that moment. I looked at my patient. *"I'm sorry,"* I said weakly. *"I'll keep trying."*

The next day, I was back on the phone. Another obstetrician was on-call. I pleaded with him. I guilt-tripped him. I groveled. I tried to convince him that waiting for complications would cause him a lot more trouble than if he just induced her. *"All right, send her up,"* he said finally. *"I've got to be here anyway."* My patient delivered a healthy baby boy. But I aged a few years in those 24 hours, and that kind of stuff happened every day. Our clinicians on the front lines of caring for the marginalized burn out fast. And if we don't burn out, we build up a lot of scar tissue. I've aged in my soul.

It was a case of what Dr. Fitzhugh Mullan called "Tin Cup Medicine," "the perpetual, frustrating, quixotic, creative, and demeaning process of begging for services from others for our patients."[27] In contrast, when I myself had severe back pain and leg weakness from a herniated disk, my insurance paid for specialized orthopedic care. I recovered quickly. My uninsured patients with far worse spinal problems would never get that. I never once could get a neurosurgical or orthopedic spine consult for an uninsured patient, no matter how terrible their back pain was.

An FSU nurse practitioner colleague recently saw a young migrant boy whose hand was injured in a piece of farm machinery. It stripped skin from his fingers and tore a tendon. The emergency room cleaned it and put a bandage on it. They told him he needed a hand surgeon to repair the tendon to avoid permanent crippling of his hand. He had no insurance. His parents called for an appointment and were told to bring $500 cash to the first visit. My friend spent the rest of her day calling doctors she knew. We started raising donations. In the end, she found one of our medical school alumni who was a hand surgeon. He did us a favor and saw the child.

Orthopedics was always a challenge. One patient with a broken arm told me, *"Doc, if you don't put a cast on it, I'm gonna tie a stick on it."* By that benchmark, my casts were pretty good. Dermatology and plastic surgery were also out of reach for either Medicaid or uninsured patients. I had to do a bunch of skin surgery in our little Groveland clinic because no one else would see the patients.

One patient was albino, with white hair and white skin and a history of various skin cancers starting at age 15. She was nearly 30 years old when I first saw her. Over the next few years, I cut out a number of cancers, burned some off, and froze a bunch. I asked her to go to see a dermatologist at the University of Florida to make sure they didn't have better treatments. I was hoping for some new laser thing. They charged her a hundred bucks for the 10-minute visit, only to tell her, *"Nope. He's doing the same things we would do."* But they kept her hundred bucks.

Those patients should have gotten the same specialty care that I could get for myself or any other well-insured patient. Unless we change our health care system, we will keep on providing inadequate care with insufficient resources to those who need it most. Caring clinicians burn out standing in the gap.

For my entire first year at the migrant/community health center, I was on-call 24/7 for 365 days in a row. I admitted our patients to the hospital, did weekend rounds, and took phone calls from patients at any hour of the day or night. I even took some of the local family doctors out to lunch to see if they would be willing to help. I offered to take a night in their call schedule if they would cover for me some nights. *"Well,"* said one of the physicians, smiling devilishly as he took a bite of the steak I had paid for, *"that would be kinda like Burger King helping McDonald's, wouldn't it?"* The conversation was over. No help for the weary.

I admitted patients to a small rural hospital that had only 32 beds and a four-bed ICU. Beside the family docs, there were only two internists, one general surgeon, and one pediatrician (my wife). A few specialists would come to town once a week. When we needed something more urgent, we would move our cars out of the doctors' parking lot so that the helicopter could land and med-evac our patients to larger hospitals in Orlando.

South Lake Memorial was also a tax-district hospital, collecting local dollars to support indigent care. Before I came to town, the clinic doctors would just send their patients to the emergency department for acute problems. Often our patients were treated badly because they didn't speak English, were Black, or were uninsured. It was bad for our patients and bad for the hospital. That pattern of care used up their indigent care fund dollars faster than the tax revenue was coming in. The fund had run a deficit for several years.

When our clinic doctors got hospital admitting privileges, it was good news for the patients and bad news for our physicians. We took on a lot of extra hours but with inadequate backup. As medical director, I had to manage that burden among the docs in all our clinics. On a personal level, I took it on with a workaholic zeal that only Mother Teresa could love. Nothing was too much to ask in service of the mission. *Can you see why I might need healing?*

I was always on-call, so I bought myself one of the early mobile phones. It was a pay-by-the-minute contraption as big as three bricks. The handset was connected by a coiled wire to the main unit. Another cable snaked out between the seats through a rear window to the magnetic antenna stuck on the roof. Cell signals were a bit dicey back then. When I was driving between rural clinics, I could only talk when I reached the top of a hill. This was before smartphones. Ancient times. Before the internet.

I drove an old blue Subaru, a four-wheel drive SUV smaller than today's compact sedans. It was rusty and beat up. I loved it, except when the power windows stopped working and then the A/C broke. I would drive down highway 50 to Groveland through the Florida heat with my door cracked open, desperately sucking air from the outside breeze.

When I drove to meetings in Orlando from Apopka, there was an old dirt farm road that wasn't on any maps. It was my shortcut and my adrenaline release. For a few moments, I could pretend I was racing the Baja 500 in my off-road machine. I could even catch a little air when the rough dirt road launched me skyward. It was a little dangerous and a little irresponsible. It was just what I needed.

One day I was driving the backroads from Apopka to Groveland when the hospital ER nurse called me. A patient of mine was a young woman with a history of severe asthma attacks. She was breathing hard when she came in, and the meds weren't turning things around. *Status asthmaticus*—a severe asthma exacerbation that wasn't responding to the usual nebulizers and IVs and oxygen. At first, I wasn't too concerned. The ER was mostly staffed with young, well-trained physicians contracted from an emergency medicine group.

"OK, let the ER doc manage her. I'll come by and see her upstairs after clinic."

"No, you need to come now!" the nurse fairly shouted in a fierce voice. Then her voice dropped to a near-whisper. *"Dr. Bob is on today!"*

Dr. Bob was a wonderful old doc, a general practitioner who had seen everything in his years in practice. He had retired, but he picked up occasional shifts in the emergency room. Great guy, great doc, but he had one Achilles heel. He couldn't intubate a patient to save his life. Or theirs. My patient was pooping out fast. Rapid breathing had turned to barely breathing. The patient was slipping in and out of consciousness. My patient needed that breathing tube. *Stat!*

I goosed the Subaru like I was kicking an old mule. I raced on backroads through the frozen-out orange groves and mobile homes. *"Be there in ten minutes,"* I said, picturing the 12 miles I needed to cover and hoping an old carrot truck wouldn't slow me down on the winding two-lane road. My thoughts were racing even as I tore through the hills, between sawgrass-edged lakes and marsh.

In residency, I had placed lots of endotracheal tubes. You had to slide the heavy metal instrument between the teeth and over the tongue, watching the light find its way to the back of the throat. I would lift the lower jaw with force but carefully to avoid breaking teeth. It was easier in the neonatal unit, with preemie babies who had no teeth and whose larynx was easy to find.

Here I would be looking for the upside-down V-shape of the vocal cords. The goal was to slip my tube smoothly between the cords and into the trachea. I hadn't had to do the procedure in several years, and now I wished I had brushed up on it. I would be rushing into the ER for a patient who was rapidly losing consciousness and unable to breathe.

I called the nurse back from my big-brick mobile phone. I wanted to make sure the tray was set with all the equipment and supplies. I was still seven minutes out. I had one last thought. Give her half a milligram of atropine in the nebulizer machine to breathe. I knew it could be absorbed through the lungs. I was free-styling my anticholinergic pharmacology.

I hung up the brick-phone and raced the rest of the way to the hospital. I pulled up at the ambulance entrance and jumped out of the Subaru. As I came through the door, I was ready to grab a laryngoscope to intubate. The nurse met me at the door. I feared the worst. Then I saw that she was smiling. *"I don't know if we're supposed to use atropine like that,"* she said, *"but it was magic!"* Dr. Bob pulled the curtains aside and came out of the ER bay beaming. *"Didn't have to intubate after all,"* he said with more relief than bluster. He shook my hand vigorously, as if I had just graduated or had a baby.

I slipped in to see my patient. *"How are you doing?"* I asked.

"I thought I was dying," she said. Her breathing was steady and not rushed. *"But I'm doing fine now,"* she said calmly. *"I think I'm ready to go home."*

"I think we should keep you overnight to make sure your breathing doesn't get worse when the medicine wears off."

"*No,*" she said. "*I'm good. I've already got a big bill here. They'll send me to the collection agency again.*" She held out her hand to shake mine as well as for me to help her off the stretcher. "*Thank you,*" she said sincerely. "*Really.*" She started walking to the door. A nurse chased after her with paperwork to sign. Dr. Bob looked at me and shrugged.

It turned out that when we cared for our own patients in the hospital, they did better. We got their chronic conditions under better control. They had fewer visits to the emergency department. When they did show up in the ER, I would get a phone call. The patient with a blood sugar over 500 who might normally be admitted could get some IV fluids and some insulin and be sent home. I would see them later that morning in our clinic. The savings were substantial. The tax-district hospital ran a surplus in its indigent-care funds for the very first time that year. It turns out that caring for people properly actually has a concrete, bottom-line financial benefit. Go figure.

The win-win-win strategy of health care for all is still waiting to be harvested for America. In six-sigma terms, variation is inefficient. Variation in outcomes, whether by race or by insurance status, is not only bad for the patient but also economically wasteful. In 2018, health care economists estimated that the cost of illness and premature death due to racial disparities nationwide was at least $421 billion every year.[28] It costs taxpayers' money to allow preventable suffering. It would save money to do it right. Why don't we?

Healthy People 2000 focused on "reducing health disparities." Sadly, a 2012 progress review showed "a significant lack of progress in reducing or eliminating health disparities."[29] Over 30 years ago, an article published in the *Journal of the National Medical Association* had a table that listed racial health disparities in the United States.[30]

- Black infant mortality rate 2 times higher than that of white infants
  [now 2.3 times higher, which is even higher than it was in 1916]
- Black maternal mortality rate 3.3 times higher than that of white mothers
  [now 2.6 times higher]
- Black death rates for diabetes 2 times higher and kidney disease 3 times higher
  [same or higher now]
- Black non-elderly death rates 2 times higher than whites
  [same or higher now]

Compare that to Dr. Martin Luther King Jr.'s assessment from over half a century ago:

> When the Constitution was written, it declared that the Negro was 60 percent of a person. Today, another formula seems to declare that he is 50 percent of a person. Of the good things in life, the Negro has approximately one-half those of whites. Thus, Negroes have half the income of whites, and half of all Negroes live in substandard housing. Of the negative experiences of life, the Negro has a double share: there are twice as many unemployed among Negroes, and the rate of infant mortality is double that of whites.[31]

There's a saying in the African American community that when white folks get a cold, Black people get pneumonia. That was certainly true during the first few years of the COVID pandemic. I lived it on the front lines in my role as a local public health department medical director. Wearing my N-95 mask and face shield and double gloves, I leaned in through car windows in the COVID-testing drive-through lanes. I slid long swabs up people's noses and deep into the recesses of their nasopharynx as they coughed in my face.

When vaccines became available, I took students to community outreach events. At the fire station, we held a COVID vaccine drive-through. We vaccinated over a thousand people per day. I was on conference calls with hospital administrators who struggled to find ventilators and adequate supplies of oxygen. They also struggled to replace nurses who were burning out seeing hundreds of COVID deaths. In South Georgia, hospitals rented refrigerator trucks as temporary morgues for all the bodies.

Initially, our political leaders supported testing and vaccine efforts. The community-wide response saved lives. As is the way of the world, the advantaged took advantage first. The appointment slots for vaccines were quickly filled by people with the best education and computer skills. Cadillacs with older white people were overrepresented at the early drive-through events. Special outreach events were held at senior-care facilities. We saved lives.

Disparities were a real concern. My Morehouse colleagues have found a significant association between racial segregation and COVID vaccination rates.[32] Here in Tallahassee, we worked hard to prevent those disparities. Historically Black Florida A&M University (FAMU) set up a COVID testing center and then a vaccine distribution center. We coordinated our efforts. African American physicians and opinion leaders promoted the vaccine. Townhall sessions addressed community concerns and trustworthiness issues. We saved lives.

And then politics happened. Or maybe it just took an ugly turn. The president, who had authorized Operation Warp Speed to develop an effective vaccine in only one year, suddenly caught the wave of "populist" antivax passions. Distribution faltered. White, conservative, evangelical MAGA voters became the group at risk of being hospitalized and/or dying from COVID. Their devoted following of a leader betraying their best interests was killing them.

Our Florida governor also could have claimed a great success in saving so many lives. Early on, we achieved a 95 percent vaccination rate in our elderly population. Instead, he bailed on his success and chose to ride this angry "don't trust the scientists" political wave. Public health officials were not allowed to speak with media on actual science or facts related to COVID. We weren't allowed to engage in effective public health measures like using geographic hot-spot maps to target high-risk neighborhoods. These maps had been essential to public health ever since John Snow's 19th-century mapping of the London cholera epidemic. It became harder and harder to do our job. Harder and harder to save lives.

Instead of hiring a state surgeon general with actual public health credentials or experience, our governor went out of state to bring in an antivax, ideologically driven, academic hospitalist who could create pseudo-science rationalizations for the governor's decisions. Suddenly treatment with antibodies for people sick with COVID became the preferred public policy. Was it ignorance or ideology? Or was it because of political donations to the Republican Governors Association from those who sold the antibodies or ran the infusion centers? One thing I do know—favoring treatment over prevention was certainly not public health. And for that, people suffered and people died.

More than three decades earlier, small-town Groveland had been where I saw patients with preventable suffering. I saw late-stage cancer. I saw leg amputations from diabetes and strokes from uncontrolled hypertension. I saw the impact of untreated depression. I saw the lack of resources for alcohol or addiction recovery. I saw both fatalism and faith. Both assumed that we could not change such inequities in this fallen world.

Stalin once said that "one death is a tragedy; a million deaths is a statistic." As a health outcomes researcher, I know the statistics. As a family doc serving low-income and uninsured people, I know the tragedies. Cervical cancer, for example, is rarely seen at advanced stages in white, well-educated, well-insured patients. Once the Pap smear was widely adopted, cervical cancer went from being a leading cause of death for younger women to being a preventable, treatable condition. When a Pap smear comes back abnormal, the patient gets a minor procedure. The cancer never develops.

One evening, I was called to the emergency department to see one of my patients who was having profuse vaginal bleeding. She was from the dirt-poor enclave of Stuckey Still, once an old turpentine work camp outside of Groveland. The emergency physician thought she might bleed to death. She had been previously diagnosed with cervical cancer and treated with radiation implants by a specialist in Orlando. Perhaps because our patient didn't have good insurance, the GYN oncologist refused to have her transferred to the larger specialty hospital. *"I don't really have anything else to do for her,"* he said blithely. *"Just pack her with gauze, and maybe get her some hospice care."* Images of Pilate washing his hands flashed through my mind.

I examined her gently. With a lighted speculum, I tried to see past the blood that was pouring out. A normal cervix looks a bit like the tip of a nose, pink and round with a small hole at the center. Instead, I saw what appeared to be a huge stalk of rotting cauliflower where her cervix should be. Blood was leaking from multiple sites. *What the hell could I do?* I'm not a surgeon, and none of the specialists wanted to help me. I was alone in another moment of powerlessness that would age me prematurely.

I ordered blood transfusions to replace the blood she was losing so quickly. I packed sterile gauze up against the bleeding cauliflower cancer. I kept packing until the vaginal canal was full of bloody gauze, hoping that the pressure would staunch the bleeding.

I spoke gently with my patient. *"You know what's going on?"* She nodded. *"I got the cancer last year and they put the radiation seeds in me. But they said it was pretty far gone. I never had the Pap smear. Never really went to doctors at all. . . ."* I pause to let the wave of grief and sadness pass over me.

"The specialists, they say. . . ." I stumbled for words.

"I know," she said, trying to comfort me more than I was comforting her. I felt inadequate and powerless and sad. *"I've done everything I know how to do. We'll keep you here tonight and see if we can get the bleeding to stop."* We both knew how this would end if we couldn't. She expressed her faith in God and her sense of peace, whatever the outcome might be. My faith was a lot less adequate. We held hands for a bit, as I tried to give her my spirit and my compassion, even as she gave me her strength.

The next morning (a few hours later really), I came back to the hospital to check on her. The bleeding had stopped. Her blood count had stabilized with the transfusions. Later that day, we changed the packing. With old clots of blood came pieces of the cauliflower, the cancer that was trying to kill her. She was having a late response to the radiation. The cancer was dying more quickly than the patient. *"Tissue necrosis with hemorrhage due to erosion into a blood vessel,"* I wrote in the chart. But in my soul, I know it was a miracle. *Can't it be both?*

I came to understand that beyond each individual, the community was also my patient. I was practicing the specialty of community health,[33] and my community was ailing. It had a sick, abusive, dysfunctional history, largely based on race and poverty. I was trying to make a sick, dysfunctional health care system work for the uninsured and for the poor, for people of color and for immigrants.

The patients all needed healing, but so did the community. And the longer I worked there, the more I needed healing too.

FOR FURTHER READING

Agency for Healthcare Research and Quality. *2021 National Healthcare Quality and Disparities Report Executive Summary Agency for Healthcare Research and Quality.*

Caraballo C, Massey DS, Ndumele CD, et al. Excess mortality and years of potential life lost among the Black population in the US, 1999–2020. *JAMA.* 2023;329(19):1662–1670.

Injustice at Every Turn: A Report of the National Transgender Discrimination Survey.

LaVeist TA, Pérez-Stable EJ, Richard P, et al. The economic burden of racial, ethnic, and educational health inequities in the US. *JAMA.* 2023;329(19):1682–1692.

Satcher D. *My Quest for Health Equity: Notes on Learning While Leading.*

Satcher D, Fryer GE Jr, McCann J, Troutman A, Woolf SH, Rust G. What if we were equal? A comparison of the Black-white mortality gap in 1960 and 2000. *Health Aff (Millwood).* 2005;24(2):459–464.

Unequal Treatment: Confronting Racial and Ethnic Disparities in Health Care. National Academies Press; 2003.

Villarosa L. *Under the Skin: Racism, Inequality, and the Health of a Nation.*

3.

Unmentionable History
The Foundational Roots of Structural Inequities

I've been an MD for over 40 years now. I've seen some stuff. I've lived the history of modern medicine advancing into the 21st century. When I say, *"Before HIV . . ."* or *"Before we had beta-blockers,"* the students give me a look like I gave my older professors who said, *"Before we had penicillin. . . ."* Maybe for these students it will be, *"Before the AI robots took over."* But the amazing advances I have witnessed over the past 40 years came with echoes of America's troubled history.

My first day of medical school in 1977 was a flurry of activity. There was financial aid paperwork and trying to find an apartment. I went to pick up my course handouts for anatomy in the office of the department chairman. *"Hello, I am Dr. Zitzelsberger,"* he said with his distinctive German accent. I reached out and shook the chairman's hand. Just as I said, *"Hi, I'm George Rust,"* I fumbled my cup of coffee. *Bloosh!* Right onto his pristine tile floor. I was mortified. I awkwardly mopped up the mess. I slunk out of the room, hoping that he would not remember my name.

He was a passionate teacher of anatomy, who eschewed gloves. He would thrust his ancient bare hand deep into the abdominal cavities of our formalin-preserved cadavers. We didn't know his backstory, so stereotypes took over our imaginations. German accent, dead bodies, hand plunging ungloved into open corpse.... None of our fears or stereotypes were true, but that's how bias works sometimes. Somehow, we knew at least vaguely of Nazi medical experiments. But no one ever taught us the history of American medical atrocities.

In our OB/GYN rotations, we were taught surgical techniques pioneered by Dr. James Marion Sims. Statues have been erected to honor him, but now we know more. His research involved incredibly painful and invasive procedures on the most sensitive parts of slave women's bodies. It was all done without anesthesia.[1] On slaves, because, well, who else? Consent was obtained not from the slaves but by their owners. He himself was a slaveholder.[2] "The first one he operated on was 18-year-old Lucy, who ... during the procedure, ... was naked and asked to perch on [her] knees and ... elbows."[3] He did not use anesthesia, in part because of the stereotype that Black persons did not feel pain. But his own descriptions belie this belief: "Lucy endured an hour-long surgery, screaming and crying out in pain, as nearly a dozen other doctors watched. As Sims later wrote, 'Lucy's agony was extreme.'"[4]

He knew. The other doctors knew. Sims did not perform the procedure on white women until he had perfected it. Never without anesthesia. Recently, Virginia Republicans voted against issuing an apology for such historic atrocities. One argued that there would be "no end" to the number of apologies needed.[5] No end indeed. Dr. John Kenney of the Tuskegee Institute said this in 1941, "I suggest that a monument be raised and dedicated to the nameless Negroes who have contributed so much to surgery by the 'guinea pig' route."[6]

Dr. Kenney also described how Black surgeons had to overperform. He described the surgical scrub technique of the barebones operating room he worked in. They started by scrubbing their hands with boiling hot water and laundry soap and a stiff brush. The hands were then turned purple by immersion in potassium permanganate. Then there was a burning solution of oxalic acid. Bichloride of mercury came last, before the rubber gloves. He was proud of their abdominal surgeries in that rustic operating room, saying that "there was not a single infection that originated there."

How many students of color and of non-male gender have felt this pressure to overperform, just to be seen as equal? How many have felt the need to prove that they were not an affirmative action admission? How many have been asked by a classmate, *"How did you get here?"*

Non-white and non-male health professionals experience this every day. They are already swimming upstream against majority culture and microaggressions. Theirs is a different reality. On top of that, they feel pressured to overperform just to be perceived as equal. Is it any wonder that students of color, or those who are trans or queer, experience excess stress? Are we surprised that they drop out at higher rates than do their white cisgender peers?

As recently as 2015, only 6 percent of US medical graduates were African American. Only 5 percent were Hispanic or Latine.[7,8] Native American physicians are also grossly underrepresented.[9] These groups make up a third of young adults in the US population. In my medical school class, one of only a handful of students of color dropped out. He felt like he *"just didn't belong there."*

Gender inequities also abound. In 1949, only 1 in 20 physicians were women. By the time my wife was admitted to medical school in the early 1980s, a third of our class were women. By 2008, women had achieved near equality with men. Yet women are still grossly underrepresented in senior faculty and leadership roles.

Dr. Damon Tweedy writes of the challenges of being *A Black Man in a White Coat*. He attended medical school at Duke and trained in neurosurgery at University of Michigan. Dr. Tweedy reminds us that it's not just Black patients who need Black doctors. He quotes one of his white patients in Michigan who said, "I would like to thank you for two things. One, for saving my life, and two, for changing my point of view. Before you took out my brain tumor, I didn't like Black people."[10]

In one of my years at Morehouse, Georgia's public medical school matriculated only one African American student in an entering class of over 120. At the same time, the state's population was over 30 percent Black. The student dropped out of the nearly all-white medical school after only a few weeks. Black legislators who had approved state funding for the Medical College of Georgia (MCG) were outraged.

I was in our school president's office when Dr. Louis Sullivan took a call and put it on speakerphone. The state legislator who led the Georgia Association of Black Elected Officials was outraged. He had had enough. In quite angry and slightly profane language, he assured Dr. Sullivan that Morehouse School of Medicine (MSM) would get extra funding that year. By God, Black physicians would be trained in Georgia. That extra million dollars in our state appropriation also sent a message to MCG. Diversity was not optional.

Although new at the time, MSM was still known as a "historically Black" institution. It was born out of Morehouse College, and it continued to build on the legacy of other historically Black colleges and universities (HBCUs), training new generations of Black physicians and leaders. It's what Meharry Medical College and Howard University had done in the century following Reconstruction. Morehouse College alumnus Dr. John Silvanus Wilson described the difference between learning at an HBCU versus going to Harvard: "At Morehouse, they held a crown over my head and expected me, challenged me, to grow tall enough to wear it. When I came to Harvard, they held a question mark over my head. I felt the institution was causing me to ask, *'Do I belong here?'*"[11]

Would having more persons of color in the medical profession improve care and outcomes? Sometimes. Often a Black doctor seeing a Black patient gives more empathetic care and is trusted more. Citing recent research, the *Washington Post* reported this: "Mortality rate for Black babies is cut dramatically when Black doctors care for them after birth."[12]

But sometimes not. Doctors of color can internalize the mind-set of the historically white male institutions they trained in. Patients can internalize a racism that says that Black doctors are somehow "less than." I was a Morehouse physician practicing at historically Black Southwest Hospital in the Black Mecca of Atlanta. Still, African American patients would call the clinic and ask for an appointment with the *white* doctor. It broke my heart to realize that it wasn't because of me. It was internalized racism, and I was complicit.

In the 1960s, one young Black medical student stood up at Case Western Reserve University to protest low-income Black women being coercively subjected to students practicing pelvic examinations.[13] The future US Surgeon General walked out, rather than being complicit. The dean considered kicking young David Satcher out of medical school the very next day. To their credit, the other students backed him up. But he had been the only student who saw the patients as women who could have been his sister or his mother. He saw their essential humanity when others did not.

HBCUs and tribal colleges have Black, Indigenous, and other People of Color (BIPOC) in power all the way from their governing boards to their presidents and deans. It extends down through their faculty, staff, and students. White people are there and have a voice. Yet the organization is overbalanced from the top-down toward minoritized people having the power. They define the institutional culture and priorities.

Where is the historically white institution that has made such a transition? When will we see a 21st-century historically white medical school begin to fully reflect a Black–Brown majority, multilingual, multigendered America in its leadership, its culture, its budget, and its curriculum? Spend a day in the leadership meetings of institutions that claim to have diversity. Watch how people interact with one another. Look at their curriculum. It's a last-century, white male-dominated culture, with a little "diversity-icing" on their organizational cake.

I find myself now as a white male professor in a historically white-majority university in the no-longer-purple state of Florida. Tallahassee is a progressive college town surrounded by rural Deep South communities. Our state's capital city is ground zero for the battle between progress and regress, between woke and anti-woke, and between justice and "just us."

A member of the Florida Board of Governors singled out FSU for having "a DEI ideology" that has "embedded itself everywhere in the university."[14] That one actually made me feel proud! Our university has achieved four-year graduation rates that are equal not just across all racial-ethnic groups but also for young people who are the first in their families to attend college. That's equity.

For all who are against DEI, let me ask—"*what are you for? If you're against* inclusion, *whom would you like to exclude? If you're against* equity, *which inequities do you favor? And if you're against* diversity, *are you advocating white supremacy?*" I'm proud that I work for a medical school that regularly receives awards for the diversity of our students. Still, I do wonder, relative to what? Compared to HBCUs, we have a long way to go.

Sometimes someone will ask, "*Why do we still need affirmative action? Why do we need DEI initiatives? Why do we still need*

HBCUs?" And I answer with my own question. *"When exactly did racism end in America? When did structural inequities get repaired? When was there truth and reconciliation and recompense for all that has gone before?"*

I love my country, but it's complicated. In my home I have an American flag that was folded and presented to my mother at my father's grave. I put it in a triangular frame with a bronze marker. It is a dedication to the military service of my son (Air Force), my father (Navy), and my two grandfathers (Army Medical Corps and Marine Corps). When I place my hand over my heart during the national anthem, I do it to remember and honor them. I do it to honor what America aspires to be.

In a Fourth of July speech, Dr. Martin Luther King Jr. said, "On the one hand, we have proudly professed the noble principles of democracy. On the other hand, we have sadly practiced the very anti-thesis of those principles."[15] More than a hundred years earlier, Frederick Douglass had asked, "What to the Slave is the Fourth of July? . . . Are the great principles of political freedom and of natural justice, embodied in that Declaration of Independence, extended to us?"[16]

For me, I love the aspirational ideals that define us as a nation. I also hate that we have not yet been able to live up to these ideals. I hope that somehow, in fits and starts, we're still making progress. In our generation, Colin Kaepernick knelt during the National Anthem to protest police violence and racial injustice. It was a sacred act of patriotic protest. A generation earlier, baseball hero Jackie Robinson had said, "I cannot stand and sing the anthem. I cannot salute the flag. I know that I am a Black man in a white world."[17]

There has been progress. John Meacham's history books describe those standing up for justice "from Seneca Falls to Selma to Stonewall." He cites John Lewis, who saw this progress firsthand.

Lewis said, "If you think nothing's changed in the past 50 years, ask somebody who lived through Selma or Chicago or Los Angeles of the 1950s."[18]

In 1970, Ralph Ellison said that "today it is the Black American who puts pressure upon the nation to live up to its ideals."[19] More than 50 years later, from Black Lives Matter to Tennessee state legislators, African Americans are still having to call us out to live up to our American ideals. To do so, we must keep ratcheting up our actions to match our ideals. Our walk must match our talk.

America is like a dysfunctional family that is struggling to grow out of its own contradictions. I honor my father's father, a World War I war hero whom I met only briefly as an infant. He died from lung damage caused both by mustard gas in the trenches and by decades of heavy smoking. I honor his sacrificial service. He received commendations for evacuating wounded men on stretchers from some of the most bloody and horrific battles of World War I. He got a Purple Heart for his lung injuries. I also know that he was an alcoholic, posttraumatic, war-scarred veteran. Military records show that he once was docked a half a month's pay for "negligently" getting syphilis. His unpredictable fits of rage led him to violently abuse my grandmother.

I know of him as the scary man that my father stood up to at the age of 12. The brave, trembling little boy stood with a baseball bat to protect his mother. For the rest of his life, he blamed himself for their divorce. My dad could never acknowledge how that trauma had hurt and scarred him. He never understood the pools of anger and mistrust it left deep inside him. He had no sense of where his unpredictable fits of rage came from. When he had a series of small strokes, I prayed that they might erase his pockets of pain and hurt and bitterness. I grieve that he found so little healing.

Addiction counselors say that we are only as sick as our secrets. I know what it is to be part of a family that does not speak of those secrets. We dare not acknowledge our shame. We only pretend that our ancestors were good and true and noble.

I also know what it is to walk on eggshells to avoid poking the bear. We step carefully to avoid unleashing the pools of rage. Yet I know now what it is to find healing in looking honestly at the hard truth of my own strengths and failures. I look clearly at both my family's proud accomplishments as well as its hidden shames. We move forward by cleansing our wounds, in honest and sometimes painful healing.

Can America face its own history? Our history is hard because it goes against the grain of American mythology, of our idealized Founding Fathers and of the reasons for America's success. How we see America is like a Rorschach test for the experience of disadvantage versus advantage, of oppression versus privilege. Langston Hughes lamented that "there's never been equality for me, nor freedom in this home of the free. . . . Who said the free? Not me!"[20]

Growing up, I thought I knew what a "race riot" was. By the time the Watts riots occurred in Los Angeles in 1965, it had come to mean an uprising of people angrily demanding racial justice. But from the 1900s through the early 1960s, the term "race riot" meant a violent attack of a white mob on a Black neighborhood. Race riot really meant race massacre.

A white-on-Black massacre occurred in Tulsa, Oklahoma, in 1921, when white people violently assaulted Black Wall Street's people, buildings, and economic power. Threatened by the election of Black local officials in 1898, white people in Wilmington, North Carolina, overthrew a democratically elected local government. They killed dozens of African Americans in a "white declaration of independence." In any other context, we would call it terrorism. Such *race massacres* were numerous throughout the 20th century.[21]

The tired trope of immigrants coming to steal white people's jobs has also been part of our history. It often led to state-sanctioned violence. When a Chinese immigrant was shot and killed by a white man in 1854, the California Supreme Court deemed testimony from Asian people inadmissible.[22] In 1871, 17 Chinese men and boys were lynched in Los Angeles. In Wyoming in 1885, vigilantes killed 28 Chinese mineworkers and burned 79 homes. In World War II, more than 110,000 Japanese people were held in internment camps.

Similar atrocities were perpetrated against Native peoples in America. Many of us have heard of Wounded Knee but may not recall that 150 Sioux people were massacred there in 1890. In school, I never learned of the killing of 130 Cheyenne people in 1864 or of the Bear River Massacre of 350 Shoshone Nation people.

After World War I, the 1920s saw a spike in racist violence. Many congresspersons, the president, and even Supreme Court Justice Oliver Wendell Holmes explicitly endorsed white supremacy. In those years, many statues were erected to Confederate "heroes." It is when the Confederate flag found a resurgent role, becoming the *f***-you* flag of aggrieved white men of the South.

Some of this hard-truth history was almost entirely erased, just as the town of Rosewood was erased from the Florida maps I grew up with. The town of Rosewood was destroyed by a white mob in 1923, and its African American citizens were massacred. The Black population in Ocoee, Florida (just west of Orlando), was also decimated. People died as their homes burned in 1920. The catalyst was that a Black man had tried to vote. In the 1980s, I was medical director for community clinics that cared for patients who had moved to Apopka after fleeing the race massacre in Ocoee. This hard history was never taught in our schools. It was never spoken of by white families.

Now, a century later, my Florida governor and legislature seem intent on making sure that Florida's children are protected from ever learning this history. There can be no arc of history connecting past oppression to modern racial inequalities. Because of the

"Stop Woke Act," the Disney film *Ruby Bridges* was banned in Pinellas County schools, all on the objections of one white mother. She thought her child could not deal with a movie about a brave little girl who had courageously walked through a racist mob to attend elementary school.

Meanwhile, children of color are being subjected to white denial of their reality every day.[23] How will all our children understand the strength and resiliency of African Americans if they do not understand what they were up against? What good is it to teach about Harriet Tubman and the Tuskegee Airmen during Black History Month if we do not also teach the realities of slavery and race massacres and the Jim Crow South?

Florida laws aren't needed to protect the white children. Children are fine with learning about the realities of our nation. They're not fragile. They are way better at having honest conversations about race and culture and gender and sexuality than we are. How does it serve even white children to restrict their learning? Will protecting them from critical thinking really prepare them for college or the job market? How can those protected children possibly be effective in the non-white rainbow America we are becoming? And how will they ever be competitive in a global economy that needs both workers and leaders to be multilingual, multicultural, and forward-thinking?

Archbishop Desmond Tutu and his daughter cite research on resilience in children. "The more children knew the stories of their family's history—the good, the bad, and the ugly—the more resilient the children turned out to be."[24] The researchers said that knowing their families' tragic history turned out to be "the single best predictor of children's emotional health and happiness."

In Florida, we live in the state of denial. Governor Ron DeSantis has said that Florida is "where woke goes to die." Many who slur the term "woke" can't even say what it means. The governor's communication director said simply that "woke" was "a slang term for progressive activism." In court, the governor's general counsel said that it referred to "the belief there are systemic injustices in American society and the need to address them."[25]

Being woke can mean different things in different settings. For people of color, *"Stay Woke"* can mean to sleep with one eye open. There are always those (individuals and systems) that mean to do you harm. For me as a white guy, it means to constantly be aware of others' reality. To be woke is to see the world through others' eyes. See the injustice. To be woke is to stand up for what's good and right and true.

The point of honest teaching about race and history is not to foster white guilt. It's to learn factual American history. It's to see both our glorious aspirations and our tragically imperfect implementation. It's a gap analysis, understanding the gap between our ideals and our reality. It's honest and true and necessary. A district court judge recently suspended some of the Stop Woke Act's provisions, saying, "Defendants argue that, under this Act, professors enjoy 'academic freedom' so long as they express only those viewpoints of which the State approves. . . . This is positively dystopian."[26]

We see history and society and even theology through race-tinged lenses. Tom Skinner, an evangelist of Black liberation theology, said one day that he "realized that he'd gotten Jesus wrong. Jesus wasn't in the Rotary Club, but instead was 'a radical revolutionary . . . with dirt under his fingernails." He said, "Any gospel that does not speak to the issue of 'enslavement' and 'injustice' and 'inequality' . . . or does not want to go where people are hungry or poverty-stricken and set them free . . . is not the gospel."[27]

White evangelical authors labeled Tom Skinner "the prophet of Harlem."[28] As a college student in the 1970s, I heard Skinner speak. He said that the score in the ballgame we call America was 27 to 3. The white team and the umpires were cheating for the first seven innings. Suddenly, the white team captain stands up and says, *"Hey, everybody. From now on, nobody cheats, okay!"* And the Black team may score in the eighth and ninth innings, but the Black team will almost certainly lose. The white team will say that the game ended fairly. Skinner challenged us all to see through new eyes the white frame on which evangelicalism was being defined.

This now is also the white frame of American political conservatism. In Virginia, Governor Glenn Youngkin restricted any public school teaching of race in America. Dana Milbank called it "Glenn Youngkin's No-Guilt History of Virginia for Fragile White People."[29] Like textbooks from the 1950s, it portrays slavery as a genteel and mutually beneficial relationship between Black slaves and their white masters. In 2023, Florida set new curriculum standards to institutionalize this very notion. It required teaching the *benefits of slavery* for Black slaves.

This simply institutionalizes white denial. It reinforces false narratives of a benign "happy plantation" history that ended with the Civil War. The claim is that to revisit that past, or to connect it to ongoing structural inequities, is to propagate a racialized view of America. It's the ultimate projection. "I'm not racist. You are, because you keep bringing up race. Who's the racist now?"

Such white denialism also extends to ideologues such as Youngkin's public health director. He denied that racial health disparities are real, as well as the structural inequities that drive them.[30] But if no system-level inequalities have persisted from our history, and if there is no overt discrimination now, then how do we explain all the disparities suffered by communities of color? Is it somehow their own fault?

The key to understanding systemic racism is to trace the arc of current inequities to their history. Many were codified in law.[31] Ta-Nehisi Coates wrote that "there exists, all around us, an apparatus urging us to accept American innocence at face value and not to inquire too much."[32] What gives America plausible deniability now is that these structures and systems act almost invisibly to produce racial (and gender) inequalities. They don't require any explicit bias or overt discrimination. They are insidious. Racism without racists. Community development leader John Perkins described the system born of this history well. He cited "the whole structure of economic and social cages that have neatly boxed the Black man in, so that 'nice' people can join the oppression without getting their hands dirty—just by letting things run along."[33]

Our history in health care is especially complex. For the entire century following the Civil War, hospitals and clinics were segregated. Older African American physicians often describe their interest in becoming a doctor in terms of a tragic experience of a family member. The ambulance that would not carry Black patients. The doctors who would not treat them. The hospitals that would turn them away.

This was not just a phenomenon of the South.[34] Blueprints of many northern hospitals also showed specific intent to segregate care between the races.[35,36] There were separate wards, separate operating rooms, and even separate historically Black hospitals. Describing a patient as a 30-year-old Negro male made clear which ward a patient would be sent to or whose blood could be used for transfusions. Segregation of hospital wards was enforced every day by doctors and nurses. The banality of evil, of racism, was the way in which it was so casually internalized by doctors and patients alike.

Nor was this just an issue of hospitals. Physicians of our day like to pretend that they had nothing to do with this ugly racial history. But until the mid-1960s, doctors' offices throughout the country were built with two separate waiting rooms. That is, if they would allow African American patients to be seen at all.

In the 1960s, the federal government forced hospitals to change. First, they prohibited the use of Hill–Burton funds for the construction of segregated facilities. Then Medicare reimbursement was withheld from hospitals that persisted in racial segregation. In response, many hospitals sued to fight what they called government overreach.

But eliminating racially segregated hospital wards did not suddenly end racial discrimination. It did not end explicit and implicit bias. Nor did it end disparate care for persons of color or of non-male gender or of non-English language. History and progress occur gradually, not in sudden discontinuities. Colleagues of mine called it "Medical Apartheid" more than 30 years ago.[37] In 2021, a medical resident described *"the segregated care provided within our academic institutions"*: "To the right were the 'resident' clinics, where Medicaid patients were seen. To the left were the 'attending' clinics for privately insured patients. I watched as Black patients turned right and White patients turned left. It was 2020, but it could have been 1950."[38]

Harsh truths make history hard but no less true. Authors of a paper on racial disparities said that "physician leadership helped to establish the slaveocracy, create the racial inferiority myths, and build the segregated health subsystem for Blacks and the poor."[39] *Ouch!* But what if we were to embrace this hard history? What if we could acknowledge that we are a complicated people who can only grow if we learn from our past? What if we could embrace the language of recovery, that we are only as sick as our lies and denials? What if honest transparency could lead us to healing?

Archbishop Desmond Tutu said that the past "will return and haunt us unless it has been dealt with adequately. Unless we look the beast in the eye, we will find that it returns to hold us hostage."[40] I have seen the beast of our past all throughout my career. I trained in Chicago, the "progressive" North. At Cook County Hospital, I cared for African American patients from the Great Migration, people with strong Mississippi and Alabama roots. They came north to find work in the steel mills that offered salaries and a middle-class life. But many didn't find the good jobs. Janitorial jobs or construction work didn't provide health insurance. That's how they came to be my patients at Cook County Hospital.

These patients had left to escape the oppression of the Jim Crow South. Each of them knew deep in their bones what it was like to live in that reality. Lynchings. Beatings. Legal segregation. Humiliation. Colored and white bathrooms and water fountains. Sundown towns, where the siren went off at 6 p.m. to remind all people of color (and, in western states, all American Indians) that it was illegal to be there after dark. After dark, your very personhood was illegal. Before the Great Migration, 90 percent of African Americans lived in the South. At its end, nearly half lived in the North or West.

But Chicago had its own flavor of oppression. Chicago was the city where a march for fair housing was disrupted by 700 angry white people in Marquette Park. Dr. King was hit by a rock. Others were injured by bricks and bottles. The North could no longer pretend that racial animosity was a southern thing. "I have to do this—to expose myself—to bring this hate into the open," said Dr. King.[41] Afterward, he said, "I have seen many demonstrations in the south, but I have never seen anything so hostile and so hateful as I've seen here today."[42]

To call out housing discrimination, Dr. King moved into a run-down third-floor apartment in the North Lawndale neighborhood of Chicago. By the time I worked at Cook County Hospital 16 years later, North Lawndale was still a low-income Black neighborhood. Nearby South Lawndale was a low-income Latine neighborhood. I knew South Lawndale and the Pilsen/Little Village neighborhood (La Villita) because that's where Dr. Jorge Prieto had started a clinic for first-generation Mexican immigrants. It was the small, crowded facility where I saw my own clinic patients for three years in the early 1980s.

Vice Lord and Latin King gangs enforced the separation of Black residents in North Lawndale from Latine residents in South

Lawndale. North Lawndale was where I walked to take the L from the clinic to my home. This whole area of abandoned factories and burned out neighborhoods was described in the *Chicago Tribune* like this—"Drive west . . . out past the hospital complex [where I trained]. . . . The overwhelming sensation is emptiness . . . What's left is literally nothing."[43] The unemployment rate was almost 60 percent.

North Lawndale was one of the neighborhoods in which Jonathan Kozol documented the *Savage Inequalities* of US public education. There he visited schools serving some of Chicago's lowest-income kids. Poor educational outcomes fed a culture of low expectations. Kozol looked at kindergarten kids, and despite their hopeful faces, he read their future: "More than half will drop out of school; fewer than one in five will go to college, and less than one in twenty will graduate from college. One in four of the boys will spend time in prison."[44]

A few miles north, my grandmother had lived out her days on the near north side of Chicago in the house where she had been born. In her day, the phrase was "white flight." Neighborhoods fought hard to keep even one "Negro" from moving in. Banks and federal lending programs such as the Veterans Administration and Federal Housing Administration redlined neighborhoods. They worked to make sure that loans were only given to people in "desirable" white neighborhoods.

The racial discrimination was explicit and institutionalized. When African American families moved in, there was white fear. In a self-fulfilling prophecy, property values declined because white people fled the neighborhood. Central urban areas became more Black and more poor. Wealth and whiteness moved to the suburbs.

What do poverty and residential segregation have to do with health? Measures of neighborhood poverty are associated with physical changes in people. There are measurable changes in metabolic indices. Cells show markers of stress and aging. We call it racial weathering, or allostatic load. The stress of poverty also causes profound changes in the developing brains of infants and children.[45,46] For adults, cognitive bandwidth for decision-making is consumed by the day-to-day uncertainties of living in poverty.[47,48]

Internationally, countries with greater social support systems and greater equality consistently have the best survival rates.[49] They also perform better on metrics of well-being, such as literacy, trust, and social mobility. They experience lower rates of homicide, imprisonment, teenage births, obesity, and mental illness. In the words of a recent book title—*More Equal Societies Almost Always Do Better.*[50]

In our second-year neuropsychology block, I co-teach a session with Ms. Miaisha Mitchell. She is a friend and community advocate, formerly a health care administrator. The session is titled *How Poverty Gets into Our Heads: The Neurobiology and Psychology of Poverty*. Ms. Mitchell tells the story of the Smoky Hollow community here in Tallahassee where she grew up. She had 13 siblings, raised by her mother (a teacher) and her father (a skilled laborer). There was no stove, so they cooked in the fireplace and used kerosene lamps. Schoolbooks were handed down from white schools.

It was dirt-poor poverty. And yet she describes with fondness the strength and resiliency of the extended Black family. She speaks of the sense of community connectedness she felt. Everyone in the neighborhood looked out for the children.[51] Then suddenly, urban renewal forcibly displaced African Americans from their cohesive neighborhood communities. Valuable downtown land was taken. Black families were forced to find housing in other segregated areas or in public housing projects. The poverty was re-concentrated, while the community strengths and cohesiveness were disrupted.

Cascade Park is now beautifully landscaped with fountains and water features that seemingly wash away that history. Millennials walk and jog in the park. The idealized snapshot of white and Black children playing in the same fountains nurtures the illusion of living in a postracial society.

But when everyone goes home at night, the neighborhoods are not the same. Resources are not the same. Public schools are not equal. Crime and policing are experienced differently. Employment opportunities, family wealth, business ownership, and home values all differ dramatically by neighborhood, often defined by race. Racial inequality without visible racists. Nice people like me, benefiting from the oppression without getting our hands dirty.

Segregation in the small town of Groveland, Florida, was just a little more obvious. My wife and I moved there in July 1985. Groveland was the two-stoplight town where I would see my patients. They were not just farmworkers but anyone who was poor or uninsured. The town had one general practice doctor, a family-owned pharmacy, and a family-owned funeral home (same family). There was a Black side of town and a white side. Guess where the roads were paved? Groveland was the kind of Deep South town where my Chicago patients would still have been living if they had not moved north in the Great Migration.

My Latine farmworker patients and their families were the "invisible community." They typically lived in trailers and small homes outside of town. They lived even beyond the low-income white enclave of Mascotte and the Black hollows of Stuckey Still. Many found seasonal work in the orange juice processing plant. During harvest season, they picked Hamlin oranges or Minneola tangelos. In summer, they drove north to Georgia or the Carolinas to harvest fruit or vegetables. Or they drove south to pick tomatoes in Immokalee. Sometimes they drove and found only rainstorms. Then there was no work and no income.

Groveland still had Old South racism. My patients still experienced structural inequities and discrimination every day, but now it was thinly papered over with polite denialism. We had become that next-generation dysfunctional family who dared not speak of it. History included lynchings and sheriffs who openly supported the KKK. Black families had had to run into the woods to escape white mobs shooting and burning down homes. It was all part of the well-known but unspoken shame of this little town.

That history is part of our American family's story. It is our ongoing dysfunction. It is passed down across generations. The intergenerational legacy of this trauma is both psychological and epigenetic. It changes our basic DNA expression regulating stress responses.[52] None of us escapes. The family dysfunction accrues to not only the children of the oppressed but also the oppressors. It is most insidious for the children of those who stood by and said nothing.

We cannot achieve the ideal of America until we honestly confront all that we have inherited. We cannot have reconciliation without truth first. We cannot find redemption without repentance and recompense. And we cannot heal ourselves or our nation unless we work through the trauma and the ongoing dysfunction.

And so, inevitably, we must talk not just about race, but racism.

FOR FURTHER READING

Bronshi M. *A Queer History of the United States for Young People.*

Dunbar-Ortiz R. *An Indigenous Peoples' History of the United States.*

Dunn M. *A History of Florida Through Black Eyes.*

Kozol J. *Savage Inequalities: Children in America's Schools.*

Nehisi-Coates T. *Between the World and Me.*

Pickett K, Wilkinson R. *The Spirit Level: Why More Equal Societies Almost Always Do Better.*

Rothstein R. *The Color of Law: A Forgotten History of How Our Government Segregated America.*

Wilson DE, Kaczmarek JM. The history of African-American physicians and medicine in the United States. *J Assoc Acad Minor Phys.* 1993;4(3):93–98.

Zinn H. *A People's History of the United States,* by Howard Zinn.

4.

The Unspeakable R-Word: Racism

Am I a racist? Is our nation racist? Are these questions even helpful?

Let's start with the first question. Am I a racist? On one level, my answer is, *"Of course I am."* I was raised with an internalized white bias in a racialized America. I have both ignored and benefited from white privilege with only occasional guilt. White postracial denial is still a part of me.

On the other hand, I never belonged to the KKK. I don't use the n-word. I reject white nationalism. I don't carry racial animus. I have Black friends. I can have conversations about race without getting all squirmy and defensive. By white people's definition, I am not a racist.

One scholar said that for white people, *"Racism is like murder. . . . Someone has to commit it in order for it to happen."*[1] It is defined by intentionally committing a heinous act. If you don't do any blatantly racist evil things, then in white-world, you are not a racist. Whew! By that definition, my fellow white folks, we are not racists, and America is not a racist nation. Rest easy.

But . . . if we define racism as the following:

- Having a white frame of reference in a racialized nation
- Having conscious and unconscious (implicit) bias buried deep inside us
- Living in white privilege (even if we faced enormous life challenges)
- Being passively okay with racial inequities in health and wealth
- Engaging in white postracial denial
- Failing to confront racism in our families and our work and our communities

Then yeah. We are kinda racist. Maybe a lot racist. And our country is kinda racist. Maybe a lot racist.

A key dimension of bias is my frame of reference. As Robin Di-Angelo says, "I was not taught to see myself in racial terms. I was made aware that somebody's race mattered, . . . [but] it would be theirs, not mine."[2] That's what I mean by a white-normed frame of reference. It's a privilege of living in white-world. In the imperfect metaphor of racism as an addiction illness, I sometimes think of myself as a recovering racist (also a recovering chauvinist, homophobe/transphobe, etc.). I have a lot of work to do. I need healing.

Hi, I'm George. I'm a racist. Celebrating two hours of un-racist sobriety. My recovery is imperfect, incomplete, and day-to-day. I am a walking contradiction in racism recovery. One day, I speak passionately about health justice at a conference. An hour later, I may choose not to confront an overt statement of white postracial denial. I'm avoiding the conversation because I've had it a thousand times before and I'm just too damn tired today. That's white privilege in action. I can choose my own moments of engagement.

I'm also a very imperfect antiracist. I sometimes purposely avoid the word "racism" when I'm trying to get white people to hear me. In those moments, I understand white denial all too well. I also understand what the word "racism" means in white-world.

For me to call out speech or policies as racist means that people hear me calling them racist in the ways that white people understand the word. I am lumping them with KKK-loving, n-word-using, white nationalist segregationist racists. The word "racism" is kryptonite to white people. Their sphincters instantly clamp down in a protective spasm of every bodily orifice. It closes their ears and brains as well. There is nothing else I can say to influence them from that moment forward. Their defensive shields are up.

Maybe I'm catering to their/our white fragility by coddling them. But if I can get a white hospital executive or political leader to commit to achieving racially equitable outcomes, then I'm good with it. If I can get them to do what it takes in policy or structure, then I'm okay. I'm willing to forego the moral satisfaction of calling it out with such a loaded word. Racism.

In his book, *How to Be an Antiracist*, Ibram X. Kendi says, "Only racists shy away from using the R-word."[3] So by that definition, in those moments, I'm a racist. I accept that. I wrestle with it, but I still choose my moments. Professor Kendi goes on to say, "The only way to undo racism is to consistently identify and describe it—then dismantle it."

Over some decades of work, my research teams have quantified a wide range of health inequities. We have described paths to health equity.[4] We have put forward a vision of what racially equitable outcomes would look like.[5,6] I have called for the dismantling of racially unbalanced power structures in hospitals and medical schools. I've argued for untipping the scales of diversity in leadership positions. Sometimes I use the word "racism," and sometimes I don't. Sometimes my audience just can't hear it.

Maybe it's a compromise, taking the easy way out. But maybe it's also about speaking their language, in institutions where the culture and leadership are still majority-white. Some white men who would otherwise be sympathetic can be turned off simply by using the term "white privilege."[7] Start with where they're at. Walk them through the minefield of talking about racism. Help them move beyond the safe haven of *"not all white people. . . ."* If they can't deal with the word "racism" but are open to working on racial inequalities, then we're moving forward. If it leads to change, I can live with that.

Does calling people or institutions racist sometimes break through denial? Can it lead to transformative change? Maybe, but not very often. It feels like refusing to help someone until they say the magic words, *"I'm an alcoholic,"* or *"I'm an addict."* Stubborn people and well-defended institutions rarely have that road-to-Damascus moment of epiphany. They don't fall to their knees saying, *"God, forgive me for I am a racist! I see it now!"* Nor did I. People of love and generous spirit and truth and justice walked with me and shared their lived experience. They helped me see the world through their eyes. And by grace I began to heal.

In primary care practice and in life, I have found that the three S's (shaming, scolding, and scaring) are not effective in getting people to change their behaviors. Instead, I choose to enter into a relationship with people who have self-harming behaviors. Whether it's smoking or alcohol or heroin or racism, I will walk with them on their journey. I try to understand their choices. I try to help them in whatever ways they're willing. If they begin to see how their mindset and behaviors can hurt others and themselves, they can find their own motivations to change. Only then can they perhaps find a path to healing and recovery.

Words do matter. I once kicked a patient out of our community health center practice for referring casually to my colleague as the *n____-doctor.* The patient was an old southern white guy with a grade-school education who couldn't read. He was poor and uninsured. He had nowhere else to receive care. He eked out a living selling ears of corn or watermelons by the side of the road. Eventually it was our African American nurses and doctor who convinced me to take him back. That's grace.

The patient I should have refused to see was the state senator who came to me for a cheap shoulder injection. He could have gone to the private specialists who often refused to see my patients. He was too shrewd to be caught saying the n-word in public. Still, the bills he supported in the state legislature did far more harm to the African American community. More harm than ever did a simple, ignorant white man who had grown up in a family that used the n-word. To my knowledge, after that moment, my poor illiterate farmer never used it again.

I choose to believe that no person is inherently racist, or at least that they are not so hardwired for life. We all can make choices. We can all have more antiracist moments and less racist moments. We all can seek to learn. We can all begin to heal. Intentionally. Imperfectly. One day at a time.

I once was asked by students of Atlanta's elite historically Black institutions to give the keynote address on health care reform. It was our culture there to speak openly about the nuances of race and racism, about health and poverty. The students had also arranged a panel of respondents, most of whom I knew as colleagues with progressive views.

One panelist I didn't know. She was invited specifically to represent a diverse perspective. She was a white, conservative, suburban state legislator with free-market, high-autonomy, white racism–denying views. I gave a straightforward presentation. I showed images and graphs that documented racial and socioeconomic health disparities. I offered international comparisons of what America spends on health care (the most) versus where we ranked in health outcomes (pretty poorly).

I reminded us of the history of racism in American health care. I mentioned specifically the racial segregation of hospital wards and operating rooms. I connected the dots between the racism of the long-ago past to the current pattern of Black–white health disparities. I spoke of structural racism, enforced now through poverty and uninsurance and Medicaid policies.

Then it was the legislator's turn. To her, my talk had been pure anti-white, anti-American socialism. It was a stick in the hornet's nest of her white conservative denial. I could instantly see that her anger had overwhelmed any facts or logical train of thought. Her face was red. As she spoke, her words came out spitting rage. *"I don't know why you invited me here,"* she fumed. *"If this is what you are teaching here and if Dr. Rust is the kind of professor you're hiring, I'll make sure that Morehouse School of Medicine never gets another dime of funding from Georgia again!"*

Ruh Roh. I had no concerns about her attacking me personally. But she was a state legislator on the budget committee that decided our state funding. She could cripple or even kill our institution. The students asked eagerly if I would like to respond to her comments. *"No,"* I shook my head weakly. *"I would very much* not *like to anger the legislator again, thank you very much."* Dr. Camara Jones was a Morehouse colleague and is still a leading voice for antiracism in medicine. She's also a great human being. At the end of the program, she approached me with great compassion. *"You look like you need a hug,"* she said. I really did.

The next morning, I found myself sitting in the office of our school's president. Dr. John Maupin had played a key role in creating the original vision of our National Center for Primary Care. He had always been supportive. *"Dr. Maupin, I'm sorry,"* I said. *"I didn't know who she was, didn't know she was on the panel . . ."* as my voice trailed off. *"I'd never want to do anything to hurt Morehouse,"* I offered lamely. He smiled and waved away my concerns. *"I know. The dean says your talk was mom and apple pie. Just lay low for a little while, okay?"* he said with a fatherly smile. And that was it. That was Morehouse.

For months I turned down media interviews and kept good on my promise to lay low. Almost a year later, I was asked to speak at the annual legislative dinner of our Atlanta Medical Society. I hesitated. Was this conservative legislator going to be there? She was indeed. I went to our school's president. No hesitation. He gave me a quick green light to do the talk. No cautions. No request to review my slides or my speech. Just a full measure of support. That was the Morehouse School of Medicine.

So, I gave myself a challenge. Could I find a way to articulate racial health inequities so that a conservative white legislator could hear it? Could I communicate in a way that would make them want to do something to improve outcomes? I decided to use the language of business. *Six sigma . . . defects per million opportunities . . . the cost of variation in outcomes. . . . . Fix the system, don't fix the blame.* What if a factory was producing a thousand cars a day where a third of the red cars had only three tires? You'd shut down the factory and fix it, right? Because the cost of fixing defective cars over and over again would far outweigh the one-time cost of fixing the factory.

I presented all of my usual graphs and charts. But I also included slides of the estimated costs of racial variation in hospitalizations to payers in the state of Georgia. Then I framed it not just as a cost but as an opportunity. *"We could save over 100 million dollars each year in Georgia if we eliminated this racial variation in outcomes."* I paused and let it sink in. The Chamber of Commerce folks and conservative legislators were with me. And then I described the opportunity for human savings. *"We could save a baby's life every day in Georgia, if we eliminated the Black-white gap in infant mortality."* The image on the screen morphed from a premature Black baby struggling on a ventilator to a smiling Black toddler. The whole crowd was with me.

Afterward, some of my colleagues gathered around me. Distracted, I scanned the crowd for the legislator who had gone off on me the year before. Suddenly she appeared at my side. *"Nice talk,"* she said simply. And over the following years, our institution saw annual increases in our state funding.

What I was describing was systemic racism. We have a health care system producing racially unequal outcomes that everyone says they don't want. Racism without racists. Here's the rub. If we know this to be true, and if we don't do anything to fix it, aren't we part of the problem? If we do only trivial, ineffective things, don't we just strengthen inertia in a system that is consistently producing inequities? Systemic racial injustice is not really racism without racists. It just requires us to embrace the passive racism of white denial. And sorry, folks, but that's racist.

Don't get me wrong. Overt individual racism is still quite real. A conservative Republican member of the Orange County, California Board of Supervisors recently described his experience as a young Vietnamese refugee. He described a constant fear of violent racism, "extreme hostility," and physical assault.[8] He said he stopped participating in sports in his last two years of high school. *"I didn't want to walk home alone after practices and be harassed, and beat up, and strangled."*

But hovering just below the surface is subconscious or implicit bias. We can measure it with psychological tests such as the Implicit Association Test. We can even demonstrate it with neuroimaging. The emotion-processing amygdala lights up more when we see facial images of people from different racial-ethnic backgrounds.[9]

The brain response is not your fault. It just is. But what we do with it is critical. Does a biased sense of threat make a white police officer more likely to draw their gun on a Black man? Do I and other doctors have racial biases? Misogynistic or homophobic thoughts? I hope and wish not. But I do. Most of us do. Most of us need healing, deep healing.

Racism can be pictured as an iceberg.[10] Overt discrimination and white bias are only the tip of the iceberg. But in the downstream wake, we see all the swirling effects that reveal a massive iceberg underneath the water. Black women dying at a threefold higher rate from pregnancy-related causes and Black babies dying at twice the rate of whites. Tens of thousands of Black and Latine and American Indian adults being disabled prematurely due to complications of diabetes. Income and wealth inequality. Educational inequities. I could go on and on. What is beneath the surface in this massive iceberg of inequity?

The scaffolding and strength of this iceberg is structural racism and genderism. It's the myriad ways in which schools and banks and legislatures and health care organizations operate. They have evolved as institutions that are not overtly discriminatory. Instead, they have whitewashed all superficial signs of their historically explicit racism. Still, their policies and structures consistently produce unequal outcomes. As Bonilla-Silva says, these systems and processes "are invisible to most whites."[11] System-level racial inequality (i.e., systemic racism) is real. And it's deadly.

Beyond structural inequalities, institutions and policies and people *work together*. Complex dynamic systems generate these unequal outcomes. Societal relationships and networks of influence all have racial and gender dynamics. The good old boys' network always hires the same contractor. He has a track record. But he also goes to my church, and we play softball together. It was never about race or gender. Or was it?

So where did I learn about race? How did this social construct of race get into my head? Is racism a virus like chickenpox that infects everybody? Does it then stay in our bodies, only to burst forth unwanted as a painful and ugly case of shingles? How do we learn our notions of race and racism? And who is our teacher?

Zora Neale Hurston said that she remembered "the very day that I became colored." She said, "I was not Zora of Orange County anymore, I was now a little colored girl . . . the granddaughter of slaves."[12] Immigrants to America often describe the moment they discover this racialized identity. Boyah Farah put it this way in the title of his book—*America Made Me a Black Man*.[13] Our society teaches Black kids that they are Black.

Somewhere, I learned whiteness. More accurately, I learned to define non-white people as "other." Whiteness was unmentionable. I spent many of my childhood summers in small-town Illinois. For us kids, it meant vacation with all my aunts and uncles and cousins. Summers meant fishing and swimming and messing around in little boats. One uncle was loud and gregarious and fun. He was also a loud and happy drinker, whose cocktails started early in the afternoon. The other uncle was quiet and seemingly unaffected by all the chaos around him. Both taught me to fish and to love the outdoors. Both were pretty tolerant of noisy kids having fun. And both were racist as hell.

One day, we were with my uncle at his house in the ironically named Normal, Illinois. We were watching the Chicago Cubs play an afternoon game. He was making jovial commentary on the game with a drink in one hand. He perked up when a beer commercial came on. Men were drinking beer together at a backyard gathering for a cookout. Some were Black and some were white. *"I don't need to see that crap!"* yelled my uncle. "What?" I asked, truly confused. "I don't need to see white guys drinking beer with those *j*_____. Damned *n*____." He had a dozen racial slurs that he seemed to use interchangeably. I was in junior high school the first time I heard this, and I had no response. I didn't expect it. I didn't know what to do with it. But those words are still stuck in my brain.

My other uncle wasn't as vocal or animated in his overt racism, but in a way, he was a lot scarier. When he spoke of race, his eyes grew distant, and he got real quiet. In the end, southern Illinois racism was no different from Chicago racism or South Georgia racism. "White folks is white folks, honey, South or North, North or South," said a character in a Langston Hughes story.[14]

My parents each had their own flavors of racism. As many men do, I think of my mom as an angel incarnate. She was sweet, impossibly positive, and optimistic. She overflowed with unconditional love. She had grown up white and privileged as one of three daughters of an orthopedic surgeon in Springfield, Illinois, the home of Abraham Lincoln.

The emotional abuse Mom took from my father, the difficulties in her marriage, and racial tensions in the world were all covered up in denial. She saw the world through rose-colored glasses. She believed or pretended that there was no conflict. She was the yogi master of walking on eggshells, while my dad was balancing on the edge of rage. We learned to deny our family dysfunction from my mom. We learned to deny race-awareness from Mom and from our white-normed culture. We could just pretend that we lived in a postracial world. The Civil War was over. Let's just all get along. Golden rule and all that good Sunday School stuff. And yet, there were limits.

One summer in our tween years, we were on vacation at a fishing cabin in Wisconsin with my grandfather and uncles and cousins. My brother met a girl named Pat, and everyone could tell they liked each other right away. Call it puppy love, but when you're 12 or 13, it's very real. But Pat and her family were Japanese. Asian. Other. And my angel-on-earth mom, who *"just treats everyone the same,"* felt the need to pull my brother aside and have a talk with him. Maybe it was pressure from my uncles and grandfather, but it was sad and confusing.

My dad had his own flavor of racism, one that was complicated. If he hired someone to help with yardwork, he would hire a Jamaican man. Dad would praise the man's work ethic and the way he sharpened his tools continuously as he worked. My father would say that there are *n____* and there are Negroes. He had learned racial stereotypes and disrespect from his own alcoholic, abusive father. He made it his own by adding the nuance of Black exceptionalism for hardworking Afro-Caribbean men.

Growing up in the 1960s, we engaged explicitly in discussions about race. *"What do you think about MLK?"* he would start. Over time, he evolved from seeing civil rights leaders as agitators or communists. He began to see their point, but only as long as they weren't *disruptive*. He became one of those white people Dr. King wrote about in his letter from the Birmingham jail, "the white moderate, who is more devoted to 'order' than to justice; . . . who paternalistically believes he can set the timetable for another man's freedom."[15]

My dad never fully escaped his racial upbringing, but he lived part of my "white-guy healing" journey vicariously through me. He had his faults, but he was proud to say, *"my son the doctor."* Over time he even grew proud of my bent toward social justice. Late in life, my aunt and uncle came to visit my parents in their Florida retirement community. My uncle made a wisecrack about *"that n____-lover son of yours."* Bad idea. My dad might not have known a lot about expressing love (my wife had to teach him to hug his sons), but he could be a powerful beast if someone threatened his family. Dad responded. Angrily, he defended me.

"I guess he's turned you into a n____-lover too," my uncle said. Uh-oh. My father had immeasurably deep pools of rage to tap into. He cursed and called my uncle a racist and turned him out. *Really? My father calling another man a racist?* I smile to this day when I think about all the ironies and contradictions that came together in that moment. In some small way, in that moment, my dad could be a white guy healing too. Baby steps.

Let's get a few things straight. White people—we are never allowed to use the n-word. Not ever. We are also not allowed to use the word "racism" to describe what happens to white people when we have to face up to racial inequities. It's intentionally obtuse. It ignores the directionality of racism. It ignores the centuries of slavery, Jim Crow laws, policing, economic barriers, laws, rules, regulations, and culture that continue to make being Black very different from being white in America.

So, I call bullshit on this notion of "reverse racism." It starts from the assumption that we're all equal now. It suggests that to bring up race is not only impolite but that it somehow victimizes white people. Trump advisor Stephen Miller sponsored a television ad saying, *"stop left-wing racism"* and *"end anti-white bigotry."*[16] Every white man in America needs to call bullshit on this every time it is spoken.

Why do white people buy into this stuff? It's complicated, but President Lyndon B. Johnson nailed one version six decades ago. He said, "If you can convince the lowest white man he's better than the best colored man, he won't notice you're picking his pocket. Hell, give him somebody to look down on, and he'll empty his pockets for you."

Do white people sometimes have struggles in their life? Sure. Can white people be poor or live in rough neighborhoods? Absolutely. Can we experience unfairness at the hands of employers or landlords? Do we sometimes grow up in abusive or dysfunctional families? Of course. Does that mean that if a company intentionally chooses to build a diverse leadership team, then every white guy with better technical qualifications has been discriminated against? Nonsense.

Denial or pretending that race is no longer an issue doesn't help anyone. Dana Brownlee once wrote, *"Dear White People: When You Say You 'Don't See Color,' This Is What We Really Hear."* She quotes Theresa M. Robinson, who says, "When I'm on the receiving end of it, it feels like . . . the person is erasing the part of me at the source of their dis-ease, of their discomfort."[17] Too many of us want the past to be forgotten and to pretend that everything's okay now.

In teaching, I often use a whiteboard with colorful dry-erase markers. I draw diagrams of social complexities or population health or even cardiac EKGs in all different colors. And when I erase the whiteboard, I can start all over again because it is a blank slate. Or is it? What color remains? It's white. It's always white. That's the baseline. Guante Tran Myhre said that "white supremacy is not a shark; it is the water."[18]

Race-denialism is the opposite of being race-aware, race-sensitive, or race-conscious. It perpetuates racial inequalities. It is a tool of oppression, whether conscious or unconscious, implicit or explicit. It's racist. As Don Lemon says, "Racism is a cancer . . . [that has] persisted because the right people had the luxury of ignoring it."[19]

The experience of being a Black or Latine or trans medical student is dramatically different from that of a white guy going to medical school. I may have struggled with biochemistry, but I was never mistaken for the janitor. Dr. Yaa Oheema created a TikTok video detailing her many experiences of racism, ranging from being told "Get me a real doctor" to being mistaken for *a cleaning lady* to being called "a Black bitch."[20] Patients often left her in tears. While we may imagine that these are only occasional occurrences, she said that "there's always at least one moment or situation every shift."

Unfortunately, science and medicine got tangled up with racism a long time ago. Angela Saini summarized much of this history in a podcast titled *The Racist History of Race Science*.[21] She describes European scientists of earlier centuries living in a context of hyper-racialized politics and ideology. Justifications for slavery were "part of the air that they breathed."

The biologist Carl Linnaeus, celebrated for his development of biologic taxonomies, also created a taxonomy of race. American, European, Asian, and African became Red, White, Yellow, and Black subspecies. These in turn were labeled as having specific temperaments (Impassive, Hearty, Melancholy, and Lazy). Some of these persist in stereotypes to this day.[22] Sadly, medicine and anthropology often served as the core sciences used to dehumanize African Americans.[23] Skulls were measured and categorized by shape to draw conclusions about differences in intelligence. Skulls of African origin were compared to those of various primates to endorse the subhumanity of people of color. If "Black" persons from Africa could be thought of as a different subspecies, then they could be subjected to slave ownership. Property, not humanity. Livestock, not people.

The threads of history carry on as a viral strain infecting society even today. In 2016, Michelle Obama was called "an ape in heels" in a Facebook post shared by a local town mayor in West Virginia.[24] Subhumanizing persons of color is a historic and ongoing threat, often used also against LGBTQ people. Throughout World War II, Asian people were also subject to dehumanizing characterization. It appeared in *Bugs Bunny* and other TV cartoons I grew up with. It helped justify killing Japanese people in war and imprisoning Japanese American people in internment camps.

This constant barrage of dehumanizing messaging aimed at minoritized people is deeply underestimated by white men. In her book *Caste*, Isabel Wilkerson identifies *Dehumanization and Stigma* as pillar number six in the systems that establish hierarchies and marginalize certain groups. She calls dehumanization "a standard component in the manufacture of an out-group against which to pit an in-group."[25]

To deny or degrade a whole group's humanity demands a response. Silence is complicity. White commentators mocked Jesse Jackson for leading crowds to chant, "*I am somebody.*" They missed how powerful that statement could be to someone who had lived their whole life hearing that "*no, you're really not.*" Students of color or non-male gender often have to overcome feelings of being "less-than." It feeds the belief that they have to overachieve just to be recognized as being enough.

How do these threads of history connect to the modern practice of medicine? We teach our students that race is not a biological framework but rather a social construct. And yet, millions of people pursue DNA tests to identify their "genetic ancestry." We should remember that all racial groups share more than 99 percent of their genome. There are more within-race genetic differences than can be found across racial groups. In fact, East Africans are more genetically different from West Africans than Europeans are from Asians.

From the earliest days of medical school, I learned that case histories always began with an introduction of the patient by age, gender, and race. If it was a 22-year-old Black male, we could assume that the case was going to be about sickle cell disease or syphilis. We were taught by repetition to recognize these as diseases associated with patients of Black race. We were also taught to associate specific racial-ethnic backgrounds with genetic proclivities toward specific diseases (e.g., Ashkenazi Jews with Tay-Sachs disease or Fanconi's anemia).

These are epidemiologic associations, but in individual patients, they lead to what the Institute of Medicine called cognitive shortcuts.[26] These shortcuts include *gestalts* (the way we put together clusters of information) and *heuristics* (rules-of-thumb). We use both in clinical decision-making when we are under time pressure and have limited information. But filtered through my implicit and explicit biases, these cognitive shortcuts can lead me to practice bad medicine. I'm biased toward overdiagnosing Fanconi's anemia in an Ashkenazi Jewish infant. I also might miss sickle cell disease in a patient who doesn't look "Black" to me.

Our biases can hurt and kill people. Schulman did an experiment with videotaped vignettes of patients with chest pain who had identical cardiac risk. He showed that the likelihood of being sent for cardiac catheterization was strongly associated with how the physician saw the patients' race and gender.[27] Our technology can even have a racial bias. For example, the pulse oximeters that measure a person's blood oxygen level were being used during the COVID-19 pandemic to show when a patient should go to the hospital. The problem? They overestimate oxygen levels in people with darker skin. People could think they were okay when they really were not.

In medical school, I was taught to evaluate lung function tests using race-normed algorithms. These were developed in the 1800s, in part to justify how African Americans could tolerate the harsh demands of slave work. Those race-normed algorithms are still in use today. Similar pseudo-science studies were done to prove racial differences in heat tolerance and sensitivity to pain. Many medical students and even physicians still hold the false belief that African Americans are less sensitive to pain. It's as if the social construct of race had created a biological "thick skin." What started as a rationalization for slavery has become a driver of disparities in modern-day pain management.[28]

The *New England Journal of Medicine* published a list of 13 medical equations that still use race correction in modern medical decision-making. These include estimates of kidney function from common blood tests. In aggregate on a population level, the race-based algorithms are accurate. But poorly interpreted at the individual level, the algorithms could imply that African Americans have higher-functioning kidneys than they really do. African Americans have twice the rate of kidney failure as whites, but this algorithm may lead to later diagnosis, inadequate treatment, and lower priority for kidney transplant.[29]

The NFL Players Association has even had to sue the NFL to stop its use of race-normed cognitive tests in evaluating former football players for chronic traumatic brain injuries. The cognitive test algorithms just assumed that Blacks as a group would achieve somewhat lower scores. The practical effect? Fewer Black players would receive the care and financial recompense they needed and deserved because their cognitive deficits were being redefined as "normal for their race." In the 21st century.

Sometimes a conversation that starts about Black–white inequities gets sideswiped by various forms of "what-about-me?" advocacy. Women still get paid less than men and experience ongoing sexual harassment. Trans people are experiencing incredible political bullying, oppression, and violence. Asian people are the target of violent hate crimes and all manner of hateful tropes. There's no check-box on race for those from the Middle East. Islamophobia is still rampant. Anti-Semitism is on the rise again. American Indians suffered occupation and genocide at the hands of colonists in America's first original sin. Yes, yes, yes, and yes.

But we need to make sure that the Black–white racism conversation can be fully explored without comparing it to other types of inequity. People need to be fully heard. One form of oppression is not the same as others. They all are real and need to be addressed. Chairing Georgia's Minority Health Council, I sometimes found myself saying, *"That's another really important issue. But at the moment we are talking about race and racism on the Black–white axis. We'll make sure to circle back to your issue in a bit."* The Black–white racism conversation must not be co-opted by others who don't want to be left out.

Then we must indeed create those additional safe spaces for conversations about all the rest. We need to talk about sexism, transphobia, anti-Asian discrimination, anti-Latine discrimination, and anti–American Indian oppression. There must then be a safe space and time to address issues of intersectionality across all these dimensions.

In leading the Council, I learned that each group needed to have an uninterrupted time to be fully heard. Their lived experience had to be affirmed and validated by others. To get sucked into the competition of *"my oppression is worse than your op-pression"* or to say *"I understand your oppression because of my oppression"* are both destructive. Both fail to recognize the uniqueness of each form of marginalization that America has created for various peoples.

Christopher Rivas describes the moment when he decided to write his book, *Brown Enough*.[30] He was at an event where Ta-Nehisi Coates was speaking, and he had an opportunity to ask a question. "All I hear is Black and white," he said. As a Brown man, a Latin man, where does that leave me?" The answer was short and cold. "Not in it."

Not in it. That's how it can feel to be anything other than Black or white in conversations about race in America. In Groveland, Florida, Latine farmworkers and their families were the invisible community. My colleague is a nurse practitioner who cares for migrant children every day in a school clinic in Quincy, Florida. It's a majority-Black community, but Quincy also has a significant migrant and seasonal Latine population. She found herself having to defend serving immigrants when there were so many African Americans in need. She said, *"Caring for others doesn't mean we care any less for all of us. It doesn't take away; it adds."*

Black–Brown racial tensions are not new but often spin off from the Black–white dynamic of the United States. Recently, the Los Angeles City Council president resigned after audio was leaked of her racist conversation with other city officials. She demeaned a white councilmember's Black son as a *"changuito,"* or little monkey.[31]

Race is more complex in Latin America. The term "pigmentoc-racies" has been coined to describe the complicated intersection of race and class and ethnicity and indigenous heritage in Mexico. It includes notions of *la raza* and *mestizo* and *la mezcla*.[32,33,34] These were all framed by the history of colonization and still correlate with socioeconomic status.

Social caste systems based on skin color and education and wealth and prominence also have within-group complexities in the African American, Afro-Caribbean, and Asian communities. We need to have three-dimensional conversations about all of these complexifying intersectionalities. There are commonalities of marginalization, commonalities of resiliency, and commonalities of community empowerment. But we also need to understand differences and avoid false equivalencies.

For white men who see this as a zero-sum game and fear being "replaced" in a non-white world, power comes from leveraging these divisions. This is at the core of politics in Miami, to pit one minority group against another. But for those of us who embrace living in the kaleidoscopic wonder of a non-white world, power comes through finding common ground. Can we not become that beautiful Rainbow Coalition described by Reverend Jesse Jackson? Can we ever become Dr. King's beloved community?

If we learned racism, can we unlearn it? Be intentional. Spend more time with people from different backgrounds. Research shows that it can increase empathy. But we need to go much farther. An hour of cultural competence training and a privilege walk aren't nearly enough. We need to recognize and confront our own whiteness.

Sadly, our nation's increasing polarization and permission structure for expressing bias are pulling us backward. Says Barbara Gross, "The truth is, doing this work is like riding against gravity. The gravitational pull is back to racism and white supremacy culture."[35] Knowledge must be linked to personal action. It takes hard, disciplined work over many years.

In the end, we're all in this together and forever. It's not someone else's job to fix it. It's a "we-all" job. Michelle Obama reminds us that "race and racism . . . can't just be on people of color." She goes on to say that "it's up to all of us—Black, White, everyone—no matter how well-meaning we think we might be, to do the honest, uncomfortable work of rooting it out." She even describes the path. "It starts with self-examination and listening to those whose lives are different from our own. It ends with justice, compassion, and empathy that manifests in our lives and on our streets."[36]

In the language of addiction recovery, the first step in AA's 12-step programs is to acknowledge the problem. We have to admit that we are powerless over our weakness (alcohol, opioids, internalized racism, etc.). Steps four and five require us to make *"a searching and fearless moral inventory of ourselves"* and *"admit to God, to ourselves, and to another human being the exact nature of our wrongs."* And then we move on, seeking to lessen our shortcomings and to make amends to all that we have harmed. There's also an ongoing, one-day-at-a-time component to this healing. We must (step 10) *"continuously take personal inventory and promptly admit when we are wrong."* One day at a time. For the rest of our lives.

Family healing doesn't happen without honesty and transparency and a willingness to set things right. Healing requires repentance, honest remorse, and open acknowledgment of past transgressions. We need inner healing first. Only then, in a spirit of honesty and humble grace, can we move on to reconciliation among our diverse peoples. Finally, we can begin structurally to tackle the complex dynamic systems that produce unequal outcomes. In the last section of this book, I will offer specific chapters on each of these levels, encouraging each of us to do the hard work of inner healing, of relational healing, and of structural healing.

Just imagine, though. What if America could take these healing steps every day, in a spirit of truth and beloved community?

FOR FURTHER READING

DiAngelo R. *White Fragility: Why It's So Hard for White People to Talk About Racism.*

Hurston ZN. *You Don't Know Us Negroes.*

Kendi IX. *How to Be an Antiracist.*

King ML Jr. "Letter from a Birmingham Jail."

Lemon D. *This Is the Fire: What I Say to My Friends About Racism.*

Rivas C. *Brown Enough.*

Telles E. *Pigmentocracies: Ethnicity, Race, and Color in Latin America.*

Wilkerson I. *Caste: The Origins of Our Discontents.*

FEELINGS

5.

Fear and Oppression

In white-world, police serve and protect me. In minoritized communities, they may or may not.

A physician colleague here at FSU brought it home to us in the early days of the COVID pandemic. *"I had put on my mask to go in the store at the gas station,"* he said. *"I got out of my car and got halfway across the parking lot. I thought, 'Omigosh, I'm a Black man walking into a Circle K wearing a mask.'"* He laughed, and we laughed. *"I took that daggone mask off."* That's a choice I never had to make as a white man. We live in the same community, but we live in different worlds. His burden, my privilege?

Our kids' childhood caregiver is an African American woman with a radiant personality. My grown-up daughter still thinks of her as her second mother. To get to our house, she often had to drive through Avondale Estates, a tiny enclave known for aggressive police enforcement of minor traffic infractions. She told us she waved and smiled every time she passed a police car in that town. She wanted them to get to know her so that she posed no threat. What white guy even thinks about having to do that?

Anne Helen Peterson calls this form of white privilege "ease of movement." She quotes Alison Désir, who says, "The general pass of whiteness remains in place: the understanding that in a white body, I will almost certainly be given the benefit of the doubt, and that my presence in a space will not be immediately understood as threatening or suspect."[1] It's another example of the law *"that protects but does not bind"* an in-group (white guys like me) and at the same time *"binds but does not protect"* out-groups such as people of color or trans people.

Driving while Black has almost become a cliché in our country. Research on over a hundred million traffic stops nationwide has documented the increased risk for Black drivers.[2] In January 2023, five police officers were charged with second-degree murder for the fatal beating of Mr. Tyre Nichols. He was a young man pulled over on a traffic stop, but these officers weren't focused on traffic safety. These were police of a special unit called SCORPION, an Orwellian acronym for Street Crimes Operation to Restore Peace in Our Neighborhoods. The purpose of the unit was to patrol "high-crime neighborhoods" and to help people feel safer.

But to do their job, they needed to find reasons to pull cars over, including trivial traffic violations. They especially stopped those fitting their profile of potential criminals (e.g., young Black men). It's a vicious cycle of circular bias. Young Black men are profiled more, stopped more, arrested more, and convicted more. Therefore, more young Black men are criminals. Ergo, young Black men fit the profile of a criminal . . . and so it goes. Tyre Nichols was pulled over in that traffic stop. In a move that can only be understood by those who have experienced such policing, he fled. He was beaten until he was unconscious and then left for a time with no medical attention. He died in the hospital.

The good news is that authorities in Memphis acted swiftly to terminate five police officers. Within a month, they brought charges that included second-degree murder. Was it easier because the officers were Black? What form of racism is that?

Police encounters don't have to end in death to be dehumanizing or traumatic. The NAACP says that "a Black person is five times more likely to be stopped without just cause than a white person."[3] A third of Latine and Asian adults have felt targeted because of race. So now even old white guys like me and President Joe Biden know about *"the talk"* that African American parents give their teens about how to behave with the police. It's the talk we never had to give our kids. The only guidance I ever remember receiving from my parents was to call the police if you needed help. Dad also said, *"If they take you to jail, I'll bail you out in the morning. You're going to spend the night learning a lesson."*

One Black father wrote an entire book about "the talk."[4] Others share on social media all the steps they take to decrease their risk. They turn on a camera and put their wallet on the dashboard. They keep an image of their insurance and registration documents on their phones.[5] Boyah Farah said in the months after George Floyd was killed that "driving while Black at this moment is not a neutral act. I'm fully aware I'm in genuine danger. . . . Every cell of my body is getting ready."[6] Hyper-vigilance. Constant fight-or-flight adrenalin. Racial stress. Racial weathering.

Don Lemon describes it as the same adrenalin rush a sprinter gets waiting for the starter pistol. Ready . . . Set . . . "You rise up, chest tight, every muscle flushed with acetylcholine, every neuron firing . . . That hovering edge of hypertension just before the crack of the starting pistol—a perpetual state of SET!—that is where I, as a Black man, spend most of my waking hours, and having White people deny that this dynamic exists only serves to pour another tablespoon of fight-or-flight acid into my stomach."[7]

During the writing of this book, there was a soul-crushing series of police killings of African American citizens. George Floyd. Breonna Taylor. Rayshard Brooks. Andre Hill. Others too numerous to name. Every year, over a thousand people in the United States are killed by police.[8] A third of these are African American. At least one-quarter are unarmed.[9]

If you're a white guy leading a diverse health care team, what do you say on the day after George Floyd's killing by police? Can you understand the fear and the rage? What do you do? Can you create a safe space for people to feel what they feel? Can you be an ally in this moment? Ta Nehisi Coates said this to his son: "Sell cigarettes without the proper authority and your body can be destroyed. . . . Turn into a dark stairwell and your body can be destroyed. The destroyers will rarely be held accountable. Mostly they will receive pensions."[10]

Sadly, this has gone on throughout my lifetime and for too many generations. In 1963, Freedom Rider, Civil Rights warrior, and future congressman John Lewis said, "We are tired of being beaten by policemen. We're tired of seeing our people locked up in jail over and over again. And then you holler, *'Be patient.'* How long can we be patient? We want our freedom, and we want it now."[11]

One of our medical students recently told other students that she had a version of "the talk" with her four-year-old son. He was starting preschool in a predominantly white setting. *"You can't act up like the other children,"* she said. *"They'll treat you different."* She's not wrong. What would lead to timeout for one child might lead to police being called for a child of color. Half of the 250 children expelled from preschool every day in America are Black boys.[12] In Georgia, there were more children receiving mental health care in juvenile detention than there were in the community mental health system.

And it's not just Black men and Black boys. Black women face their own strains of abuse, violence, disrespect, and discrimination. Brittney Cooper describes "the effects of oppressions on Black women's lives as . . . multiplicative." She goes on to say,

"Our class position, sexual identity, and many other vectors of power . . . determined how many boots there were on our collective necks."[13]

LGBTQ people have also been harassed and abused by police throughout the 20th century, with gay bars being a special target. The issue came to a head in New York City in 1969 when New York City police raided the Stonewall Inn, a gay bar in Greenwich Village. Initial resistance was followed by six days of protests known as the Stonewall Uprising. It catalyzed the formation of organizations that were the founding pillars of the gay rights movement. The first day of the uprising, June 28, is still memorialized in celebrations of International LGBT + Pride Day.

Police harassment is an "ongoing and pervasive problem in LGBT communities."[14] Trans people often face the greatest threats. According to the Anti-Violence Project, "Transgender people were seven times more likely to experience physical violence when interacting with the police."[15] White, straight, cisgender men like me have no clue as to how a trans woman feels when people tell her to *"just call the police"* after she has been beaten again.

In Michael Eric Dyson's *Sermon to White America*, he says gently, "Beloved, to be Black in America is to live in terror."[16] He pleads with us to understand. "We do not hate you, white America. We hate that you terrorize us and then lie about it and then make us feel crazy for having to explain to you how crazy it makes us feel. . . . Can you truly say that you can't understand why most Black folks fear, sometimes hate, the police?"[17]

There was a time in the South when police, sheriffs, and the KKK all blurred together as a force keeping Black men in their place. When we moved to Groveland, I knew it was a typical small southern town, segregated by neighborhood. What I didn't know was the specific history of Groveland. I didn't know all the racial violence that this small town had seen. I didn't know the specific role that Thurgood Marshall had played in trying to effect justice there or how it all still affected my patients every day. I didn't see it. I didn't ask.

I learned the details years later when I heard about the Groveland Four. I read *Devil in the Grove*, chronicling the case of four innocent young Black men accused of raping a white woman. I learned of the sheriff who accused the men and eventually shot two of them. I learned of the white racist mobs that threatened to lynch them and to burn entire neighborhoods. I also learned of the white reporter who initially wrote stories applauding the arrests, only to say, later in life, *"I was wrong."*

I once spoke with an older African American woman who was my patient in Groveland. She asked me what she could do about her constant worries. *"What do you like to do? What relaxes you?"* I asked.

"I like to go fishing in the pond back behind the orange groves," she said. *"But it's been a long time. I can't afford to get my fishing poles back."*

I looked confused. *"They're in the pawn shop,"* she said. Her son was caught up in cocaine addiction. When he needed cash, he would steal and pawn her fishing poles. And this is when my naive I've-got-an-answer-for-everything idiot-self kicked in.

"Why don't you just call the police? Maybe he really needs to hit bottom."

There I was, a young, white, Chicago-trained doctor telling an old Black woman in Groveland, Florida, to turn her son over to the police. *How stupid could I be?* This was a woman who had lived through decades of lynchings and KKK intimidation. She knew specific police officers as enforcers of Black oppression. Police were the protectors of white folks who would do violence against her community. This was a woman who, years earlier, may have had to run into the woods when a white mob was burning down homes in her neighborhood.

I was seeing the police and the justice system through white eyes. I had no idea how many African American sons had been taken away by police over the decades. I was ignorant about what it felt like to be a Black grandmother in Groveland. Ignorant about what it was to be a Black man in the South. So. Damned. Ignorant.

As white men, we have no idea. To begin to understand, we have to follow the threads of history. We have to trace the role of police and sheriffs in controlling the Black community from slave-times to the present. By 1860, 73 percent of the Leon County (Tallahassee) population comprised enslaved people. Their dollar value far exceeded the value of the land they worked on.[18] Leon County led the state in cotton production. Although the Emancipation Proclamation was signed in 1863, it wasn't proclaimed in Tallahassee until May 20, 1865. We celebrate it a month before Juneteenth, the date when federal troops finally brought word to Texas.

The white population now faced a new reality. How would they maintain control over a formerly enslaved Black population that was three times larger than the number of white folks who used to be in charge? There was already a template and a precedent. Black codes were laws designed to restrict the freedom of "free" Black persons even before the emancipation of slaves. Indiana's constitution in 1851 and the Illinois Black Code of 1853 actually banned Black people from settling in their respective states.

After Reconstruction, even more Black code laws were passed to maintain racial apartheid. They also served to provide a Black labor force for plantations. Police used sundown laws and vagrancy laws to incarcerate Black men. Eight southern states explicitly allowed convict leasing. The 13th Amendment, which abolished slavery and involuntary servitude, also included this clause—"except as a punishment for crime." Slave labor became convict labor, under contract to the very plantations on which they had been enslaved. In 1871, the Virginia Supreme Court declared that an incarcerated person is "a slave of the state."[19]

For those who were not incarcerated, sharecropping relationships had the same result. White landowners made up all the rules. Sharecroppers were charged exorbitantly for tools and seed until they were hopelessly indebted. In one description, "For newly freed people, many of whom worked the same land, lived in the same housing, and worked under close supervision of the same overseers, sharecropping was like slavery under another name."[20]

Tallahassee neighborhoods now carry the names of those slave plantations, with no sense of remorse or irony. Generations of Tallahassee white folks have chosen to get married on the grounds of the Goodwood Plantation. Winthrop Park, Chaires Road, Eppes Drive, and Bannerman Road—all have plantation slaveowner family names for their streets and neighborhoods. Some homeowners in those neighborhoods still have deeds to their houses showing restrictive covenants. Those in Betton Hills require that "no person of other than the Caucasian race shall own, use or occupy any property in said subdivision."[21]

By the 1880s, Jim Crow laws were expanded to enforce segregation in public parks, theaters, and restaurants and on public transportation. Residential segregation was enforced to protect white neighborhoods. And segregation was enforced in health care, from hospital wards to doctors' offices to nursing homes and even to blood banks.

Throughout the Jim Crow era, police and sheriffs enforced these immoral but official laws. In parallel, the KKK and White Citizens Councils enforced the unwritten law that Black people were less than full citizens. White supremacy groups surged after the *Brown v. Board of Education* decision on school segregation. A similar backlash occurred after passage of the Civil Rights Act and Voting Rights Act in 1964–1965.

Lynchings accelerated at the end of World War I with veterans returning home to fewer opportunities than they expected. They needed someone to blame. During the summer of 1919, at least 25 white-on-Black race massacres took place. The Great Depression further increased racial resentments and white grievance, with another rise in lynchings.

In Florida, we had the Ocoee and Rosewood massacres. Forty miles to the northeast of Rosewood, there was a mass lynching in Newberry, Florida. Six people lost their lives in a series of escalations starting with two boys accused of eating a watermelon from a farmer's field. It escalated with the failed arrest of a man accused of hog-stealing. Six bodies from the lynching were displayed publicly. Hundreds of white Floridians drove 20 miles from Gainesville just to see it.

This is all "hard-facts" history. Read Marvin Dunn's *A History of Florida Through Black Eyes*.[22] He cites Tuskegee University's "lynching list," in which Florida lynchings alone take up 15 pages.[23] This is the history that our governor and state legislature do not want to be taught. They fear that some tender white child (or their ironically named "Moms for Liberty") might feel some sense of guilt or shame. Better to be the dysfunctional family that hides its shame and keeps its secrets.

This history is what makes Black resiliency in the face of oppression so profoundly moving. As a Morehouse College student, Dr. Satcher trained in the discipline of nonviolence. He learned how to minimize his injuries and to maintain his nonviolence while being punched or thrown down a flight of stairs. He led students to participate in lunch counter sit-ins. When he was jailed with MLK's brother, they engaged in a hunger strike. The late congressman John Lewis was beaten within an inch of his life during a peaceful march for voting rights on the Edmund Pettus Bridge. Hundreds of others were hurt in various protests, small and large. And still they persisted.

Women such as Rosa Parks didn't just sit in the front of the bus. They played active leadership roles in the civil rights movement at their own peril. Emmett Till's mother insisted on an open casket for the mutilated body of her son so that the world would know what violent white men had done. Some white people also stood up for civil rights and freedom. Six members of the original group of 13 Freedom Riders were white. They were all beaten as their bus burned in Anniston, Alabama.

Arrest and prison continue to be tools of oppression in my lifetime. The modern era of mass incarceration began in the 1970s with Richard Nixon's war on drugs. It expanded in the 1980s with tough-on-crime laws and mandatory minimum sentencing. Racial bias was baked into these laws. For example, there was a five-year mandatory minimum sentence for possession of just 5 grams of crack cocaine. The same sentence for powdered cocaine required possession of 500 grams. Crack was a common cause of arrest of African American men, while powdered cocaine was for upper-income whites. It was a racially biased, 100-to-1 differential in sentencing guidelines.

In 1970, the US prison population was just under 200,000. By 1985, it had more than doubled to over half a million people, fueled by the 1994 crime bill. Incarceration finally peaked in 2009 at over 1.6 million persons. This paralleled a trend in the corrections industry toward privatization of prisons. There was now a business imperative to increase the customer base (incarcerated persons), supported by state spending on incarceration. It also built a politically valuable, job-creating prison industry in poor, rural small towns.

America has built the necessary infrastructure for excessive incarceration and specifically for the disproportionate incarceration of Black men. A Black person is much more likely to be convicted of a felony than a white person for the same crime. Black Americans are incarcerated in state prisons at nearly five times the rate of white Americans. In 12 states, more than half the prison population is Black.[24] More African Americans are in prison, on parole, or on probation than were enslaved in 1859.[25]

Bias permeates the justice system. Hispanic and Latine individuals are subject to higher rates of arrest, incarceration, and police violence. Just to the east of Tallahassee is one of the rural counties I cover in public health, where a damning document was recently exposed. It showed that Jefferson County prosecutors made it their policy to seek harsher sentences for "people with criminal histories *and/or Hispanic*" arrestees. The whistleblower who discovered the document said, "Oh my God, they wrote down the racism policy!"[26]

An Oklahoma sheriff was caught on tape talking with other county officials about killing two journalists and hanging Black people. When confronted, he doubled down. He suggested that felony charges might be brought against the journalist for obtaining the recorded conversation.[27] Sure. The recording was the bad part.

Incarcerating Black men also benefited whites who felt their economic and political power slipping away. Convicted Black felons could no longer compete in the job market. They were also stripped permanently of their right to bear arms and their right to vote. In Florida, Kentucky, Tennessee, and Virginia, more than one in five African Americans can no longer vote because of a felony conviction.[28] Florida voters passed a state constitutional amendment to restore voting rights to convicted felons. In response, our legislature passed new laws to impede these rights. The governor sent the voting police to arrest former felons who attempted to vote.

Current Republican strategies explicitly endorse voter suppression and racial gerrymandering. In the 2013 *Shelby County v. Holder* case, the Supreme Court weakened the Voting Rights Act. It allowed discriminatory state laws on election rules to stand. The goal of all of this was to diminish the voting strength of young adults and low-income and minority voters. Understand this— suppression of Black voters gives white votes disproportionate weight. Privilege. One person, one vote? Not exactly.

Beyond police violence, minoritized individuals must fear for their lives all across America. James Byrd Jr. was an African American man who was chained by the ankles and dragged for three miles behind a pickup truck by white supremacists in Texas in 1998. After his arm and head were severed by hitting a culvert, they dragged his body another mile to dump it in front of a Black church.[29] In the first year of the COVID pandemic (2020–2021), more than 9,000 anti-Asian incidents (hate crimes, assaults, etc.) were reported.[30]

A third of lesbian, gay, or bisexual youth report being bullied at school. Nearly half have considered suicide.[31] LGBTQ people are nine times more likely to be victims of a violent hate crime.[32] Matthew Shepard, a 21-year-old gay college student, was beaten and tied to a fence and left to die in Wyoming.[33] As a result, the Matthew Shepard and James Byrd Jr. Hate Crimes Prevention Act amended federal hate crime law to include gender, sexual orientation, gender identity, and disability.[34] The law forever connects the dots between racial hate crimes and LGBTQ hate crimes.

Hate-driven mass shootings have become an almost uniquely American phenomenon. In 2022, we saw the mass shooting that killed 10 people in a grocery store in a predominantly African American neighborhood of Buffalo, New York. The shooter was a 19-year-old white male who believed in white grievance theories such as "white genocide" and "the great replacement."

In 2019, a young white Anglo man shot and killed 23 people in a Walmart that served mostly Mexican Americans. He had driven 650 miles to El Paso to open fire with a civilian version of the AK-47 type military assault rifle. He posted online that his attack was "a response to the Hispanic invasion of Texas." His greatest fear?

That immigrants could "replace" white Anglo Americans.[35] Replacement theory kills.

Some men are threatened by women, and when their views become extreme, violence ensues. More than 4 in 10 women experience intimate partner violence or stalking at some point in their lives. A survey showed that one in three German men found violence against women to be "acceptable."[36]

Here in Tallahassee, the shooter was a white man who identified as an *incel*, an involuntarily celibate young man. He had been banned from our FSU campus for groping female students. In 2018, he drove to Tallahassee's Hot Yoga studio. He put on hearing protectors and then pulled a Glock pistol from his bag. He kept shooting until two women were dead and four others were injured.

That one was personal. My retired pediatrician wife is now a yoga instructor. She knew some of the individuals present that day. One of my FSU faculty colleagues was killed. The Nancy Van Vessem M.D. Center for Healthy Aging is now named in her honor, but a new generation of students and patients will never get to know her.

In all of these cases, the targeted victims of the mass shootings were people with a demographic profile that was the polar opposite of the shooter. It was the object of the shooter's hate. White shooter, Black victims. Anglo shooter, Mexican American victims. A white sexually rejected "incel" male shooter targeted women exercising gently in a yoga studio.

Mass shootings have targeted the LGBTQ community as well. Straight men who hold rigid beliefs about gender and sexuality can be dangerous. In Orlando in 2016, a young man killed 49 people and injured dozens more at a gay nightclub called Pulse.[37] The Pulse shooting only ended after a three-hour standoff with the police. At the time, it was the deadliest mass shooting in US history (sadly, that record has since fallen to other mass shootings). More than 300 people inside the club were traumatized for life. Millions of other LGBTQ Americans were reminded once again that their very personhood put them in danger.

Racial violence is purposeful, yet random. White men from South Georgia chased down and shot an unarmed Ahmaud Arbery as he was jogging through the neighborhood. In Florida, a 17-year-old high school student was shot by an aggressive neighborhood watch captain, George Zimmerman. Trayvon Martin's only crime was walking through his neighborhood with dark skin. He was seen by his assailant only as a young Black man in a hoodie. In 2013, President Barack Obama said, "When Trayvon Martin was first shot, I said that this could have been my son." Hiding behind Florida's "Stand Your Ground" law, George Zimmerman was acquitted by a mostly white jury. The US Justice Department declined to bring federal civil rights charges. President Obama called for national soul-searching.

Both the historic and modern-day oppressions send fear-waves throughout our communities even today. One of my Morehouse colleagues is a trailblazer in her own right. She once tried to describe to me the feeling of driving down a country road at night in rural Georgia. She was driving through a county that still had a small KKK presence and pathetic little white power rallies but much more prevalent racism. Confederate flags were a common sight.

"I was driving to get home from speaking at a conference, and I knew I had no business being on those roads at night. An old pickup truck came up behind me and pulled up very close. I tried to go faster but he just stayed on my bumper. I thought, Oh my god, what is this man going to do to me? They might never find my body." She told the story in a humorous way, and we all laughed nervously with her. I knew her well enough to know that her fears were real. I knew Georgia well enough to know that the risk was real.

In epidemiology, we use terms like absolute risk, relative risk, and perceived risk. My colleague's perception of risk was off the charts. She felt a very real sense of danger. There is a white part of me that wanted to say, *"He probably was in a hurry and knew those old roads well enough to want to pass you."* In other words, my instinct was to discount her fears. I wanted to insert my assessment of the "actual risk" of the situation into the narrative. That would be gaslighting.

African Americans live in a world of disproportionate *actual risk.* In the exact same situation, her risk is very different from mine. What might be overreacting and irrational fear in my world would be realistic risk assessment, survival instincts, and learned cautiousness in hers. One colleague called it learned paranoia. And even if I know it in my head, I find it almost impossible to feel it in my gut. The best I can do is to believe. All I can feel is empathy. I can't say, *"I know how you feel,"* because I don't. All I can say is, *"I'm with you."*

The current politics of Florida public schools has also created an environment rife with fear and oppression. Cameron Driggers wrote an article titled, "What It's Like to Be an LGBTQ+ High Schooler in DeSantis's Florida."[38] "As part of the LGBTQ+ community myself, it was terrifying to see members of my own school board proposing banning books, simply because they were written by authors who speak to my very existence." When the students stood up to it, their protest attracted radical opponents from a white nationalist militia group called the Three-Percenters. The militia wore masks and tactical gear and brought weapons to school board meetings. Then they followed *high school students* home to intimidate them.

Children growing up in poor neighborhoods are much more likely to be exposed to violent or traumatic events. In Immokalee, Florida, Haitian and Latine children are traumatized by the fear of parents being seized by immigration authorities during the school day. Some of their classmates now have no parents to go home to. Wajahat Ali wrote a "Helpful Guide to Becoming an

American" for immigrants, saying, "The Whiteness doesn't want us to be American. But since it can't remove all of us, it will always find ways to dominate the rest of us and make our lives uncomfortable."[39]

It's not just in poor neighborhoods in the South. Margo Jefferson writes of growing up among the Black elite. Her world was among educated and upper-income African American families in the Hyde Park neighborhood of Chicago. She calls this land of contradictions *Negroland*.

"Life in Negroland meant that any conversation could be taken over by the White Man at any moment. 'When he's not lynching you, he's humiliating you,' said the men at the dinner table." It wasn't just a problem for Black men. Jefferson described the framing of race in her own mindset. "A Negro girl could never be purely innocent. The vengeful Race Fairy always lurked nearby. . . . Work hard, child . . . Internalize The Race. Internalize both races. Then internalize the contradictions."[40]

In researching racial disparities in survival and health, we see the effect of a lifetime of racial oppression. We use terms like "allostatic load" and "racial weathering" to describe chronic racial stress and repetitive racial trauma. Researchers can even measure it inside the cell's machinery through shortening of telomeres (a sign of accelerated aging). A research review found that high allostatic load was associated with a 22 percent increased risk of all-cause mortality and 31 percent increased risk of cardiovascular mortality.[41] Being under constant threat wears on both body and soul. It can literally break your heart. It can kill you.

The converse of Black fear is irrational white fear. CNN called it the "fear of Black men in public spaces."[42] In New York's Central Park, a woman called 911 and said, "I'm going to tell them there's an African American man threatening my life." The man was a bird watcher and had asked the white woman simply to put her dog back on its leash. A CNN reporter said, "All those incidents have a depressing familiarity to many Black men. It's part of the ambient racism of our everyday lives."

Another example was an African American man stopped for simply walking through a white neighborhood in Houston. Police told him that they had already received three calls from local residents describing him as a suspicious person. In *Dying of Whiteness*, Jonathan Metzl tells two stories of our different realities as Black and white people in America. Imagine that you live in a state allowing "open-carry" of guns. A white man casually shopped in a Walmart in Winder, Georgia, with an AR-15 assault rifle strapped to his back—no problem. But when an older African American man wore a legally owned pistol in a Walmart in Tampa, Florida, he was tackled and held in a choke-hold by a white customer yelling, "He's got a gun!"[43]

This deep-rooted fear of Black men is woven into our history and our national consciousness. The fear of plantation owners started with slave rebellions from Haiti to the American colonies, personified by Nat Turner. These fears broadened into the image of Black men as aggressive and violent and sexually dangerous to white women. *The Birth of a Nation* (originally *The Clansmen*) codified this imagery in a 1915 silent movie. It was the first movie screened in the White House by a sitting president (Woodrow Wilson). The film even offered up familiar tropes that are now being recycled, such as Black men stuffing ballot boxes.

How many lynchings were born of white fears? How many race massacres were started by untrue allegations of a Black man or teen sexually assaulting a white woman? Newspaper articles in Atlanta had linked sexually aggressive Black men with "uppity Blacks." They called both a burgeoning threat to white supremacy.[44] In 1906, the result was the Atlanta massacre. W. E. B. Du Bois wrote an anguished prayer called "the Day of Death, 1906." He prayed, "O Silent God, . . . Bewildered we are . . . mad with madness of a mobbed and mocked and murdered people; . . .

Surely, Thou too art not white, O Lord, a pale bloodless, heart-less thing?"[45]

White fear is a dangerous animal. It's born of generations of prejudice. It's the deep instinctive primal fear that made my sweet loving mother unconsciously reach over and lock her car doors when she drove through a Black neighborhood. Much racial fear is a subconscious lizard-brain fear. It's an emotional reaction we have even without conscious thought. Why else would a white neighbor shoot through her front door to kill a Black mother of four in Ocala, Florida, in 2022?[46]

The more limited our interactions are with people of another race, the more likely we are to have irrational fears. But the more we have diverse relationships, the more we can free ourselves from those fears. Here's an example from my own life.

I once was robbed at gunpoint. I was leaving my office next to our Morehouse Family Practice clinic on the back side of South-west Hospital. It was one of the last remaining historically Black hospitals in the nation, surrounded by Black neighborhoods. I was leaving the office late. The clinic was closed, and everyone else had gone home. I was wearing a coat and tie, carrying a briefcase. I looked like the whitest person in a three-mile radius.

A red truck suddenly sped loudly through the parking lot and jumped the curb onto the sidewalk, where it screeched to a stop. The passenger window was open barely a foot in front of my face. I stepped back, confused, as my brain processed the fact that there was a large silver revolver pointed straight between my eyes. Strange, the details we notice in those moments. I can remember to this day the tips of the bullets that were visible in the revolver's chambers. I remember their teal-green hue and the small grooves carved in their tips. I had tunnel vision. I saw only a big chrome gun and groove-tipped bullets in each cylinder. I was only vaguely aware of an African American man with a shaved head telling me to throw my wallet into the truck.

As the red truck sped out of the parking lot, I tried to be a good citizen. I strained to see the license plate. Two shots rang out, as he fired into the air or maybe in my general direction. *"Time to go, time to go, time to go . . ."* I said as I ran around the small hill up to the front entrance of the hospital. I told my story breathlessly to the front desk receptionist, who quickly called the police. By the time they arrived, I was calm.

I began to realize how little I could do to help catch the robber. *"Red pickup truck,"* I said. *"I'm not sure the license number—I think it started with a DZ or a QZ, but. . . ."* They asked what he looked like. *"Umm. . . . Male. African American. Shaved head or bald. Thirties, forties? Maybe older? I'm not sure."* How tall? *"Don't know, he was sitting."* How much do you think he weighed? *"No idea."* No way would I be able to pick him out of a mugshot book or a lineup. But I remembered the gun and I remembered those bullets.

I went to work on campus at Morehouse the next day, aware that I was still processing a scary experience. I worried a little bit that my fight-or-flight neural pathways would be organized around some vague archetype of a bald-headed, middle-adult Black man. One of my African American colleagues passed me as I entered. Black man, no fear response. Maybe I'll be okay. I went to a meeting. Lots of African American faculty and staff. At least three were bald-headed, middle-adult Black men. They were my friends and my colleagues. I knew each of them as individuals. We had laughed together and worked hard together.

I went to a grocery store and again worried that maybe my fear pathways would generalize to African American men whom I didn't know. White fears and racial archetypes are so deeply embedded in the American experience. Lots of people were there, Black and white, men and women—no response. *Whew, I must be strong.* No traumatic fear response for me.

I walked blithely out to the parking lot, where a loud red pickup truck suddenly roared straight toward me. I jumped back instinctively, heart racing. My mouth was dry. My eyes were scanning for danger, pupils undoubtedly dilated. The red pickup truck was nowhere near me, but I was scared as hell. That was my neural trauma pathway, now centered on an archetype of loud red pickup trucks. The fear pathway had been formed. Until that moment, I had no conscious awareness of it. Red pickup truck, or Black men? What if I had only ever lived and worked in white-world? What if I hadn't known dozens of African American men with bald, shaved heads?

White fear is pervasive and powerful. It's dangerous. In its extreme, it is the fear of being replaced, whether by people of color, Jewish people, or immigrants. Sometimes, these are just vague fears, a sense of unease. Our fears are only unmasked when our white male dominance is undermined.

White fear is political dynamite. Politicians have figured out how to weaponize these racial-ethnic fears. When public schools lose their white majorities, or when their teachers embrace diversities of gender and sexuality, politicians can stoke fears. They talk of "losing our way of life" at the hands of "enemies of traditional values." These are similar code words used in the 1950s when white America reacted to the Supreme Court's decision mandating school desegregation.

Version 2.0 in 2022–2023 is to stoke fears of the radical left. Fear "the woke mind-virus." In Florida, Governor DeSantis and others have mobilized "Moms for Liberty." They describe themselves as "moms on a mission to stand up for parental rights." Not surprisingly, these are all heterosexual, cisgender, conservative white women. Their vision of parental rights is to affirm their [white/straight] liberty to ban books in school. With no sense of irony, the Indian River County School Board banned a book called *Ban This Book*.

The anti-woke folks also want to make teachers afraid to teach about our racial history. They bully transgender kids and their parents, trying to erase their visible presence. Freedom to re-strict freedom. The right to constrain rights. Restricting liberties redefined as liberty. What fresh Orwellian hell is coming next?

If you're trying to preserve white control of schools in a state whose nearly five million children are 31 percent Hispanic, 20 percent African American, and 3 percent Asian, good luck with that!

We have to overcome our fears. We have to take the first steps. A father was standing with his child in the crowd outside the courtroom in Minneapolis when the George Floyd police trial verdict was announced. In an on-the-spot interview by CNN, he said, "I had a moment of awakening. . . . I became aware of my privilege." And then, he took the next small step. He said, "I actually googled, 'what can a white person do to help Black Lives Matter?" He wanted to become an ally, but he didn't know how.

That's how we start.

FOR FURTHER READING

Alexander M. *The New Jim Crow: Mass Incarceration in the Age of Colorblindness.*

"American History, Race, and Prison," Vera's Reimagining Prison Web Report.

Dyson ME. *The Tears We Cannot Stop.*

Martin R, Lakins L. *White Fear: How the Browning of America Is Making White Folks Lose Their Minds.*

Matthew Shepard Foundation. *Matthew's Story.*

Norris DM, Primm AB. *Mental Health, Racism, and Contemporary Challenges of Being Black in America.*

Parker HW, Abreu AM, Sullivan MC, Vadiveloo MK. Allostatic load and mortality: a systematic review and meta-analysis. *Am J Prev Med.* 2022;63(1):131–140.

6.

Anger and Rage

When the trial of a police officer in the murder of George Floyd came to a close with three guilty verdicts, my instinctive white response was, *"Finally, the system works."*

In 1991, I had come to work at Morehouse School of Medicine. It was only a few months after we all saw the video of Los Angeles police officers savagely beating Rodney King. A year later, I remember exactly where I was when the trial of those police officers ended with verdicts of "not guilty."

African American communities across the country erupted. I had been doing hospital rounds at the historically Black Southwest Hospital with our Morehouse resident physicians. Soon we took another admission through the emergency room. The patient had suffered a severe beating. He was a white student from Morris Brown College, one of the historically Black colleges of the Atlanta University Center.

The student had found himself in the middle of a spontaneous protest. It had erupted after the community heard the not guilty verdict for the officers who had savagely beaten Rodney King. The protest crowd was filled with rage that could not be expressed in mere words. It was a rage directed at hundreds of years of injustice and oppression and inhumanity of a white-majority system that still held them down. It flowed out of all the personal experiences of disrespect and indignity that these students and their neighboring communities had experienced at the hands of white people for all of their young lives. The pools of rage were deep and hot. On this day, they blew their gaskets.

This rage was not specifically directed at our white student-patient. He was in the wrong place at the wrong time. He also responded in the wrong way. He could have acknowledged the pain and affirmed the rage and then gotten the hell out of there. Instead, he felt threatened and shifted into a fighting posture, trusting his martial arts skills as his defense. Despite what you see in the movies, no black belt or kung fu wizardry is any kind of match for an angry crowd of young people. They beat the snot out of him.

The story did not end there. Along with this student, whom we decided to keep in the hospital overnight for observation (and protection), came his African American college roommate. He stayed at his side in the emergency room and came up with our patient to his hospital room. Other Morris Brown students showed up as well and spent the night in chairs next to his bed. *"We want him to feel safe,"* they said. And to a person, the African American doctors, nurses, aides, and techs who staffed this hospital all gave the same affirmation. *"He's safe with us."*

I felt this depth of concern very personally. Colleagues from Morehouse had called to find out where I was. They wanted to make sure that I was safe. They didn't want me driving back to our Atlanta University Center campus, where the demonstrations were escalating. One colleague called my intern to say, *"Make sure he doesn't come over here." "It's not safe, and he doesn't know any better. Not everyone's going to treat him like we do, especially today."*

We have to understand the depth of the pain and the burning rage that have been building over generations. How else can we understand just how heroic it is for African Americans to choose civility and working within the system? I understand the spiritual strength it took to offer me (and my patient and my country) such grace or unmerited kindness in that moment. After the Rodney King verdict, more than 11,000 people were arrested. Two thousand people were injured, and 55 people died.

That day, a truck driver named Reginald Denny found himself driving through a neighborhood where spontaneous riots had burst forth. He was pulled from his truck and beaten senseless by four Black men. Moments later, four other Black men jumped in to rescue the truck driver. They helped him back into the cab of his truck while defending him from further attack. One of those men drove him to the hospital. Acts of rage and, in the same moment, acts of heroism and grace.

Over the years, a federal agency often asked me to provide consultations to community health centers around the country. I especially remember my California visit to the Watts Health Center, in the lobby of which there was a round globule of glass in a display case. The orb represented molten glass from the windowpanes of businesses burned to the ground during the Watts riots of 1965. As with the Rodney King protests, the Watts rebellion was triggered by the arrest of an African American man during a traffic stop. A crowd had formed. Officers began fighting with onlookers. Things escalated. More and more highway patrol units arrived. The crowd grew in size. Batons were used, and shotguns were brandished to control the crowd. Police believed that a woman in the crowd had spit on the officers. The pregnant woman was physically subdued and dragged into custody. And so it began.

More crowds formed. Rocks and bottles were thrown. A community meeting was held to quiet things down. It was overwhelmed by people describing various incidents of police mistreatment of Black people in Watts. Rather than de-escalating the situation, the L.A. police chief called in the National Guard. When violence and flames were engulfing the community, he referred to the rioters as "monkeys in a zoo."[1]

In contrast to race massacres in the first half of the century, this was a modern "race riot" led by members of the African American community itself. Over a thousand buildings were destroyed, often businesses that served the Black community. From the outside, it seemed senseless. But for the 30,000 or more people caught up in it, the riot was an emotional expression of pent-up anger and rage. It was in a way self-destructive, even community-destructive; senseless but making perfect sense.

I think as a white guy, I will never fully understand racialized trauma or rage. We underestimate the impact of our American family's racial abuse and dysfunction. Linda Villarosa summarized it as "Strong, Loud, and Angry: The Invisibility of Black Emotional Pain."[2] At the 2023 Academy Awards ceremony, Will Smith went on stage and slapped Chris Rock for telling a joke that insulted Smith's wife. Later, he apologized, saying this—"Hurt people hurt people." He went on to describe his experiences growing up in his own dysfunctional family. Our American family is filled with hurt people who hurt people.

In 1968, Grier and Hobbs published the book *Black Rage*. They subtitled it, *Two Black psychiatrists reveal the full dimensions of the inner conflicts and the desperation of Black life in the United States.*[3] That's a mouthful and a mind-full. While the book focuses on the Black psychological reaction to racism, the white source of the dysfunction is clearly understood. "How come there's so much hate?" the authors ask.[4]

We think of Dr. Martin Luther King Jr. as the moderate and nonviolent advocate for racial justice, especially in contrast to Malcolm X or Black Panther leaders. We forget just how frustrated and angry MLK could be with America's slow pace of progress. In an interview with Alex Haley, he said this: "Why do white people seem to find it so difficult to understand that the Negro is sick and tired of having reluctantly parceled out to him those rights and privileges which all others receive upon birth or entry in America? . . . This . . . has begun to generate a fury in the Negro."[5]

Cornel West reframes Black rage as a "Black affirmation of self, a Black desire for freedom," indeed a "Black psychic conversion—the decolonization of the mind, body, and soul."[6]

I can understand intellectually, but I know that I will never fully understand with my heart and in my gut. Anger frightens me. It has psychological roots going back to my own dysfunctional family. I often withdraw in the face of anger, like the scared child I was when my father would rage. I can never truly *feel* Black rage. In this context, we must never say that we "understand" another person's experience of racism or marginalization, especially if it has not been ours to experience.

One of the cool things about working at an HBCU is how openly we talked about issues of race and poverty and marginalization. Early in my time at Morehouse, one of our conversations had begun to get a little heated. It was when our department faculty had recently become more white than black. Feelings were being expressed openly, and they included anger and frustration. One of my white colleagues, somewhat naive in this space, made two mistakes in short order. She had no idea that she had done it.

"*I just treat everyone the same,*" she said.

Strike 1—color-blind racism.

She continued. "*No, I get it. I'm a woman in medicine. I know what it feels like to be discriminated against.*"

Strike 2—false equivalencies.

Another white colleague of mine flinched. Robin and I looked at each other, instinctively wanting to duck because we knew a response was coming. Our African American colleagues were visibly angry. It was unusual, given their ability to maintain "the mask" in most of these conversations with white people. But in an HBCU, they were in their own house. *"You have no idea what it's like,"* said a colleague, controlling his anger. *"There is nothing in your experience that can relate to being Black in America. Or to being a Black doctor. You have no idea."*

In the summer between my junior and senior years of high school, I attended a journalism summer program at Northwestern University. We learned about writing and the newspaper business but also discussed issues of the day. At the end of the program, the counselors (themselves journalism majors), gave each of us a book as a gift. The book I received was *A Special Rage*, written by Gilbert Moore about his experiences of racism in America as a Black man and as a reporter.

The inscription my teacher had written on the cover was in itself grossly racist. It also implied that I (being from the South) was starting from a position of explicit racism. I could have taken offense at someone assuming that all Southerners are racists. I could have just thrown the book away. But for whatever reason, I didn't. I read it. I learned from it. I took it to heart. And the parts of myself I could recognize in it, I started to try to change. It's okay. We're all starting from somewhere. We all have stuff to learn and stuff to let go of. No need to be defensive. None of us are perfect, and all of us need learning or growth. Or we can just be stubborn and rigid. Our choice.

I read it cover-to-cover. I had always thought of myself as being clean and pure in the racism department because I had two Black friends in high school. I still worked on a mostly Black janitorial crew. But I began to see just how shallow my under-standing of "the Black experience" might be. My teacher was right. I didn't get it. And because I still haven't experienced it, I will never get it. But I keep trying and learning and growing, and each year I come a little closer to "getting it." At least a little bit.

Don't take offense but also don't beat yourself up. If you're ac-knowledging gaps and seeking to grow, then be at peace with it. Stand up for others as the best ally you can be at this stage of your growth. Just don't get too comfortable, because tomorrow brings new light, new insight, new growth to achieve, and new paths to follow. We're all peeling back layers of the onion, unless or until we choose to stop trying.

What I have learned a thousand times since from my patients and colleagues of color is that they have experiences every day that would make any of us angry. These assaults on a person's hu-manity both tap into and replenish a pool of anger and rage. It can either be consciously subdued or unconsciously repressed. If it flares even for a brief moment, it can reinforce a stereotype of "the angry Black man" or the angry Black woman.

Growing up in a home where anger and rage could be scary and dangerous, my inner child has always been uneasy with anger. I have learned a thousand ways to avoid it, to minimize it, to smooth it over, or to talk it down. Give me an angry patient or staff mem-bers shouting at each other, and I'm your man. I have an innate capacity for peacemaking and conflict de-escalation.

I also know that anger avoidance can be self-destructive. An-ger turned inward can lead me to depression or alcohol. Anger can only be used for good if its energy can be harnessed. I've learned over some decades to allow others space for that anger. It's not my job to fix it or smooth it over, but to be present and supportive. If I can, even if just a little bit, I try to acknowledge and understand.

I needed these skills in 2016. During that election year, then-candidate Donald Trump unleashed a wave of overtly racist and misogynistic sentiments across the country. He gave permission for people to use racist and anti-immigrant words they had previously learned to suppress. He was openly abusive to women.

Our students of color felt like they were under constant assault, whether through mainstream media, social media, or the various aggressions of their daily lives. Even their interactions with other students became fraught because of all the implicit bias and the white-norming and the race denialism. The little things that just pick at you day after day seemed amplified. People were walking on eggshells, trying so hard not to say the wrong thing. We were once again being the dysfunctional American family that we had tried so hard not to be.

Student after student came to my office or stopped me in the hallway to express their sense of frustration, their anxieties, their fears, and their anger. Feelings bubbled up like a volcano. Some felt overwhelmed and out of control. Some cried, some vented, and some shouted. I felt once that one of my favorite students wanted nothing more than to punch a hole in the wall. And that was okay. They needed that space. They needed to know that it was good and right to feel angry at injustice. It was good and right to feel angry at the overt insults and the unintended micro-assaults. It was good and right to feel angry at always having to be the one to fit in.

Desmond Tutu and his daughter Mpho Tutu co-wrote *The Book of Forgiving*, built on experiences of profound oppression and even genocide in South Africa. They have spent their lives seeking healing through truth and reconciliation. They remind us that "victims need to feel they are being heard and affirmed."[7] They then give us a very specific to-do (and not-to-do) list for "How to Acknowledge the Harm":

- Listen.
- Do not try to fix the pain.
- Do not minimize the loss.
- Do not offer advice.
- Do not respond with your own loss or grief.
- Keep confidentiality.
- Offer your love and your caring.
- Empathize and offer comfort.[8]

Over time, our students figured out how to cope and survive. Eventually, they channeled the angry energy into something good and positive. Entirely on their initiative, they came up with a program they called RAW: Racism Awareness Week. They garnered the enthusiastic support of our old white-guy dean. Speakers, lunch-and-learns, and activities were designed to help us all understand better. We learned to explicitly name the racism that had always been there. We are learning to recognize marginalization in all its different forms and to call it out.

Since then, each class of first- and second-year students on our Tallahassee campus has re-created and added to RAW week. They have added layers of learning about national origin, gender and sexuality, and intersectionality and institutional or structural racism. What a gift these young people are! But the gift started with the honesty of their emotions.

Brittney Cooper calls it *Eloquent Rage*. She talks about using our rage to destroy things like white supremacy and homophobia "and a whole bunch of other terrible shit." She says, "May your rage be a force for good."[9] So during the peak of Black Lives Matter protests, our white College of Medicine faculty and deans marched to a very tame rally on Florida's Capitol steps. We sought to express solidarity with our students and our community. Baby steps.

Black lives do matter. The psychology of constant aggressions, socioeconomic hurdles, and dehumanizing messages desperately needs healing. Dr. Joy DeGruy calls it "Post-Traumatic Slave Syndrome," America's legacy of enduring injury and healing.[10] Starting from slavery to the modern day, she asks, "What do repeated traumas endured generation after generation produce?"

In a recent NPR interview, one person who experienced the Selma march as a child remembered all of the violence inflicted on the marchers. He noted sadly how "they never had psychologists or counselors" come and talk with us. Amid terrible trauma, they were expected just to go on with their normal lives. He said that it didn't turn out well for some of them.

A young girl described being so scared she ran out of her shoes. When civil rights leader Hosea Williams tried to carry her to safety, she said, "Put me down, you're not running fast enough." She ran all the way home and straight to her bedroom. Hosea Williams continued to fight for civil rights his whole life. He worked tirelessly to feed the hungry and the homeless. But over many decades, his own psychological struggles with this trauma could not be hidden.

Anger and rage are the natural consequences of any abuse or oppression. Patriarchy and misogyny feed anger for women as well. Soraya Chemaly describes women's anger as the last taboo. She asks this: "'What do we lose, personally and as a society, by not listening to women's anger or respecting it?' Answer: the true voice of half of humanity."[11] Gloria Steinem added, "How many women cry when angry because we've held it in for so long?" The #me-too movement helped release some of that anger in a sentiment that women were just not going to take it anymore. Women spoke out, and men were convicted of crimes that had gone too long unpunished.

Sometimes anger will be directly expressed at me. Sometimes I deserve it, for something I did or said or didn't say or do. Sometimes I've done something trivial, but it unleashes a suppressed pool of anger that finally boils over on me. The patient who unloads on me for keeping them waiting a half-hour may have just spent the previous three hours going through the dignity-stripping experience of applying for Medicaid. It's okay.

Sometimes I receive anger because I represent an institution involved in historic inequities. It starts with listening. The Tutus remind us not to argue or justify our actions or even our own motives when listening to community pain. Instead, we must "listen and acknowledge the harm you have caused."[12] How I wish that hospital CEOs or university presidents could do just that in community *listening* sessions tied to public apologies.

Sometimes white people see Black anger even when it's not there or not expressed. Whether we're carrying buckets of white guilt or white grievance, we may project it onto those of another racial group. I feel guilty about racism in our workplace, so *they* must be angry about it. I feel grievance that I was left behind for promotion, so *they* must be celebrating my loss. A student seems guarded, or doesn't smile easily, and stands stiffly in our learning sessions. So a white preceptor notes on their student evaluation that they *"have a chip on their shoulder."*

Because of white fears, Black men in particular must be careful not to provoke. One former football player described to me how he would try to hunch over and shrink himself. He would even soften his deep voice, just to make sure that his large Black physical presence didn't frighten white folks. In 2010, CNN published an article, "Why Obama Doesn't Dare Become the Angry Black man."[13]

And a Black man with a gun? It scares the stew out of white folks. As one author noted, "Even the NRA Supported Gun Control When the Black Panthers Had the Weapons."[14] During the late 1960s, the Black Panthers for Self-Defense openly protested on the California Capitol steps armed with pistols and shotguns. They said it was time for Black people to arm themselves. To prevent police violence against Black community members in California, they conducted "police patrols."[15] They followed police cars and made themselves visible (with their weapons) in a non-threatening stance. They offered advice on legal rights to African American people who had been pulled over. Soon California passed a bill prohibiting the open carrying of loaded firearms under super-conservative, pro-gun Governor Ronald Reagan. The federal Gun Control Act of 1968 also passed, with political support from the NRA. Black men with guns? No way!

The emotional responses of white people are hard to see in ourselves. I almost understand white guilt and maybe even white fear as a projection of white guilt. But white rage is a concept that is hard for me to comprehend. Similar terms include white backlash, or the politics of white grievance. The meme of the angry white man. It mystifies me, yet there it is.

A colleague says that when you're used to privilege, equality feels like oppression. Someone is taking something away from you. We justify it because none of our lives are perfect. Some of us have experienced our own traumas, whether by poverty or loss of a parent or living with alcoholism or abuse. Maybe a parent lost a job in a recession or maybe we even experienced homelessness. We ask the universe, *"How the hell is that privilege?"* But I ask each of us who engage in this self-pity talk, would our lives really have been easier if we had been Black while we were having all these other traumas?

In a commentary in *Forbes* magazine, Dana Brownlee said this: "When racism deniers reject the very real existence and impact of white privilege, I simply ask them why there has never been a Black female governor [or] . . . why there have only been 22 Black CEOs throughout the entire 67-year history of the Fortune 500 list."[16]

She says people inevitably go silent in response, so she offers only two possible answers. One is that Black people are somehow "fundamentally deficient" or inadequately qualified, which seems racist on its face. The second is that "somehow the system and the selection process itself tends to disadvantage Black people (particularly Black women)." Okay, racism-deniers—which is it?

Still, a former advisor to twice-impeached President Trump has formed a legal firm explicitly to fight "racism against white people" and "anti-white bigotry."[17] They run ads on TV asking, "When did racism against white people become OK?" They cite Biden administration efforts to provide COVID relief funds first to high-disparity communities.[18] Trump even vowed retribution at the opening bid of his 2024 presidential re-election campaign in Waco, saying, "I am your warrior, I am your justice." In a recent speech to the Conservative Political Action Committee (CPAC), Trump said this—"If you've been hurt, if you've been betrayed . . . I am your retribution!"

What, really? Retribution? Betrayal? Clearly not retribution for America's multicentury history of hurt and abuse and oppression against people of color. Nor for the immigrants who are the constant object of his hate speech, nor for the genocidal seizing of Native American land or the forced taking of their children for culture-washing. Certainly not for the abuse of gay parents or the targeting of trans teens. No, in the context of President Trump speaking at CPAC, the "you" in "if you've been hurt" can only mean white people. Especially white men, whose privilege is slipping away. Victimized white men of grievance. "I am your retribution!"

This is another example of the intentionally obtuse choice to ignore the directionality of racism. In a pretend world of no racial inequalities, any consideration of race to level the playing field must itself be racism. The very notion of reverse racism requires a substrate of white denialism, an intentional setting aside of the facts of racial disparities in health and wealth and justice in America. Poor little white men just can't catch a break. Sorry, but that's just stupid. And immoral. And wrong.

Roland Martin says that "whenever there is Black progress, there is white backlash." In her book *White Rage*, Carol Anderson chronicles the history of white backlash against progress toward full human rights of America's non-white citizens.[19] She documents how the underlying emotion begets structural inequalities. "The fear of a multicultural democracy" seeks to institutionalize white privilege or racial inequality through laws and policies.[20]

She also connects our present struggles to the history of white responses to the *Brown v. Board of Education* decision. Those included the Southern Manifesto and a variety of ways in which communities sought to maintain segregation in their schools. Some communities even went so far as to shut down their public schools in favor of funding (white-only) private academies. Twenty-first-century efforts to outlaw affirmative action in education are just the newest flavor. There is a common thread in history between Jim Crow laws designed to prevent African Americans from voting in the 1950s with 21st-century voter suppression laws designed to target cities with high minority voter turnout. "That's white-rage policy," Anderson says.

Race and gender backlash are connected as well. Michael Kimmel is a sociologist who studies the connections between masculinity and far-right movements around the world. He says that the one thing all angry white men have in common is a sense of "aggrieved entitlement."[21] It is the reaction of some white men to the rise in women's rights, civil rights, and racial progress. It's a fear-based response to the shifting demographics of a pluralistic society.[22] He details the rise of the "manosphere" on the internet, an echo chamber where men harboring grievances find a community of supportive peers. It becomes a brotherhood of sorts. Says Kimmel, "These are guys that really think that they don't matter in the world and have been tossed aside." Notice the overlap as well between racial grievance and male grievance. White-guy grievance.

In her classic "Ain't I a Woman" speech, Sojourner Truth summed up the white guy's dilemma. "I think that 'twixt the Negroes of the South and the women of the North, all talking about rights, the white men will be in a fix pretty soon."[23] Supporters of the racial hierarchy and patriarchy are threatened by those who would seek progress. One used the term "freedom shriekers" to describe advocates for true equality and racial justice. In the 1950s, the strategy was to label advocates as Communist sympathizers. During my lifetime, they have pigeonholed us with labels that have evolved from "socialists" to "social justice warriors" to the current favorite, simply "woke."

On Veterans Day in 2023, thrice-indicted President Trump made a campaign speech with not-so-subtle echoes of Nazi fascism. He said that threats from abroad were "far less sinister, dangerous, and grave than the threats from within." He went on to promise veterans that he would "root out the communists, Marxists, . . . and radical left thugs that live like vermin within the confines of our country."[24]

This dehumanization of people with whom we have policy differences is incredibly dangerous. It ultimately became the rationale for exterminating people by race in 1940s Germany. Does DeSantis really mean that Florida is where "woke" goes to die? He says he plans to defend our border with deadly force, in speeches that describe Mexicans "ending up stone cold dead at the border." In Trump's America, am I to be rooted out like vermin from the country I love?

Dr. King was often accused of being a Communist or Marxist. He even called himself "a drum major for justice," so the pejorative label of social justice warrior is okay by me. I'll even accept "woke" if you'll acknowledge that the opposite is to be un-woke, asleep, unconscious, oblivious, or purposefully unaware. Follow the arc of history. See where this is headed. Look back at the trajectory from slavery to Black codes to civil rights legislation to the increasing diversity of our society and our leaders. Look at the current antiracism movement in the arc of our history. Look at our push for health equity and social justice. Celebrate the passage of marriage protection for LGBTQ couples with sometimes grudging but bipartisan support. Progress will prevail!

Think about where the anti-woke folks stood in the 1950s, yelling "segregation forever" at kids trying to go to school. *Would you stand with them now?* Think about the homophobia and LGBTQ bullying that we all saw and may have participated in during our school years—*are we proud of that now? Would we teach it to our kids now?* How many of us have discovered that we have friends or family members (or our own selves) who are gay or non-binary? How many of us are trying now to get everyone's pronouns right out of respect for who they are? How many of us are trying so hard to shed our layers of bias? How many of us just want to show love and acceptance? What if we all tried really hard?

The march of progress is often slow and uneven, two steps forward and sometimes two steps back. But it marches on. Demographics are driving us forward. Communicating openly about who we are as diverse humans is driving us forward. The complexity of modern families is driving us forward. Civil rights advocates and social justice warriors and democratic socialists and allies and woke people are all leading us forward. We can all be drum majors for justice. And the aggrieved, privilege-hoarding, change-averse, gender-insecure, status quo anti-woke shrinking minority will have the same experience as all those who came before. They will live to see the progress. Perhaps one day they may see this brave new world as an opportunity for learning and growth. It is our moment for both giving and receiving love and grace. It is our moment for healing.

If we so choose.

FOR FURTHER READING

Anderson C. *White Rage: The Unspoken Truth of Our Racial Divide.*

Chemaly S. *Rage Becomes Her: The Power of Women's Anger.*

Cooper B. *Eloquent Rage.*

Grier WH, Cobbs PM. *Black Rage: Two Black Psychiatrists Reveal the Full Dimensions of the Inner Conflicts and the Desperation of Black Life in the United States.*

The Autobiography of Malcolm X, as told to Alex Haley.

Tutu D, Tutu M. *The Book of Forgiving: The Fourfold Path for Healing Ourselves and Our World.*

7.

Trust and Mistrust

"Why should I trust you?" she asked. I was shocked and hurt and offended all at the same time. *What had I done?*

I had recently taken a leadership position as medical director of the Morehouse Family Practice Center, where she was a nurse-educator on the clinical faculty. To give it context, the older physicians on faculty were all Black, while the recent hires (including me) were white. The nurses were all Black women. The front desk staff were all Black women. The non-physician faculty (nutritionist, psychologist, etc.) were all Black women. A new, young white-guy physician (me) had been put in charge of the clinic. To a small extent, I had been given control over my colleague's schedule and her workload.

The instinct to distrust a white man with power was deep and visceral. It was a distrust that had been earned by many white men in positions of power before me. It was distrust built up over generations and reinforced almost every day. Of course people of color shouldn't give their trust freely to white people. Let white people earn it. Do I frame the problem as hers, as a problem of her distrust? Or is it my challenge to become and to be known as trustworthy?

But really, what had *I* done to lose *her* trust? Nothing. This was the beginning of a new insight that took a while to grow. I had done nothing to lose her trust, but I had also done nothing to gain her trust. I was starting from an assumption that trust was something I started with and that I could lose if I behaved badly. She (and many of our colleagues of color) started from an instinct of caution and skepticism. Some scholars call it "a hermeneutic of suspicion."[1]

Mistrust was the logical conclusion of knowing that "we've been burned too many times before." Mistrust is a rational response to an irrational world. Think of all the good historic reasons to mistrust white people. Start from slavery. Move on to Jim Crow oppression to lynchings to race massacres to voting suppression (then and now). Think of redlining in housing and of employment discrimination. Wrap your head around the massive attempt to dehumanize African Americans. Think about it in health care, from torturous surgical experiments on slaves to the psychological diagnosis of "runaway slave syndrome." We segregated hospital wards and doctors' offices. We ran government-funded syphilis experiments. We still have disparities in treatment for pain and cancer and heart disease. Then multiply those by a thousand demeaning experiences and microaggressions that people of color experience every day in their own lives. Why should they trust me?

In 1990, *Essence* magazine published an article titled "AIDS: Is it Genocide?" It asked, "Could AIDS be a virus that was manufactured to erase large numbers of us?"[2] African American celebrities ranging from Spike Lee to Will Smith to Bill Cosby all endorsed some version of the HIV genocide meme in the 1990s.[3] What sounds extreme to my white ears seems reasonable through the lens of lived experience in the Black community. The statistics on health disparities remind us that it's not paranoia if they're really trying to kill you.

White leaders or professionals must pay attention to this dynamic. We are either building trust or destroying it. If we grew up white, we may not understand this instinct to distrust. Our white privilege, the unseen tidal flow that carried us along effortlessly, made it easier to trust. Not that life was always easy. Just easier.

If we experienced abuse as a child or trauma as an adult, we may have our own trust issues. It's not the same, but it's a start. I had a little bit of dysfunction in my growing-up years. I've learned to tap into it to empathize with, if not to fully understand, these deep-rooted feelings of racial mistrust. In those moments, our brokenness is our strength.

At Morehouse, I had to work to earn the trust of patients and staff and fellow physicians. Dr. Lonnie Fuller was my department chair. He took a risk. He gave me the grace of trusting me before he had good reason to. He asked me to write grants that would build and define new programs for our department. He asked me to lead some of those programs. He engaged me in honest but relaxed and nuanced conversations about race and health and poverty.

I came to love that man. He had an infectious smile and an ability to make me laugh inappropriately. He would whisper-curse under his breath, long and low. With a glint in his eye, he would say *bulls**** or *racist motherf****** just barely loud enough for me to hear in formal meetings. And he would maintain his composure while I would laugh out loud. I drew some funny looks, but I never gave him away. I loved Dr. Lonnie Fuller like a wise and cool older brother. I wept at his funeral.

Dr. Fuller gave me his trust before I had earned it. His department was having trouble recruiting Black physicians. Our faculty had become more white than Black. At that very moment, he trusted me to lead a strategic planning retreat. We agreed that one of the questions on the table was this: *"What is our role in being a clinical department in a historically Black medical school?"*

Within the institution and in the community, Dr. Fuller was taking heat for not having enough Black faculty. As I facilitated the conversation that day, we got to the difficult question. *"What proportion of our faculty should be African American? How much Black would be Black enough?"* I could see that my white colleagues were uncomfortable, but I couldn't gloss this one over. The faculty, Black and white together, looked at the question unflinchingly. *"Maybe 95 percent,"* said the woman who had asked, *"Why should I trust you?"* I felt like she wanted to say 100 percent.

She watched for my reaction. I didn't blink. I embraced all the responses. They were honest and raw. I was there to facilitate getting the group's real answer, even though that number might not allow room for even one white physician on the faculty. In that moment, I earned a small speckle of trust from her.

Ultimately, the group came down to a number around 80 percent, a threshold of "Blackness" below which we could not achieve the core value of being a historically Black department. We were training students and residents to provide care in one of only five remaining historically Black hospitals in the nation. Eighty percent Black faculty is what it would take to create the nurturing environment of an HBCU. It was the climate that for generations had created "Morehouse men" (now more women than men in the medical school). It had allowed just a few HBCU medical schools to train over 80 percent of the Black doctors practicing in America.[4]

It was a critical moment for the department. We had thought our strategic plan would focus on improving medical student education or enhancing the residency training program. Instead, it turned out that the rate-limiting factor was to recruit or develop African American physician teachers. At that time, the Association of American Medical Colleges estimated that there were only 43 Black family medicine faculty across all of the 126 US medical schools in the country. One-third of them were at HBCU medical schools—Howard, Meharry, Morehouse, and Drew.

If we wanted Black faculty, we would have to grow our own. As a chief resident, I had been a member of the charter class of Cook County Hospital's faculty development program. I proposed developing a similar program at Morehouse. There was no money, so we wrote a grant proposal. With the funding, we hired a wonderful program manager and staff. We reached out to community physicians. We paid them to come and learn to teach and to write grants and publish papers. The goal was for some of them to become academic physicians. Some days I was teaching skills that I had only just barely learned myself.

It took years, but we began to fill our faculty ranks with those who had come through the program. We didn't dare suggest that African American colleagues already on the faculty might also need to learn some new skills. But now they began to approach and say, *"Can we come to your program?"* One of our physician-leaders had actually completed a faculty development program at Duke. She said, *"They taught me all about this stuff, but you're coaching people through actually doing it."* And so the trust continued to build.

After some years, we had graduated nearly a hundred African American primary care faculty from our program. Compare that to the 43 Black family physicians working in medical schools when we started. We were beginning to have a national impact. Across the country, Black and Brown professionals in academic settings were facing discrimination every day. They also carried an extra burden of bridging the gap between their white institutions and their minority patients or students.[5,6]

We developed an Executive Faculty Development program to train faculty from all over the country. In feedback after completing our program, one family physician from California said this: *"I have spent many years as an academic physician. This is the first program that actually nurtured and supported my growth."* How can you feel good about such praise when it also breaks your heart?

The faculty in our program were great physicians. Many were also great teachers. But they were struggling to write papers for peer-reviewed publication, the coin of the realm in a scholarly career. They knew how to write. They often had started a number of papers. But they were stuck, because they couldn't bring themselves to share a paper with a colleague until it was perfect. Which meant never. No publications. They didn't want to show their work to others for one of two reasons. First, they had had their work stolen in the past, only to see it credited to someone else. Learned paranoia. Second, they had been torn down too many times. For so long, they had been told that they weren't smart enough to be a doctor or a scholar. Their walls were up. They would never invite someone to criticize them again. So, they were stuck. And they had no idea that it was a trust issue.

We worked hard on that. Our National Center for Primary Care developed an open-invitation research team meeting. The agreed-upon goal was to generate grants and papers. My hidden agenda was to build trusting collaborations. We created a safe space. We gave each other a lot of affirmations. We celebrated even the smallest victories. We had our own Fantasy Football League.

We created models for collaboration that felt safe. For example, we worked out the order of first author, second author, and so on transparently and concretely. The group kept the process fair. When outside collaborators were acting badly, the group could discuss how to respond without risking the scholar's career path.

We invented strategies for letting go of our manuscripts that weren't perfect yet. For example, we used the game Hot Potato to create rapid-cycle revisions. Never let the paper sit on your desk for more than three days. Change just one sentence, if that's all you can do. Then pass the hot potato to your colleague. Don't get burned. In reality, if three or four emerging scholars played Hot Potato with a manuscript for at least three cycles, it was probably close to being done.

The format of our research meetings was built around three questions:

- What are you working on?
- How can we help you?
- When is it moving to the next step?

The last one was a push toward holding each other accountable. I let it slide for the first six months because it was the toughest one. The mutual trust and safe space had to be built first. It's no coincidence that my co-leader of the group was a psychiatrist. Dr. Ruth Shim had incredible emotional intelligence and facilitating skills. She brought her own lived experience of being a Black physician-teacher-scholar. I knew it was finally coming together when a member of our group described their manuscript, and a colleague gently asked the third question. "So, you've been working on this paper for a while now—when do you see it going out the door?" Accountability. I knew the group dynamic had matured. The question wouldn't have been asked if the trust wasn't there.

I also came to understand that the instinct to distrust could be deeply internalized. It was a way of relating to the world, not just to white people. From old plantation dynamics to new corporate plantation-equivalents, some African Americans have been coerced or co-opted into playing a role in the oppression. The instinct to distrust was reinforced even for interactions within race. The instinct could generalize to distrust anyone, even Black colleagues in a historically Black institution. Colleagues had to learn to trust one another enough to share their ideas, to write papers together, and to build fair budgets for grants. It took time.

In many ways, this trust/distrust dynamic was the opposite side of the respect/disrespect coin in how we related to each other. My colleague's unwillingness to start from a baseline of trusting people she didn't know was similar to how I thought people should have to earn my respect. Her assumption was that showing respect to all people was a given. Showing disrespect was an assault on one's humanity. It was fascinating to me in that moment when my trust was questioned that neither of us was aware of how the other perceived issues of trust/distrust and respect/disrespect. We had polar opposite racial and cultural lenses.

This trust/distrust dynamic plays out in medical care every day. It manifests itself as one of the many root causes of unequal health outcomes. There is a growing body of research designed simply to find valid measures of the various domains of trust,[7,8] including trust in physicians,[9] trust in institutions,[10] and more generalized cultural mistrust.[11,12] Unfortunately, much of this research frames the issue as a minority problem of "those people," of the minority group. Blame the patient. Much less research has been devoted to the measurement of white trustworthiness or institutional trustworthiness. Not my problem.

Early in my career, I joined the medical staff of the West Orange Farmworkers Health Association. Within months, I became medical director for all the clinics, but I cared for patients in our smallest, most remote clinic. Groveland, Florida, was a town with two stoplights, no Dairy Queen, and a dark history of racial animus. My patients were not just farmworkers but also low-income and uninsured people of all backgrounds. Maybe a third were African American, a third white, and a third Hispanic or Latine. Our other clinics served Haitian and Chinese immigrants as well. All too often, my heart was broken by seeing preventable suffering. We saw late-stage cancers and extreme complications of treatable diseases that doctors serving the well-insured and well-off rarely saw. Sometimes the barriers were financial or structural and sometimes cultural or psychological. Sometimes the barrier to getting the right care was mistrust.

Michelle Obama speaks very personally about this, describing her grandfather's belief that doctors were untrustworthy. It kept him from getting an early diagnosis or treatment for the cancer that would ultimately kill him.[13] Among African American patients, there is an association between mistrust of physicians and lower rates of potentially lifesaving colorectal cancer screening.[14] Delay in diagnosis is even more common if people experience everyday discrimination.[15]

Patients who have more trust in their health care professionals are more satisfied with their treatment, have fewer symptoms, and pursue healthier behaviors.[16] In pain research, patients who mistrust the experimenter actually experience more pain. African American subjects experienced greater pain than did white subjects.[17] In contrast, roughly half of medical students at one school believed that "Black skin is thicker than white skin"[18] in a way that would lower the perception of pain.

In America, race is complicated. Trust is complicated. Skin color is a continuum. Some patients have darker skin and experience greater discrimination, even when compared to other persons of color. Some African American patients place "being Black" more centrally in their personal identity. There are also intersectional nuances. Black–white trust issues may have some commonalities, but they can be very different across the spectrum of gender and sexual identities.[19]

Whom do our African American patients trust? Some of our patients simply *"trust in the Lord."* We can affirm such spirituality if we provide spiritual support according to their preferences and not ours.[20] Meanwhile, some patients trust their nurse but not their doctor. Nurses are often more competent in relational skills. Sadly, medical schools do not select future doctors for their emotional intelligence.

The power dynamics are also different for nurses than for doctors. Power and control are central to issues of racial mistrust and white trustworthiness. As physicians, especially white-guy physicians, we must give up the need to control. Instead of the usual push-pull of trying to get my patient to do the healthy choice (i.e., what I want them to do), I've learned to practice my motivational interviewing skills. I come alongside my patient and see the world through their eyes. I need to feel as their heart feels. I walk with them toward their goals, not mine.

When I took over as medical director of the Farmworkers Health Association, my predecessor took me out to lunch. Dr. Otilia Mariña is an incredibly dedicated family physician. She had once provided care for Cesar Chavez in the United Farmworkers movement. I think she was worried that I didn't quite "get it."

As we were eating, she tried to pass along some of her passion and wisdom. *"George,"* she said, *"when I'm in the exam room with a patient, they tell me things they wouldn't even tell their spouse or their best friend."* She paused. *"I feel like a priestess."* There was a sacredness in this moment as well. She went on. *"Sometimes I can't fix it. But all they expect, all they hope for, is that I will hold their hand and walk with them on their journey."* I don't know if I ever got it in the same way that Oti did, but I took it all to heart. I share her words with every class of medical students that comes my way.

Patients see nuance. For example, one group of researchers found that people might mistrust white Anglo doctors and even the whole health care system, but still trust their nurse practitioner.[21] Maybe doctors should put on our humble hats and learn about building trust from our nursing colleagues.

In one study, Black patients given a scenario of having high cholesterol were more likely to trust a Black physician when being advised to change their diet.[22] At the same time, I have had Black patients ask for me (the white guy) in the setting of a historically

Black hospital. Some had an internalized racial bias that I might have better training or competence. Men who have sex with men (not necessarily identifying as gay) asked for me specifically. They assumed either that I wouldn't ask about their sexuality or that I wouldn't judge them. They knew that I wouldn't out them in the Black community. Other patients would ask specifically for a Black physician or a physician who was fluent in their language. Not the white guy. Not the Anglo. Race and culture matter. It's okay.

But no, it's not the same if a white patient refuses to see a Black doctor. Dekalb Medical Center found this out when they had a white patient request that only white nurses provide her care. Administrators chose a "customer is always right" approach and initially acceded to her request. At least for a day or two, until Black nurses and staff staged a walk-out in protest. Again, racism has a history and a directionality.

In refugee health and family planning, we often see women who have been raped or who have experienced other violence and trauma. Trauma-informed care seeks to give the patient as much autonomy and control as possible. Seeing a female provider is a reasonable request. But a toxic masculine male refusing to see a female provider based on bigotry is not okay. History and directionality matter.

How else can white Anglo physicians or health care leaders become effective in trying to help patients of color? How do straight, cisgender physicians help their LGBTQ and non-binary patients? How do white guys learn to lead and manage diverse health care teams? One strategy is self-disclosure. Be vulnerable. Share the biases about which you have become aware. Share your struggles. Be secure enough to show your weakness. That becomes your new strength.

Other members of the community are often more trusted than I would be as a white physician. Working with those who already have trust with our patients can move us into a zone of being trust-adjacent. If we show those community partners respect and humility, then over time, we can build our own trust.[23]

In Groveland, the Latine community we served in our migrant/community health center was mostly of Mexican origin. Diabetes was a huge problem. We saw out-of-control diabetes every day. And we saw all the long-term consequences of high blood sugars and poorly controlled diabetes. We saw the nerve damage that led to foot ulcers and then bone infections and ultimately leg amputations. We saw kidney failure. We saw patients go blind from diabetic retinal damage. We saw heart attacks and strokes from the constellation of diabetes, high cholesterol, and high blood pressure.

Working in this community taught me one thing about helping people manage their own health. *It's relational, not informational.* It's about dignity and respect. It's not about facts or graphs or data. Instead, it's about personal, relational trust. Here's an example of how it worked in Groveland. I would see a diabetic patient whose blood sugars were consistently over 300. That level would almost certainly lead to future eye, nerve, kidney, and blood vessel damage. Let's call her Señora Sanchez.

"Señora, I'm worried about your diabetes. I don't want it to hurt you. I think you should take some new medication. It's a new pill you take twice a day." Mrs. Sanchez would nod and smile. I learned slowly over the years that this did not mean that she agreed. She was just listening and wanted to show me respect. I pulled out all the stops. *"Doña Maria, I want you to be with your family and those beautiful grandbabies for a very long time. I'm worried that the diabetes will damage your kidneys or make you go blind. I want you to dance at your daughter's wedding, but the sugar is already damaging the nerves in your feet."* She nodded impassively and thanked me as I handed her the prescription.

What I didn't put together until many years later was that the decision would be made at our front desk or perhaps later in her home. Our front desk team comprised wonderful young women who had grown up in the community and had only a high school education. They were part of the extended families of many of our patients. The conversation might happen something like this (in Spanish, but translated here):

Lupe: *How did it go?*
Señora Sanchez: *He doesn't like my sugars. He thinks bad things are going to happen to me. He makes me afraid they will happen. I pray it will be okay.*
Lupe: *What did he say you should do?*
Señora Sanchez: *He said I should take this new pill* [shows the prescription].

Now Lupe does *not* say that she has seen the evidence and agrees that glycemic control is essential for preventing blindness and kidney failure. She does not cite a meta-analysis showing that the new pill is better than the alternative pills. What she could say to be helpful might be something like this:

Lupe: *Maybe you should try the new pill. He's a good doctor.*

In that moment, if I had earned it, Lupe could do something incredibly valuable. She could transfer a small piece of her relational trust to me. If she was speaking of our seasoned and much-loved nurse practitioner, Lupe might say this:

Lupe: *Maybe you should try the new pill. She's a good person.*

If I can't be trusted, at least I can build a team that has trust. I can be trust-adjacent. These were the core values. *Familismo. Personalismo. Respeto. Confianza.*

Personal, relational trust.

In a Hastings Center Report, Laura Specker Sullivan says this: "For those who have faced exploitation and discrimination at the hands of physicians, . . . and medical institutions, trust is a tall order and, in many cases, would be naïve."[24]

Therefore, our task is not just to "get patients to trust us" but to become trustable. In Sullivan's words, we face the daunting task of "establishing trust in an unjust environment."[25] This is a key point. If we frame this as a problem of Black or African American mistrust,[26] we are getting it wrong. The problem is the white failure to be trustworthy, played out over centuries. It gets repeated in health care settings and communities every day. White untrustworthiness breeds Black mistrust. The Association of American Medical Colleges recently released its 10 "Principles of Trustworthiness" to guide community engagement.[27] They tell us to stop trying to educate the community. In fact, their Principle 1 is this—"The community is already educated; that's why it doesn't trust you."

We begin to make progress when we are willing to do the hard work of dismantling the untrustworthiness of historically white institutions and white people. I earn trust when I honestly acknowledge a historic pattern of abuse and bias that is still present.[28] I earn trust when I see things through the eyes of minoritized patients and colleagues. I earn trust when I acknowledge (and repent of) my own easy acceptance of white privilege. I have to own the fact that I still benefit from systems that favor me. I earn trust when I seek to change my own implicit and explicit biases and prejudice. I earn trust when I find my voice and overcome my own silence in the face of inequity.

If I'm just a white guy trying to avoid race and treat each patient as a unique individual, then I am discounting others' racialized experience. I am pretending that race doesn't matter, while they experience the abuse of racism every day. And if my health care system is producing racially unequal outcomes, I need to own it.

Either it has structures and processes that bias those outcomes, or else somehow the victims are to blame for all the inequalities they experience.

Individual "cultural competency" is not enough. We must diagnose and fix the brokenness. Can you say the word? Racism? Can you say it out loud in front of your peers or your leadership? If not, can you at least have practical, strategic, and tactical discussions about actions to eliminate bias and discrimination? Can you strategize on how to reverse power/resource inequities and health outcome disparities? Can you make a long-term commitment to actively engage in antiracism action? If not, why should people on the receiving end of racial inequities trust you?

How do patients experience racism in our clinic or hospital? Ask them but be ready to act on what you hear. Have the right person ask them, in a setting where it is safe to express true feelings, including pain and rage. Dig into the hard and marathon work of undoing racism in your organization or practice. What would it take to achieve perfect equality of outcomes across all racial/ethnic/gender and socioeconomic strata of patients? What would it take to achieve vertically proportionate diversity, with minorities oversampled in positions of leadership and power and budget authority? The days when organizations can just hire a VP for Diversity are long past.

Can we teach doctors and nurses and health care executives to do better? The jury is still out. In one review of interventions designed to enhance patient trust, researchers found no effect.[29] Clearly, short-term cultural competence workshops are not enough. We might raise awareness, but building trust requires a deep soul commitment to being trustworthy. It means acknowledging racism and injustice while using your privilege to confront the root causes of inequity.

In the first year of the COVID pandemic, we saw a heavy impact in communities of color. Black and Latine people were dying disproportionately from the virus. There was unequal uptake of the vaccine. Pundits labeled it as "vaccine hesitancy" in the Black community. They acknowledged other reasons for vaccine disparities, such as lack of access, complex computer-based sign-ups, and lack of culturally relevant information. But somehow it always came back to mistrust.

In an article titled "You Don't Trust a Government Vaccine," researchers found that African American participants doubted the motives of government officials.[30] Among the marginalized, mistrust related to lifesaving vaccines or treatment was prevalent. A study of over a hundred HIV-positive Black Americans found that 97 percent had "at least one general COVID-19 mistrust belief, and more than half endorsed at least one COVID-19 vaccine or treatment hesitancy belief."[31] The emergence of new, recently experimental vaccines borne out of rapid-paced research was especially problematic. In a survey about medical research, African American individuals were more likely to believe that their physicians would expose them to unnecessary risks.[32]

I was discussing this with a very progressive white colleague of mine when he said, *"Oh I get it. I know about Tuskegee."* As if that explained it. In the 1950s, syphilis was still a leading cause of death in the United States. What we now know as the Tuskegee experiment kept Black US citizens from being treated with a simple penicillin shot. Instead, they were followed for decades to document what we already knew about the various disabling and deadly long-term complications of the disease.[33]

Dr. Vanessa Northington Gamble acknowledges that the US Public Health Service Syphilis Study "continues to cast its long shadow." Even so, she reminds us that this was only one event in a continuing pattern and practice of untrustworthy behaviors by white institutions, clinicians, and researchers. Dr. Gamble tells us not to treat the Tuskegee Syphilis Study "as the singular reason behind African-American distrust of the institutions of medicine and public health."[34]

Tuskegee is just one piece of the puzzle.[35] At the grassroots level, you take all of that history. Think of grandparents who went to segregated hospitals or who died because the white doctors wouldn't treat them. In 1943, when David Satcher was two years old, he nearly died from whooping cough. Local doctors and hospitals would not care for him in segregated Anniston, Alabama, except for the one local Black physician. Satcher's father convinced the doctor to walk several miles to their home to treat young David, who survived to become our 16th US Surgeon General.

Almost every family of color in America could tell such a story. And then they can build on that story with whatever racist experience of mistreatment or disrespect that someone in the family experienced "just last week." If Tuskegee never happened, there would still be a plethora of reasons for every Black family in America to mistrust the medical profession and its institutions.

Trust is crucial in other domains as well. In 2023, we had an outbreak of monkeypox (now called MPox) in the United States. I saw more than a handful of cases myself. It was a scary disease. Patients presented with a smallpox blistering type of rash. There were exquisitely painful lesions in the mouth or throat or the rectum. We wanted to reach out to the group most at risk at that moment, which was men who had sex with men. But we didn't want to create stigma. We couldn't give the public a reason to target the gay community again.

We relied on trust. Our HIV team members had earned trust in the LGBTQ community. They spoke with trusted community voices, who in turn spread the word to people who trusted them. And soon, dozens of men were coming in and getting the MPox vaccine. The outbreak soon played itself out. The epidemic self-extinguished.

Trust issues also play out in organizational dynamics, especially in building community partnerships. Over the years, I have often seen universities get multimillion-dollar grants. They plan interventions "to improve the community's health" without first asking the community what they would want. They never ask the community how they would build the program or, God forbid, how they would spend the money. In the end, universities build their research portfolio, academic researchers build their careers, and the community never sees a dime. Too often, nothing in the community's health improves. And when the three-year grant is done, *Poof!* The researchers disappear. Their concern for the community vanishes like ashes in the wind, leaving only a bad taste.

The AAMC Principles of Trustworthiness put it this way: "Mistrust is a rational response to actual injustice. The community knows what it doesn't know and will ask when it thinks you have answers it can trust."[36] Thankfully, there are research scholars who have been doing it right for decades. Colleagues at Morehouse School of Medicine worked with community leaders in specific Atlanta neighborhoods to build the Prevention Research Center. They started by listening. They spent a year facilitating community conversations to understand and codify community values with regard to research. These were summarized in a statement of core values.[37] They established a community board that had the power to define and even veto research projects that affected their community. Together, they lived the principle of "doing with," not "doing for." They built trust. Now on a foundation of trust, they are working together to improve community health outcomes.

I spent some years with other good people trying to build organizational trust between Atlanta's community health centers, county public health departments, mental health programs, homeless clinics, and our urban public hospital system. It was a group we called the Atlanta Community Access Coalition (ACAC).

Morehouse was a trusted partner in this process, while the more resource-rich, historically white medical school was not.

All these agencies were trying to accomplish a heroic mission, with dramatically less resources than we needed to do the job. We routinely competed with each other for grant funding. I learned metaphors for people fighting over crumbs in the prison yard. I learned the term "crabs in a bucket," describing the instinct to pull another individual or agency down if they seemed to be getting out of this mess while we were not.

The public hospital had also burned some trust years before when they had squeezed the community partners out of a managed care deal. We spent at least seven years doing the equivalent of family therapy in that coalition just to rebuild some measure of trust. Eventually, we built meaningful cooperation in the pursuit of having a collective impact. There's an old saying that *"trust takes years to build, seconds to break and forever to repair."* It sure felt like forever.

Within a non-white (i.e., 21st-century) institution, trust is not automatic. The instinct to distrust is reinforced by harsh racial realities every day. So how can a white guy earn trust in a non-white world? Trust is earned every day in the interactions that show respect or disrespect. Trust is earned in learning to offer that respect in the form and manner in which each person receives respect. These may be quite different from the ways in which I would feel respected. And when trust is given before we've earned it, we must honor that gift as an act of grace.

Trust is earned by not seeking control. Trust is earned in nurturing others for leadership to give away power. One practical way in which we earn trust is in seeking the advancement of others before ourselves. Some of my career accomplishments of which I am proudest are not my accomplishments at all. Colleagues who started as administrative assistants are now program directors of million-dollar programs. Individuals who had not completed college earned bachelor's degrees and then master's degrees. One brilliant leader of one of our multistate programs began to believe again in her own intellectual capacity. Our team gave her support and encouragement and flexibility in her work schedule. She dug in and worked over many years to finally complete her PhD degree. At the same time, she worked full-time to expand our programs.

Many years ago, we saw great talent in a woman who was relegated to a staff-level position copy editing grant proposals. She would fix all my misplaced commas. It was an underuse of her gifts. We asked her to help in our scholarly writing workshops for faculty development. She was good. We gave her encouragement and very specific praise, and she blossomed. She began to teach scientific writing in a master's degree program and then to teach medical students. She is now a valued member of the faculty. At least once a year I get a note from her thanking me for helping *her* to see her own potential. These are her accomplishments, but she still lets me think I played a supporting role.

What does it take? How can leaders create such a culture? Care about people's needs. Ask about their vision for their own future. *"What would you like to be doing in five years? How can we help you get there?"* Flex their work schedules. Find resources (I used my speaking fees) to support their tuition needs. Offer encouragement. Give support. Nurture. Love.

People give you their trust when they see a consistent pattern in your words and your actions and your leadership decisions. Show that you care more about their well-being and advancement than you do your own. Measure your success by how well you have helped your team members achieve their own success. Even non-white institutions will give you their trust when they see that you care more about accomplishing their mission than you do about achieving your own success. When that mission includes racial equity, it means that you care more about being an ally they can count on in a fight than you care about defending white-world.

In reflecting on my decades at Morehouse, I realized that, despite many missteps and stumbles, I did indeed gain some trust. Some was earned, and some was given by grace. The "why should I trust you" moments eventually became quite rare.

In retrospect, I am truly amazed at how generous my institutional leaders were with me. They trusted me with various leadership positions. They trusted me to manage large programs and people and budgets. They trusted me to represent the school in our interactions with other institutions. In presenting the Georgia Health Disparities report in media appearances and in town-hall meetings across Georgia, they trusted me to speak for health justice. They trusted me to tear the bandage off the raw sore of ongoing health inequities.

Dr. Louis Sullivan, former Health and Human Services (HHS) secretary and founding president of our medical school, ultimately trusted me with leading the development of the National Center for Primary Care. He called it the crown jewel of the Morehouse School of Medicine. Dr. David Satcher trusted me first to be his deputy director and then again to resume leadership of the Center. I hold him in my heart as a source of inspiration and mentoring and friendship that I treasure to this day. When I left the institution, both Dr. Satcher and Dr. Sullivan each personally donated $10,000 to a research endowment in my name.

George MacDonald said that "to be trusted is a greater compliment than being loved."[38] I know that feeling now. In the end, our leaders and my colleagues did trust me. They trusted me partly because they were generous in their trust and partly because I had a passion for helping our school build out its vision. I was an ally, however imperfect, in the fight for health justice. And I was pretty consistent for nearly a quarter-century in being a white guy who knew how to give away formal authority, titles, and control. At least for one historically Black institution's leaders, I had answered the question—*why should I trust you?*

Give away power. Build others up. Fight the good fight together. Trust will come. And in the end, you'll have gained more than you ever gave up.

FOR FURTHER READING

Association of American Medical Colleges (AAMC). *Principles of Trustworthiness.*

Covey SMR. *The Speed of Trust.*

Gould SD. Trust, distrust, and trustworthiness. *J Gen Intern Med.* 2002;17(1):79–81.

Myers JR, Baird K, Jara J. *Trust Me: Discovering Trust in a Culture of Distrust.*

Sullivan LS. Trust, risk, and race in American medicine. *Hastings Center Report.* 2020;50(1):18–26.

8.

Respect and Disrespect

Walking down the hallway to my office in the Morehouse Family Practice Center, I often passed a postal worker delivering our mail. I was typically in a hurry, filled with multitasking thoughts. I would sometimes brush past without acknowledging the man. "Good afternoon," he said one day, pointedly leaning toward me. Something in the way he said it made me pay attention. I had screwed up. He might as well have been wearing the *"I am a Man"* signboard that Black protesters carried during civil rights demonstrations in the 1960s.

White guys would never say that. We've never worried about not being counted as human, or fully a man. We never considered the possibility that we were not already "somebodies." We were never subjected to generations of racial dehumanization designed to internalize a sense of being "less than."

For this postal worker, being treated as invisible or as not-somebody touched a nerve. Somehow, I sensed that I was dancing at the edge of a man's pool of frustration. It took all the self-discipline he could muster to express it as a simple, pointed *"Good afternoon."* The subtext was clear. *"Do not ignore me. Respect me. I am a man."* Lesson learned.

The first and most basic act of respect is to acknowledge each individual as a human being. Growing up, I had learned not to acknowledge people that I didn't know. Perhaps it was white fear. Maybe it was being taught not to make eye contact with people that you don't know. Maybe somehow my cultural roots included vestiges of that old British aristocratic model I see now on PBS. They had a way of treating the downstairs servants as if they were valued only in the context of their service. The lords and ladies behaved as if servants were invisible, a part of the machinery of privileged life.

Ralph Ellison says it this way: "I am an invisible man. . . . I am a man of substance, of flesh and bone, fiber and liquids—and I might even be said to possess a mind. I am invisible, understand, simply because people refuse to see me."[1]

This was not his problem. It was mine. He was not being overly sensitive. He was calling out my inhumanity. His invisibility was not a problem of his skin color but in my capacity to see him. Says Ellison, "That invisibility to which I refer occurs because of a peculiar disposition of the eyes of those with whom I come in contact. A matter of the construction of their inner eye."[2]

In the 1990s, I would enter our one small building at Morehouse School of Medicine from the gravel parking lot. I would walk past our school's one receptionist. She was a woman of great dignity. She sat almost completely hidden in a sunken workspace behind a large reception desk. I walked by the first time without even seeing her. *"Good morning, doc!"* she called out pointedly. *Uh oh*. I was making the same mistake I had made with the postal worker. A peculiar disposition of my inner eyes indeed.

For the next two decades, any time I entered through that hallway, the race was on for me to say, *"Good morning, Ms. Strothers"* before she could say, *"Good morning, doc!"* She was a person. We acknowledge our fellow humans, no matter their roles. She had a name. She was not a first-name friend or someone of first-name low status in this historically Black institution. She would call me Doc. And I would call her Ms. Strothers. Respect.

New York Times writer Lena Williams wrote an honest and practical book called *It's the Little Things: Everyday Interactions That Anger, Annoy, and Divide the Races.* In it, she catalogs a variety of behaviors that seem simple on the surface. Still, they tap into deep-seated feelings of disrespect, dehumanization, anger, and resentment. In a preface to the book, civil rights pioneer and journalist Charlayne Hunter-Gault cites the cultural norm of white persons automatically assuming familiarity.[3] We shift to familiar names before asking permission, or we never use honorifics at all.

She tied her feelings of being disrespected to her experience watching her parents being called by their first name. She cited the long and painful history of white families using only the first names of the individuals they hire as maids, or nannies, or groundskeepers. In these settings, it often seemed that white people had no idea what the Black employee's last name was. Even though the employer might be called Mr. or Mrs., the employee was called by first name as if a child, or a servant, or someone less than fully human.

Dr. King wrote with great emotion about this in his letter from the Birmingham Jail:

> When you have seen vicious mobs lynch your mothers and fathers at will . . . when you have seen hate filled policemen curse, kick and even kill your Black brothers and sisters; . . . when you are humiliated day in and day out by nagging signs reading "white" and "colored"; when your first name becomes "nigger," your middle

name becomes "boy" (however old you are) and your last name becomes "John," and your wife and mother are never given the respected title "Mrs."; . . . when you are forever fighting a degenerating sense of "nobodiness"—then you will understand why we find it difficult to wait.[4]

I begin to understand when I acknowledge a very deeply held core value in the African American community, that all persons are worthy of respect. It must be demonstrated in all encounters. If I fail to actively demonstrate respect, it will be received as an intentional act of disrespect. It doesn't matter how I learned to give respect or how I personally prefer to receive it. It doesn't matter what my intentions are. True respect is demonstrated in the manner in which the other person receives or perceives respect.

If I like to call people by their first names, because it seems friendly and open and egalitarian, then I will continue to disrespect people who only feel respected when I call them by their title. Never mind that I didn't mean it as disrespect. Never mind that proper titles seem too formal to my sensibilities. Never mind that to react in such a way in my white growing-up world would have been seen as being overly sensitive or insecure. Show respect.

A survey by the California Endowment found that this one word—*respect*—described what a diverse sample of Californians said was missing from their encounters with the health care system. They specifically called out health professionals. In a similar vein, the National Health Interview Survey asked individuals, "Do you feel listened to by your provider? Does your provider respect your values and wishes regarding healthcare?" Not surprisingly, there were significant racial-ethnic differences in the proportion of individuals who did not feel listened to or respected.

The negative word is "disrespect." On the internet, there are ongoing arguments among white people about whether or not the word "disrespect" is even a real word. We argue about whether it is grammatically correct when used as a verb. That argument never happens among people of color. People in majority culture (white folks) often have little experience with the feeling of being disrespected. Although any of us can experience acts of rudeness or being discounted, what we lack is the generations and centuries of efforts to dehumanize us as a race.

It was critical in the justification of slavery to create the concept of a Black race and then to subhumanize it and dehumanize it, until it was somehow okay to treat Black people as property like farm animals. Every moment of being treated as "less than" taps into that generational pool of frustration and outrage and insecurity and anger of being dehumanized. Disrespect.

I cannot know what that feels like. White folks in America have a very different understanding and expression of respect. Meeting new people, especially in diverse settings, I am eager to make friends. As one colleague put it, my immediate goal is to seek shallow intimacy. I don't worry about respect, because I've never known the kind of disrespect that taps into the dark bile of feeling dehumanized. *"I'm George,"* I say. Instant first names. Smiling, I reach out and shake your hand, maybe even patting your upper arm or clapping you on the back. I want you to know I'm friendly and that I'm not hung up on titles or status. I democratize the encounter in my egalitarian instincts by calling everyone, including myself, by first name.

It's not that way in other cultures or other countries. It's certainly not that way in the African American community or historically Black institutions. When I attend meetings between folks from my historically white FSU and colleagues from historically Black Florida A&M University, I expect a culture clash. FAMU colleagues instinctively call me Dr. Rust. They use honorifics in addressing each other as well, even if they are close friends. People who have known each other for 20 years will still refer to each other in a group meeting as Dr. Harris or Mr. West.

FSU colleagues instinctively revert to first names, for themselves and for people they are just meeting. They are showing their aw-shucks humility in not being hung up on their own titles. Unconsciously, they are white-norming every conversation. They have no intention of disrespecting their colleagues or community stakeholders. But they do. Even when they promise not to.

Sometimes the disrespect is intentional. In North Carolina, a zoning commissioner persistently called a public health professional by Mrs., rather than Doctor or Professor. It was during a zoning meeting, even after she had corrected another commissioner a few minutes earlier. When corrected, he defended himself and refused to call her by her title. People of color, and women in particular, report that such disrespect for their accomplishments is a common experience.[5]

When I was growing up, respect was an attribute we reserved for individuals of high esteem. Respect could be given to an elder, a teacher, or a leader. I was not taught that it was something owed to every human being. I was not taught that it would cause offense if respect was not communicated from the first greeting. I might have heard the word "disrespect" growing up, but only in the context of a smart-alecky teenager like me showing disrespect for a teacher or person in authority.

I certainly did not worry about respect, because I had never really experienced oppression. There had been no systematic effort to treat me as less than human. There was no effort to actively strip me of my dignity. I did not recognize my freedom from these experiences as privilege. I never really thought about it. My struggles were just "normal" growing-up struggles. I was a very short, skinny kid with thick glasses and braces who was an easy target for bullies. My only defense was a smart mouth and sharp tongue. I know now that my two Black friends in high school not only experienced our shared growing-up struggles but also had pain and psychological trauma from daily experiences of racism. They knew what disrespect was, but it would be years before I began to learn.

Later, as I saw patients at Cook County Hospital, I first heard the word "disrespect" used as a verb. In this urban public hospital's emergency room, we would see young men with injuries from fists, or knives, or gunshots. If we saw an x-ray with multiple bullets, we would ask, *"Which bullets are the new ones?"* The story would be told like this—*"Who shot you? (hit you/stabbed you)? Some guy. Why? I shot (hit/stabbed) his cousin. Why? He disrespected me."*

What??? It was beyond my small-world white experience. How could a seemingly small slight, an act of disrespect, a feeling of being disrespected, lead to a physical fight, let alone a knifing or a shooting? And yet it happened every day. Now in Tallahassee and nearby Gadsden County, some teens are carrying Glocks or Mac-10s. Disrespect can be deadly.

How does a white person understand this deep sensitivity and instinct to fight triggered by seemingly small perceived acts of being disrespected? Star athlete turned college football coach Deion Sanders once walked out of a press conference because a reporter addressed him by his first name. *"You don't call Coach Saban 'Nick,'"* he said. He was demanding respect. The white reporter was baffled. *"I call everyone by their first name during interviews."* Clueless. Looking at the world through his norms, it didn't make sense.

In the movie *Respect*, Jennifer Hudson plays Aretha Franklin. She finds her voice and demands the respect that she sings of in her hit title song. Over time, she begins to assert herself in controlling her own career. "I want to sing what I want to sing," she says. A white studio executive replies, "You can sing whatever you want, Aretha." She responds assertively, "I'd like you to address me as Ms. Franklin." It's a basic starting point, but it's tied to issues of power and control. "R-E-S-P-E-C-T . . . Find out what it means to me," she sings. The intersectionality of being a Black woman in that time also worked against being shown respect. Those of us who grew up with one way of understanding and expressing respect in our white bubble need to learn what respect means across a wide range of non-white worlds. Because we didn't learn it growing up.

In the movie *In the Heat of the Night*, actor Sidney Poitier plays a big-city detective who moves to the segregated community of Sparta, Mississippi. He is subjected to repeated racial insults and all forms of disrespect. The sheriff gets angry and insecure when the detective articulates a more sophisticated analysis of a crime than he expected. The sheriff picks on his name. "Virgil? That's a pretty funny name for a *colored boy* from Philadelphia. What do they call you there?" The detective is exasperated by these dehumanizing insults. He has reached his limit, and he delivers this classic line—"They call me, MR. TIBBS!!!"

Individual and cultural groups that have experienced dehumanization place a much higher priority on being treated with respect. In a non-white world, respect comes first. Respect is fundamental to beginning and maintaining any relationship. Earning trust can come second, and only much later can friendship or a personal relationship develop. Continuing to not show respect just because doing so is not my cultural norm is insulting. When my colleague or friend keeps up their mask and does not reveal their hurt or anger, I won't even know what I've done. This can lead to broken friendships or to catastrophic failure in business negotiations.

Here's an example. At Morehouse School of Medicine, I was fortunate to be immersed in an institutional culture of showing respect. The norm in meetings and hallway conversations was to call people by their titles and last names. There were rare exceptions—people I came to know and love as colleagues and friends and even family. With such individuals, in one-on-one conversations, we would often use first names with great fondness. At the same time, the moment we walked into a meeting together or entered the clinic or the classroom, I became Dr. Rust. My friends instantly became Dr. Mack or Dr. Strothers or Ms. Cobb or Ms. Walston.

I once asked a fellow clinician to *"please call me George."* She said in response, *"Dr. Rust, if I did that, my grandmother would rise out of her grave just to straighten me out."* I'm still working on my fishing buddy to call me George or Doc, but his upbringing won't allow it. It makes him uncomfortable if I push it. *"I'm out fishing with Dr. Rust,"* he'll say on the phone to his wife. And she'll say, *"Hey, Dr. Rust."* Week after week, year after year, that's how it's been. I suspect that's how it will always be.

At Morehouse, I also had the honor of working with leaders who were held in the highest esteem, even beyond the norm of universal respect. One was former HHS Secretary Dr. Louis Sullivan, founding president of the school. Dr. Sullivan had returned to Morehouse School of Medicine from Washington and was serving again as its president. No one in our institution (except his older brother) ever referred to him as anything other than Dr. Sullivan.

One day Dr. Sullivan led a number of us to a meeting at a local community hospital. We were pursuing a mutually beneficial affiliation agreement. The hospital leaders had thoughtfully (in their minds) prepared name tags for each of the attendees. Their organizational culture was to call everyone from front desk clerk to CEO by first names, as a way of leveling the hierarchy. None of their leaders recognized that this was a very white thing to do. (The way to level the hierarchy in a non-white world is to use formal names and titles for all.)

We each went to the table and politely picked up our nametags. I found mine—"*George.*" I saw Dr. Sullivan pick up his nametag—"*Lou.*" He never showed a hint of emotion and gamely wore the nametag. A few of my colleagues gave me sidelong glances when he picked it up, but no one said anything or gave a hint of emotion. The "living in white-world" masks were up. Dr. Sullivan described our institution's desire for an affiliation agreement, shook hands heartily, and laughed easily. Only because I had come to know him over many years did I see his mask. It was his public face. His inner thoughts and feelings would not be revealed.

The whole meeting was polite and yet reserved. This one behavior can call up deep feelings of resentment, but they are often masked so that the white person will never see it. Everyone from our Morehouse team held back. No agreements were made. The affiliation agreement would take years to finally come to fruition. And no one from the hospital's white leadership team had any idea what had just happened.

After the meeting, I was walking to my car with one of my more reserved colleagues. He was a physician about my age who had already accomplished much in medicine and in leadership. Rather spontaneously, he started to tell me a story. "*When I was a child,*" he said, "*I had asthma. The doctor who treated me practiced at Georgia Baptist Hospital. One day, I had a bad asthma attack, and my mother took me to the hospital to see him. In her rush, my mother took me into the hospital through the whites-only entrance. We saw my doctor and approached him in the hallway. He gave a nervous look and walked us back outside. He walked us around to the colored entrance. He told us, 'I wouldn't want you to get in trouble.'*"

My colleague never said why he suddenly felt the urge to tell me this story, but it was clearly connected to the moment. This first-names-only meeting had just called up an early memory of being treated as less than human because he was Black. He had been triggered. And every African American colleague in that room had their own story to tell. They all had experienced the indignity of being treated as less than human because of the color of their skin. And these white leaders of a local hospital, with all good intentions and with hopes of building an institutional relationship, had just blown it. They had called up deep pain and hurt and shame and anger, without ever knowing that they had done so. And I suspect that they do not know even to this day.

This is deeply engrained from childhood. Jennifer Rittenhouse has written a book titled *Growing Up Jim Crow: How Black and White Southern Children Learned Race*. She wrote about how children were taught all the unwritten but harshly enforced rules of social interaction.[6] Said historian Ronald Davis, "The whole intent of Jim Crow etiquette boiled down to one simple rule: Blacks must demonstrate their inferiority to whites by actions, words, and manners."[7]

Glasgow has suggested that disrespect is the unifying theme around which all racism can be understood.[8] Racial discrimination in lending and homeowner's insurance is a historically explicit disrespect for racialized groups of color. He even considers our nation's colonial history of nearly exterminating native peoples in America as disrespect (i.e., seeing American Indians as not fully persons, not fully worthy of respect). He concludes that disrespect toward racialized groups is the core common element of all racism. One could modify racialized to marginalized to include LGBTQ persons and all other societally disenfranchised groups.

Glasgow also cites disrespect as the underlying theme of gender bias. For example, he connects anti-reproductive rights laws to disrespect for women. Sadly, being a woman of any race in medicine is a risk factor for being disrespected, even today. A survey of NIH-funded researchers found this—"High rates of sexual harassment, cyber incivility, and negative organizational climate exist in academic medicine, disproportionately affecting minoritized groups."[9] An accompanying editorial was titled "Disrespectful Conduct in the Medical Profession: We Have Met the Enemy and They Are Us."[10] A survey of more than 2,000 cardiologists found gender discrimination to be nearly universal (reported by 98 percent of women).[11]

In meetings, women and persons of color often feel disrespected when their ideas are not given serious weight. Sometimes a white guy will then offer nearly the same idea, and the group may act as if it's a brilliant new thought. Former Australian foreign secretary Julie Bishop said, "If you're the only female voice in the room, [men] just don't seem to hear you." She referred to it as "gender deafness."[12]

Deborah Tannen writes about male and female styles of communication as being almost cross-cultural in nature. One specific attribute of a more female style of speaking is to raise the voice at the end of a sentence. To my ears, it sounds similar to a question. In a boardroom with a male-dominant style of communication, this is interpreted as uncertainty. So the comment may be given less weight. In this moment, the woman is being disrespected. The modulation of the voice at the end of the sentence doesn't mean what most men think it means.

Another common scenario is that a woman in leadership comes into a meeting expecting what she would define as polite, respectful communication. The men behave differently. She finds herself not getting a word in edgewise. They interrupt each other constantly. Seeing that the meeting is wrapping up, the woman is forced outside of her comfort zone. *"I'd like to offer a thought,"* she says politely. But the men thought the meeting was over. They roll their eyes. *"All right,"* says the chair*man* paternalistically. *"Is there something else?"* At this point, there is virtually no chance the woman will be heard.

All of these examples underscore the importance of a concept too often trivialized by majority culture (i.e., the centrality of disrespect). Attitudes and actions of disrespect are the generic expression of saying the n-word in racialized communities. It's like a punch in the face. It's the calling up of all the insults and aggressions and stereotyping and dehumanizing treatment as "less-than" that a person has ever experienced in their life. Each further experience of disrespect calls up all that has gone before. The pools of anger and shame and oppression have collected over time to create that last nerve that I just stepped on, whether I meant to or not. *Damn, I'm sorry.*

One group of researchers has created and validated a Racial Respect Scale for Adult African Americans.[13] It really measures disrespect, often tied to daily activities. As an example, the societal subscale asked people to agree or disagree with statements like these: *"When I am at the bank or other places of business, people are helpful and pleasant toward me,"* or *"African Americans are highly regarded in America."* As a white guy, I assume that people at least should be helpful and pleasant toward me when I am their customer. That's the opposite of experiencing daily expressions of disrespect. I assume respect, and I usually get it. That's privilege. Damn.

In our next section, we focus on skills to learn and practice. We can learn how to be intentional about showing respect as the first priority in all our interactions. We can replace microaggressions with micro-validations. We can pay special attention to our interactions with individuals from racialized or other marginalized groups. We will also explore differences in cultural norms where an action or behavior or language might mean a show of respect in one culture while actively offending or showing disrespect in another. We want to avoid unintentional displays of disrespect. We want to be intentional about showing respect in culturally specific ways that will actually be received as respect.

Let's do that.

FOR FURTHER READING

Douglas PS. Disrespectful conduct in the medical profession: we have met the enemy and they are us. *JAMA*. 2023;329(21):1829–1831.

Ellison R. *Invisible Man*.

King ML Jr. "Letter from a Birmingham Jail."

Ritterhouse J. *Growing Up Jim Crow: How Black and White Southern Children Learned Race*.

Scott K. *Radical Respect*.

SKILLS

9.

Consider Culture and Show Respect

I still don't know what happened to that old woman or to her donkey.

It was our first trip out of the country. Cindy and I were doing a five-week global health rotation in Haiti. It was a medical adventure in a country with a rich culture and a tragic history. We spoke little of the language. *M pa pale Kreol* (I don't speak Creole) was the most useful phrase we knew.

At one point, we were on a public bus in the living contradiction that is Port-au-Prince. It was crowded and noisy. Cars and chickens, buses and donkeys, and trucks and ox carts were all bumping for space in the same rugged street. I took a picture of the statue of Neg Mawon, the runaway slave with legs and wrists shackled but chains broken. He was blowing a conch shell to start the first successful slave rebellion in 1791. In the background is the Presidential Palace, home at that time to the ruthless dictator Baby Doc Duvalier. His violent repression was exceeded only by that of his father (Papa Doc), who had built the heavily armed secret militia known as the *Tonton Macoute*. Hopes of freedom, realities of oppression. Contradictions all around.

I fancied myself an amateur photographer at the time. I was constantly framing images as we traveled. I looked out the window of our bus and saw the perfect picture coming into frame. There was an old, almost-ancient woman. She was riding side-saddle on a donkey with a colorful blanket against the backdrop of a brightly colored Caribbean blue wall. I leaned out the window manually focusing my Canon SLR and telephoto lens. Suddenly she looked at me and saw the camera. She let out a quick scream and jumped off the donkey. She ran faster than I ever thought this old woman could. The donkey ambled off in the opposite direction.

What the heck? What had I done? Later, friends who had lived in Haiti for decades tried to explain. *"If you had gotten that picture, you would have captured a bit of her soul. You would have had power over her. Understand?"* No, I did not understand. But over time, I would begin to get a hint. They explained using phrases that Americans use, such as *"Haitians are 90 percent Catholic and 100 percent Voodoo."* Haitian colleagues would give more nuanced explanations of *voudon* as not so much a religion as it is life itself. *Voudon* is a way of understanding. It's a way of relating to the physical and spiritual world.

For me to have a physical photo of a person would allow me to have power over them. Americans trivialize this with our notion of "voodoo dolls." We misunderstand the depth of a wholistic spirituality. Doctors in multicultural settings often struggle to understand explanations of illness that involve bad *juju* or *karma* or *mal de ojo* (evil eye). We assume that these are an ethnic vestige of a more primitive culture. But nobody likes to be talked down to. The result of our condescension is that patients may decide not to share what they're really thinking.

My farmworker patients in Groveland would rarely tell me about having been to the *curandera* or a *bruja* for *the magia blanca* before they came to see me. Only after years of trust-building would friends teach me the practice of saying prayers and lighting candles. I learned about rolling an egg over a person to remove the bad spirits (*limpia de huevo*). The egg was placed in a glass under the bed until it grew fungus or roots, proof that the bad spirit had been taken.

As an anthropologist, Zora Neale Hurston studied many communities of the African diaspora. She found similar ways of integrating the physical and spiritual world. This holistic view of spirituality is one of the distinctive features of the Black church in America. Alternatively, we could say that a reductionistic view (separating body, mind, and spirit) is a uniquely white European American or Greco-Roman understanding of the world.

All this came back to me years later when we were beginning to confront the AIDS epidemic in Florida. Haitian people were subjected to intense discrimination in our state. The CDC had labeled "being Haitian" as a risk factor for HIV. We did not yet have effective drugs. Testing and education were our primary public health tools. At the same time, testing positive for HIV could lead to intense stigma and discrimination. In our farmworker clinics, we were blessed to have Haitian outreach workers and nurses. We also had Dr. Lionel Nau, a wonderful family physician who had trained with me at Cook County after a previous life as a national soccer star in Haiti. We spoke about how to approach outreach and testing in our Haitian community.

What would it mean to take blood from a Haitian person and to keep it in our lab? For me to have a piece of you (hair or blood or x-ray) gave me power to do you harm. Did we need to undo that belief by telling people that they were wrong? Or could we instead find a way to not disagree? Could we help people see that having a small bit of their blood would give us power to do good for them? We would honor their trust in us by treating the sample with exquisite care. Only the professionals who had deep cultural knowledge and respect could communicate such a nuanced message. And they did.

America is a multicultural society. Physicians in America serve an increasingly diverse patient population. Many clinical practices serve patients from dozens of different language groups. In our public health clinic the other day, I was doing refugee health assessments through a phone interpreter. The patient looked strangely at the telephone. *"Bad Swahili,"* the woman said, pointing to the phone. Then she pointed to herself holding her hand over her heart. *"Good Swahili,"* she said proudly. Who was I to disagree? So many heterogeneities exist across regions and accents and dialects and cultures. Diversity upon diversities, layer upon layer.

Unfortunately, the diversity of our health professional workforce does not reflect the diversity of the American people. That needs to change. In the meantime, we all must work with humility to increase our own cultural competencies. We must learn to be more effective in communicating with diverse patients, building trust, and negotiating treatment plans.

Try getting an appointment with a Spanish-speaking psychologist in Tallahassee. Would you want to get mental health counseling through a phone interpreter? This is why I am so proud to be affiliated with my FSU colleagues who practice psychology on our Immokalee campus. They are training fluently bicultural and bilingual PhD psychologists. They speak perfect Spanish or Haitian Creole, along with perfect English, in settings that serve a largely immigrant population. Where else in the country can you find that?

Health professionals do not automatically have the attitudes or skills they need to be effective in culturally diverse settings. The CRASH course is a cultural competency training program for health professionals. Our NCPC team at Morehouse School of

Medicine developed it with a large, diverse, multiethnic advisory group. CRASH is a mnemonic for these components of culturally competent health care: consider Culture, show Respect, Assess/ Affirm differences, show Sensitivity and Self-awareness, and do it all with Humility.[1] Learning and practicing these cultural principles will not confer cultural competence, but they can provide skills and strategies for being more effective.

CRASH COURSE IN CULTURAL COMPETENCY SKILLS

Culture: Considering the importance of shared values, perceptions, and connections in the experience of health, health care, and the interaction between patient and professional.

Respect: Finding ways to demonstrate respect in various cultural contexts.

Assess: Understanding that there are tremendous "within-group differences," ask clients to self-describe cultural identity, health preferences, beliefs, and understanding of health conditions while assessing language competency, acculturation level, and health literacy.

Affirm: Reframing cultural differences to affirm each individual as the world's expert on their own experience and identifying the positive values behind behaviors we see as "different."

Sensitivity: Developing an awareness of specific issues within each culture that might cause offense or lead to a breakdown in trust and communication between patient and professional.

Self-Awareness: Becoming aware of our own cultural norms, values, and "hot-button" issues that lead us to misjudge or miscommunicate with others.

Humility: Recognizing that none of us ever fully attains "cultural competence" but instead making a commitment to a lifetime of learning, being quick to apologize and accept responsibility for cultural missteps, and embracing the adventure of learning from others' firsthand accounts of their own experience.

NOTE: The framing of CRASH and its definitions was first published in *Ethnicity and Disease* in 2006; material in this chapter includes material adapted from that first publication.

What is culture? Cultures can represent a racial, ethnic, religious, or social group, a geographic region, or even a profession like medicine. The Core Collaborative cites anthropologist Edward T. Hall's iceberg model of culture, in which only superficial aspects of culture such as clothing, language, and customs are visible. But there are also invisible elements of shallow culture such as unspoken rules and social norms, as well as deeper culture that includes implicit beliefs and world views.[2]

Dr. Satcher says it this way—*culture counts* in health care settings. But the influence and expression of culture will differ for each individual. Several authors promote acronyms or mnemonics to help students to gain cultural competence skills. For example, Berlin and Fowlkes have promoted the acronym LEARN (Listen, Explain, Acknowledge, Recommend, and Negotiate).[3] Steele and Harrison put forward the PEARLS mnemonic (Partnership, Empathy, Apology, Respect, Legitimization, and Support).[4] Kleinman has promoted the model of asking nine essential questions to elicit the patient's own health beliefs and understanding.[5]

Here's just one example of how not addressing cultural dimensions can lead to bad health care. A Muslim patient came to our Morehouse Family Practice Center for prenatal care. Throughout her pregnancy, she had received care from a female physician. When she came to the hospital in active labor, she and her husband found out that the patient's physician was out of town. Only a male on-call physician was available to examine her and to attend her delivery. The patient's husband was adamant that his wife would not be violated this way. A stalemate ensued that was entirely preventable. Prenatal care should have included questions about the patient's values that might affect her birthing care.

No one is "culturally competent" in all dimensions of a culturally diverse community. Still, core values and specific skills can help us be more effective healers in a multicultural world. Cultural competency may require decades of immersion, not just in clinic

Factors That Modify Expression of Core Culture

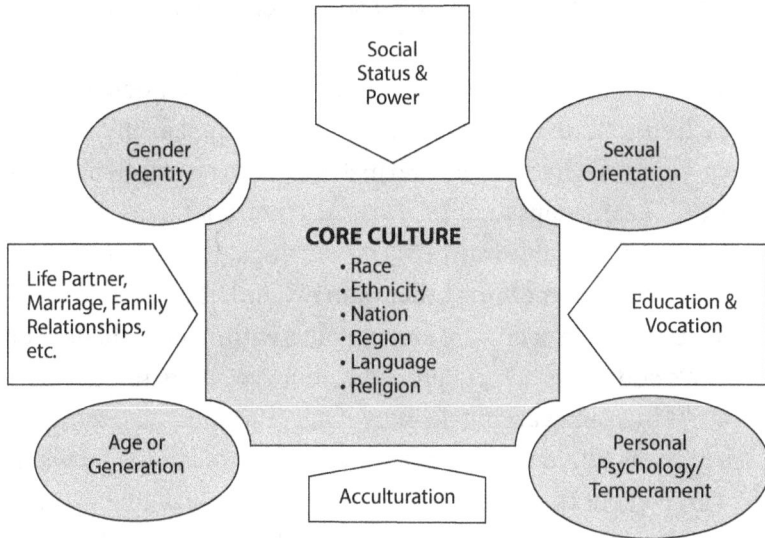

Core culture is expressed differently in each individual and may evolve over time.

but also in community. Even then, we are at best amateurs in another person's culture. A realistic goal for busy clinicians is to learn specific behaviors and habits that will allow us to be more culturally effective. We can also learn to avoid missteps that are culturally offensive or culturally dysfunctional.

Culture starts with core elements that we are born into. These might include race, ethnicity, national origin, geographic region, history, or religion. But this core culture of ours is expressed through individuals. We differ in age, gender, birth order, temperament, and sexuality. I am not the same person as my brother, even though we were born into the same family. We differ in the roles we played. He is the older brother, and I am the younger.

We also have different personalities. In our family, my brother was the confronter of our emotionally broken and sometimes abusive father. My father would say that I played the role of Ensign

Pulver, the character who hid in the shadows. I tried to remain invisible. I avoided conflict at all costs, except when trying to de-escalate family fights.

This is what has evolved in me as chameleon tendencies. I'm hardwired to fade into the background and appear invisible at times. I can walk into a room and instantly feel the emotional temperature. I can adapt to or mirror that emotional tone. This can be very useful in culturally diverse settings, but it's unhealthy when I become something other than my authentic self.

The expression of culture also changes within individuals over time. We add layers of language, education, vocation, family roles, power/status, and varying degrees of acculturation. The refugees I see at the health department speak a variety of languages when they arrive, but their children are learning English and playing video games. Those who came through refugee camps often have birthdays listed as January 1, as if they were all New Year's babies. Ibram X. Kendi describes a similar history of African Americans, "like the enslaved woman who tragically never knew exactly when she was born."[6]

Kids go off to college and learn new perspectives and new ways of being. We may gain new vocational or professional identities. The average medical student comes to our school with a vocabulary of about 30,000 words and leaves with over 100,000 words. At some point, they forget which words are medical words and which words are "real people" words. We have white coat ceremonies as a sacrament of our new professional identity. When people are hurting or dying, we have become in some ways the priests of the 21st century.

The expression of our core culture manifests itself in the relationships we form in friendships and intimacy. We may take on a spouse or life partner. Our sexuality or gender identity may put us in a marginalized group of individuals. We may feel isolated. We cling together for our own protection or sense of self. Ongoing experiences of racism can lead to internalized racial identities, which were not intrinsic to our family upbringing.

How we manage conflict can be another area of difference but also of stereotyping (e.g., assuming that all Asian people approach conflict indirectly to "save face"). Instead, we try to learn a wide range of approaches to conflict found in cultures across the world and then calibrate. To do so, we must be self-aware of how our own cultural norms and personal temperament guide our approach to conflict.

For example, I think of myself as being fairly conflict-averse. Yet, I'm also an American. My instinct is to deal with conflict gently (by American standards), but there are many cultural settings in which I may still seem blunt and overly direct. And because of my American norms, I may not even notice conflict or criticism. The sharing of a breath mint may be another person's polite, indirect, face-saving way of telling me that my breath stinks. Some people disagree so gently, I might miss it. They say no without saying no, perhaps just nodding respectfully. Or they might say, *"I will do my best"* or *"I hope to"* or *"If God wills (or 'In sha' Allah)."*[7]

One thing we often miss is the heterogeneity of people in minoritized groups. I say I'm a white guy, but my mother would describe our heritage as ¾ German, ¼ Swedish, *"and a little pinch of the Irish."* We see all the nuances and details of our own group. We identify by nation of origin, religion, region, and, these days, political alignments. And while we clearly see the granular heterogeneity within our own group, we tend to lump other people into broad-brush categories (Blacks, Hispanics, Asian . . .). I have colleagues who would say, I don't think of myself as Hispanic. I am Peruvian (or Cuban or Chicano or Borinqueña—*"and by the way, we speak the best Spanish"*).

Most of us don't just have one cultural identity. I am a white, cisgender, heterosexual, Caucasian male of mostly German and

Swedish descent. I'm a deeply spiritual but no longer overtly re-ligious Christian. I'm also a family physician, a public health professional, a health equity researcher, and a professor. My fa-vorite roles are as a father, a husband, and, more recently, a proud and happy grandpa. The combination of all of these identities is sometimes summed up in the phrase "intersectionality."

Intersectionality has special meaning when individuals have multiple minoritizing identities. To be a Black woman raises dif-ferent issues than to be a Black man. It's more complicated to ad-dress the intersections of race and gender. To be a Latina trans-gender woman with dark skin from the Dominican Republic creates three-dimensional layers of intersectionality, identity, and often oppression.

One of our challenges is to build organizational cultures and communities that affirm each individual in all of their multi-layered uniqueness. People shouldn't have to "code-switch" their style of speech or follow white dress codes. They shouldn't feel pressure to make their gender identity seem more conform-ing or even to make their hairstyle less Black. Is it any wonder that Michelle Obama only recently began to wear her hair in braids? She wanted to wear braids as First Lady in the White House but felt that the American people "weren't ready for it."[8] A 2019 study revealed that 80 percent of Black women feel like they have to change their natural hair in the workplace.

Too many of our standards are white-normed. A North Caro-lina high school student is a member of the Waccamaw Siouan Tribe of North Carolina. Wearing his hair in a long braid is con-sidered a spiritual tradition that goes back thousands of years. His white Anglo teacher told him it was "faddish." He would have to cut it to meet the school's "grooming standards." Asked by par-ents to explain, a school administrator said, "We want them all to look the same."[9]

For a quarter-century, white people would ask me about my work at Morehouse School of Medicine. *"Are all the students Black?"* And I would answer, *"It's the most diverse institution I know."* Our MD class of 2009 students made a T-shirt to reflect pride in their own diversity. It listed the following identities:

- 55 lives
- 13 cultures, 12 languages
- 1 heart, 1 family

Graduation ceremonies at Morehouse School of Medicine were always special. Being in the MLK Chapel on the campus of Morehouse College was in itself historic. Being in this sanctuary with over a thousand mostly non-white students and families was powerful. Standing there with heroes like Dr. David Satcher and Dr. Louis Sullivan was an honor. Add in a guest speaker like Archbishop Desmond Tutu on the platform singing "Lift Every Voice and Sing" with all of us, and I was transported.

When each student came across the stage to receive their diplomas, Dr. Ngozi Anachabe precisely pronounced each name perfectly, whether African or Asian or Latine or European. Names matter, and she worked hard to get it right. In white-world, many of these names would have seemed strange or difficult to pronounce. But all of our names seem strange somewhere. Family members came on-stage to carefully lift the satin velvet hoods over the students' heads. They straightened them with love followed by hugs.

Family members' outfits reflected the diversity of formal dress across the globe. There were suits and ties, formal dresses and church hats, but also saris and dhotis, kufi caps, and full-length thobes. Hats and sashes of Kente cloth. Starched white guayabera shirts. Madiba shirts and dashikis. Multicolored African royal dresses, gowns, and matching headwraps. Some reflected national or tribal origins, and some were just stylish. Glorious proud pageantry!

Grandparents and parents, some of whom had never even graduated from high school, would be bursting with pride over the child they could now call doctor. Children and sisters stood hugging their single mom. A student in a wheelchair made his way across the stage, greeted by his wife and daughter. And from the crowd came applause and whoops and hollers from family members and friends loving this moment. We were all one together, proud of our graduates and proud to be in community together. My eyes were often moist with tears of joy. I was a white guy who had found his place celebrating Dr. King's beloved community, there in the chapel dedicated to his memory.

Cultural respect does not mean merely tolerating cultures that are different. It's not just respecting cultural differences in the abstract. Respect in the CRASH course model means that each individual has a right to be shown respect in a culturally relevant manner. A certain behavior might be a signal of respect in one culture while actively offending or showing disrespect in another. We must learn to demonstrate our respect to individual patients in ways that each person will receive it or perceive that they are being respected. Showing respect and avoiding disrespect may be the single most important issue for effective physician patient communication and effective community-building.

As a child, I learned the Golden Rule—"do unto others as you would have done unto you." But this assumes that they would want what I would want for myself. So instead, my colleague Dr. Suchak teaches students the Platinum Rule: "Do unto others as *they* would want done unto *themselves*."

When I was growing up, my father was very insistent that my brother and I learn to shake hands properly. *"Firm grip, strong handshake, and look a man in the eye,"* he would say. But what if looking someone directly in the eye is disrespectful and offensive in some cultures? Or, across genders, that it can be experienced as sexual aggression or hostility? Do I continue to show respect as my father taught me? Or do I learn from diverse encounters to show respect in quite different ways, depending on culture and circumstance?

We developed several CRASH course video vignettes with the Association of Black Cardiologists. One was a 90-second video clip of a doctor entering a room and greeting a patient. The scenario opens with an older African American woman being greeted by a young white physician. The physician is smiling as soon as he enters the room. Being friendly, he holds out his hand to reach for the patient's hand. He looks her directly in the eye and cheerfully says, *"Good morning, Bessie. How're ya doin'?"* Ms. Johnson pulls her hand back, not sure how to react. The physician attempts to reassure her, gently patting her on her shoulder. *"Atta-girl,"* he says brightly.

First question: Can you identify at least three things the physician did wrong?

1. Using first name (Bessie) rather than title (Ms. Johnson)
2. Using aggressively direct eye contact
3. Moving quickly into her space and reaching for her hand
4. Touching her shoulder without permission
5. Saying "Atta-girl" to an older African American woman of her generation. She has likely seen parents of great dignity demeaned by white people using the term "girl" to keep them in their place.

Second question: "Did the young doctor intend to offend Ms. Johnson?" Or was he simply making the mistake of trying to build quick rapport in ways that would have worked within his own cultural norms? Good intent cannot overcome bad behavior.

A general rule of thumb in multicultural settings is to make sure that we use the more formal terms of address such as Mr. or

Mrs., Sir or Ma'am, Doña Maria, Deacon Jones, Reverend Wright, and so on. I also use the more formal pronoun *usted* to address Spanish-speaking patients, rather than jumping presumptuously to the informal *tu*. That's different from my own cultural instincts. If you repeatedly call me Doctor Rust, my instinctive response is to feel that you are pushing me away. Why are you distancing yourself? Call me George.

For me, the norms of showing respect across gender identities have shifted significantly during my lifetime. Saying Sir or Ma'am is hardwired into me after growing up as the son of a Naval Reserve officer in the South and spending 25 years at a historically Black institution. In racial context, it's a great way to show respect. On the other hand, some people have gender identities that fall outside of binary male/female norms. To show respect on this axis is to say, *"My pronouns are he/him/his—what are yours?"*

A colleague of mine who has taught me so much in this area identifies as agender or queer. Their pronouns are they/them/theirs. But my brain has gender ruts. I am ashamed to say how many times I have referred to them as "she" when I know better. I get it right when I'm paying attention to showing respect. When I slide into autopilot or multitask, my mouth will move forward before my brain is engaged. I still get it wrong. I apologize. I redouble my efforts to be mindful in each moment. I get it right more often now. I am growing. I am healing.

The need for respect within the clinician–patient context is not limited to culture or race. A recent review found that "most patients, regardless of their racial or ethnic identity, believe that health care personnel do not respect them."[10] Health professionals should learn culture-specific words and behaviors to demonstrate respect for individual patients. What can we do or say to make sure that this patient *feels* respected? How is it different through the filter of *their* past experience, culture, gender, occupation, and generation?

In a multicultural clinical setting, the health professional can ask patients or staff, *"I want to make sure I treat you respectfully. How do people greet an elder in the community you grew up in? How do I make sure that you feel respected in this office?"* Based on the person's response, the clinician could continue. *"Would those be similar issues for other people from your neighborhood? Are there things that our doctors or staff do that might unintentionally make you feel disrespected?"* Having this conversation with a patient begins to establish a level of trust based upon mutual respect. But only if we honor what they tell us.

In many settings, the front desk staff or lower-paid employees are more similar to our patients or clients than are the professional staff. Racially, ethnically, and socioeconomically, they are more expert than we are in the cultural nuances of people we are trying to serve. They also have become fluently bicultural, in the sense that they are also operating effectively in a white-normed organization. They can speak my language and understand my values, even as they speak the patients' language and understand them better than I do.

These are cultural bridge-people. They are my teachers and cultural translators. They can tell me when I'm misunderstanding something and help me understand. They can pull me aside when I may have unintentionally offended a patient. They can coach me on how to better show respect. I need them.

One area of concern comes when people like me from the majority culture try to shape-shift and adapt to minority cultural settings. Done with respect, a certain amount of adaptation (becoming less white) is helpful. But the risk is in stealing other people's cultural identity, without living their reality.

Does showing respect really affect health outcomes, or is it just some foo-foo huggy-touchy-feely stuff? Respect garners trust. It's associated with adherence to meds or getting screening tests for cancer. There is even a quantifiable relationship between disrespect and death. In states where collective disrespect for Blacks is high, the mortality rate for both Blacks and whites is also increased.[11] Disrespect is deadly.

In one culture, a handshake is a sign of respect. In another, bowing at the waist or a gentle dip of the head may be a gesture of respect. A business card offered in outstretched hands with head lowered may be most appropriate. The book *Kiss, Bow, or Shake Hands* offers simplistic checklists of specific, culturally appropriate behaviors for each country of the world.[12] Everywhere you go, it's a little (or a lot) different.

Eye contact is another area in which US medical training assumes that the norms of white Anglo culture are universal. When we teach students how to demonstrate attentive listening to their patients, we often teach that eye contact is essential. When participants in our CRASH course workshops describe a person who will not make eye contact, they often suggest that such persons are dishonest, or hiding something, or perhaps have low self-esteem. But the norms are different in different cultures. In some cultural contexts, eye contact may be considered disrespectful to elders. It may be aggressive or hostile to authority figures. It can even be received as being sexually aggressive.

During my training at Cook County hospital in Chicago, many of my patients had roots in rural Mississippi or Alabama. In Mississippi in the 1930s and 1940s, the simple act of a Black man passing by a white person on a sidewalk could be a moment of danger. To maintain eye contact with a white man was not submissive. It could lead to verbal abuse or a physical beating. If the Black man made prolonged eye contact with a white woman, it might be seen as lustful. The punishment could be death by lynching.

When an African American patient entered our Cook County clinic, they often had a deep and instinctive reflex to avoid prolonged eye contact. Eye contact was uncomfortable and dangerous. Now insert an eager young white medical student, sent into the exam room to interview this patient. The student would try conscientiously to achieve that elusive good eye contact. They wanted desperately to be a good listener. The patient would keep looking away. Sometimes the student would repeatedly move their head, or shift in their seat, or even physically reposition themselves. They were trying to somehow intercept the eye contact. And most of these students had no idea they were doing it, because to maintain eye contact while listening was "normal."

Often professionals think that observing an outward physical behavior like someone avoiding eye contact lets us see into that person's soul. We have a dictionary of cultural norms that is our Rosetta stone for interpreting social responses. The problem is that it's a local dictionary. It's built on narrow experiences in non-diverse settings or in settings that force people of color to live within white-majority cultural norms.

There's a simple solution in the clinic. When I sit with a patient, I try to put our seats at a 45-degree angle to one another. I look at the patient, and they may or may not look at me. We look away. To an observer, it would seem that we're sitting on a front porch, looking out over the field in front of us. I gauge how often the patient is looking at me and how comfortable they are with eye contact. I can reflexively mirror *their norms* around eye contact. In less than a minute and without saying a word, we've both racially and culturally calibrated to one another.

Another aspect of showing respect is that people have different norms around how much personal space they consider their private zone. Disney World had to do extra training for its staff to help them mediate conflicts between German tourists who had a large sense of personal space and Brazilian tourists who stood "too close" in waiting lines.

Some people don't like to be touched, especially if they have experienced physical or sexual trauma in their past. One way to show respect is to always ask permission before touching a patient.

It may seem weird, almost creepy to say, *"May I touch you?"* But there are more subtle ways to accomplish the same thing. *"May I check your pulse?"* I ask, holding out an open hand. This invites the patient to bring their hand toward mine and lay their wrist in my hand. It's subtle and often mutual, but the patient remains in control. I am showing respect.

I also need to learn to show respect in the way I communicate across genders. A male style of communication can include interrupting or finishing another person's sentence. To the interrupting man, it can mean, *"I'm right there with you. I want to build on the cool thing you're saying."* It can also mean, *"I got your point, but I need to disagree. Let's wrestle a bit."* But in many cultures, and for people (of any gender) with a more female-normed style, interrupting is rude and disrespectful.

Years ago, Roger Coleman and I traveled together to do health care management consulting visits for community health centers. Roger is a brilliant white guy, former CEO of a large health care organization, and a guest lecturer at Harvard. When we travel, we stimulate each other intellectually. We share an idea and before it's half out of our mouth, the other person is building on it and taking it to the next level. Then I interrupt and add a new thought and then he interrupts and off we go.

We were doing that in a rental car one day while the director of Georgia's migrant health program was driving us to another rural clinic site. We were talking a mile a minute, back-and-forth. We were finishing each other's sentences about what worked and didn't work in managing underresourced health centers. We interrupted each other constantly. It was awesome!

When we stopped at a traffic light, the program director finally turned and looked at both of us as if we were children. "Do you guys always do this?" she asked with an exasperated tone. *"You're constantly interrupting—it's so rude!"*

"Yeah, I guess we kinda do," we said sheepishly. Roger and I looked at each other and laughed. To us, it wasn't rude at all. She shook her head and turned her eyes back to the road as the light turned green. We could have been from another planet.

When people do this with positive agreement or affirmations, it's what Deborah Tannen calls "cooperative overlapping,"[13] like the amen choir. What Roger and I were doing was constructive or even competitive overlapping. We were actively building together toward a conclusion, in a steel-sharpens-steel style of conversation. In any other setting or in a group with diverse conversational norms, it would indeed be rude.

If we are leading a group or helping to set group norms, white guys like me need to do the shifting. Not interrupting is surely a better norm for obtaining diverse input and achieving effective group cohesion. Listen respectfully. Acknowledge what each person has said. Pace yourself. Don't dominate. Don't interrupt. Look for coherence and seek consensus, not competition.

Many people would say that this is just basic politeness or respectful communication. Until the white-guy norms change, polite people may at moments need to develop sharp elbows and assertive voices to be heard in these settings. As leaders of diverse teams, we may need to shut down the white guys (or others) when they interrupt.

In our Council on Diversity and Inclusion meetings at the College of Medicine, we start meetings by introducing ourselves. We include the pronouns we use for ourselves. Hi, I'm George Rust, he/him/his. For a time, there was an expectation that everyone would address each other by first names. We did this for lots of good reasons (eliminating titles of hierarchy, affirming an egalitarian culture, and not using gender-binary titles like Ms. or Mr.). Since chairing the Council, though, I've blurred those rules a bit.

While they are motivated by the best of intentions, they also are more characteristic of a historically white institution than they would be of a Black-normed institution. So I will use titles such as Mr. or Ms. for persons I know to use male/female pronouns. My first priority is to show respect.

This is where our language often fails us. I don't have a similarly respectful title for my colleagues who identify as genderqueer or non-binary. I default to Professor or Doctor when I can, but my binary-hardwired brain will often screw up and say sir or ma'am. In those moments, my instinct to show respect is actually the most disrespectful thing I could say. I get this wrong a lot. I am consciously, actively working on getting it right. The best thing I can do is to put myself in circumstances and settings where the new norms are the inclusive norms. Over time, the group culture can help redefine my communication style.

We can also show respect by expressing it overtly.

"That's a great idea! Would it be okay if I build on that?" (Being ready to stop talking if the person says no.)

Or with a patient—*"I really respect how you've sought help for your depression. It's really hard to reach out when you're feeling down. You've shown real strength."*

Or this—*"I don't know how things are going to go with this cancer. But I hear that you value not being in pain and having a clear mind more than you value trying to have the most possible days of life. I promise I will honor your wishes and respect your choices."*

Or perhaps this one is the most difficult, respecting autonomy. *"I hear you that right now quitting cigarettes (or alcohol or heroin or your abusive domestic partner) is not something you think you can do. I am here with you. If you decide that I can be helpful, I will be here to offer what I can. I respect you."*

I respect you.

With all of my being, in all manner of our interactions, I will do my best to show it in a way that you best receive it.

I respect you.

FOR FURTHER READING

Alvarez J. *How the Garcia Girls Lost Their Accents.*

Fadiman A. *The Spirit Catches You and You Fall Down: A Hmong Child, Her American Doctors, and the Collision of Two Cultures.*

Kowalski S. *Cultural Sensitivity Training: Developing the Basis for Effective Intercultural Communication.*

Morrison T, Conaway WA. *Kiss, Bow or Shake Hands.*

Resnicow K, Baranowski T, Ahluwalia JS, Braithwaite RL. Cultural sensitivity in public health: defined and demystified. *Ethn Dis.* 1999;9(1):10-21.

Tannen D. *You Just Don't Understand.*

10.

Assess and Affirm Differences

I once was giving a keynote speech before a diverse group of clinicians from community health centers. I was in the middle of a powerful closing story when the moderator suddenly stood up. She looked at her watch. *"That's all the time we have."* I stopped in mid-sentence and sat down awkwardly. I was miffed.

CRASH COURSE IN CULTURAL COMPETENCY

C = Consider CULTURE

R = Show RESPECT

AA = ASSESS and AFFIRM Differences

S = Show SENSITIVITY

SH = Practice SELF-AWARENESS

and HUMILITY as a life discipline

As the meeting went to break, a colleague from Puerto Rico approached me. *"That was so rude!"* he said. *"In Puerto Rico, that would never happen."* He explained it to me this way. *"If I am on my way to a 9 a.m. appointment,"* he said, *"and I run into my cousin on the street, I stop to greet him. We talk as long as we need to talk. I would be in the moment. The person would be more important than any schedule."*

I thought about it. In the same circumstance, I would do a brief greeting and check my watch. Hurrying to an appointment, I would say, *"I've got to go."* For my Puerto Rican friends, the value of *personalismo* would dictate that stopping and talking to this person was the priority. He went on to say how this posed challenges for him at times in a medical culture that is so task driven and time rigid.

Wow! It really hit me. I was part of that task-driven, time-rigid culture. But I really wanted to be a person who prioritized people over tasks. Personal connections over punctuality. I could learn and grow by seeing through different eyes. And whether I ultimately changed my behavior, I could honestly affirm what a lovely perspective he had. Assessing differences is just the first step. Affirming them, or the core values underneath them, is what leads to cultural effectiveness.

Take norms around time and punctuality. With a wink and a smile, my African American colleagues refer to CPT, or colored-people time. In the Caribbean, people refer to "island time." Similar phrases are heard in Africa. In farmworker settings, it might be Latine time. Indeed, most of the world is more relaxed about time than white Americans and some Europeans. We are the outliers. Still, we hold sway as a majority culture, so other people's values are the different ones. We should be acknowledging the weirdness of WPT (white people time).

FOCAL POINTS FOR CULTURAL EFFECTIVENESS

1. **Greetings and Introductions**

   Kiss, bow, or shake hands?

2. **Names**

   Do I prefer to be called by my first name or by my title/last name?

   Is last name or first name my family name? Which is my given name?

3. **Language**

   What language do I think in? Am I just "getting by" in English?

4. **Respect/Disrespect**

   Disrespect is universally offensive but different in every culture.

5. **Colors/Decor**

   What colors signify health? Death?

   Are the images in wall art and health education posters consistent with my culture?

6. **Religion/Spirituality**

   Mind, body, spirit separate or united? Material or spiritual view of world? Specifics?

7. **Gender Expectations**

   Can a male professional examine a female patient?

   Can a female patient make a decision without her male spouse being present?

8. **Models of Health/Disease**

   Is it epilepsy (medical culture) or "A Spirit Catches You and You Fall Down" (Hmong culture)?

9. **Basis for Health Decision-Making**

   Are decisions made based on outcomes of randomized controlled trials (data and graphs), or does Doña Maria say, *"She's a good doctor; you should do what she says"* (relational *confianza y personalismo*)?

10. **Family Involvement in Care and Decision-Making**

    How many people should be in the exam room during a patient visit?

    Who makes decisions? Who should be consulted?

11. **Sexuality/Birth/Family Planning**

    Is it okay to talk about? Do certain practices violate religious principles? What is the patient's personal view?

12. **Death and Dying**

Should we tell the patient? What are the important rituals we should honor?

Who should be present? How is death viewed?

If a student is five minutes late to a lecture, they are dinged for lack of "professionalism." But if a student shows up on time and lacks empathy, are they really more professional? It's too easy to misunderstand people showing up late. We assume that *they don't respect my time"* or *"they're disorganized"* or *"they're rude."* Behaviors don't let us see into someone's soul. My white-guy, Anglo, cisgender, medical culture norms may limit my understanding. Seeing those differences is a start, but only if I also learn to affirm core values that are different from my own.

The A in our CRASH course reminds us to assess and affirm differences. In various domains, patients may believe or behave quite differently from my norms. Some examples of practical issues and behaviors are listed in the "Focal Points for Cultural Effectiveness" box.

Assessing and affirming are two sides of the same coin. We must learn about differences without making people feel the stigma of being different or "othered." When we create environments in which differences are affirmed, people are free to be fully themselves. Only then can we gain the full benefits of our diversity.

One critique of teachers is that we praise vaguely but criticize specifically. Instead, we must learn to praise specifically. We can help our students understand not only what they did well but also precisely why it was so excellent. This also works as a cultural effectiveness skill with our patients. Brian McLaren uses the phrase "generous orthodoxy" to describe his open-minded approach to theology. He seeks to actively learn specific elements of other people's beliefs that he can affirm while still maintaining his own core values.[1] We in Western medicine could use a little more generosity in our scientific orthodoxy.

How many of us are really good at affirming others? Beyond my mother, I can count on two fingers the teachers I've known who were really good at this. One was Dr. Jorge Prieto, chair of family medicine at Cook County Hospital. Dr. Prieto was a multifaceted diamond of a man. He was the son of a Mexican leader forced into exile by political violence. He was a community activist who had worked with Cesar Chavez in the early days of the United Farmworkers movement. He was an *aficionado* of Mexican art and poetry. He was humble yet proud.

Jorge Prieto was a very small man, stooped with age and rheumatoid arthritis. He was in constant pain, yet ever optimistic. Sometimes at night, he would wake up at 3 AM in pain. He didn't want to cloud his mind with pain pills, so he would get dressed and come to the hospital. Patient cries would echo down the granite-walled high hallways. Occasionally, an aide would sing a spiritual *a cappella* for the patients. It was truly a sacred space. But every now and then at that hour, it was quiet, except for your own steps and your own breath.

Dr. Prieto would wander the hallways and find a ward where his residents were the on-call team. He'd approach the nurses at their station and ask them to *"tell me a story about my residents."* The nurses realized that Dr. Prieto was looking for positive stories about a resident who had done something good. There was the time one of my fellow residents was called to the ward to give a patient something for pain. She wrote the medication orders and then sat by the patient's bedside. It would be a half-hour before the Demerol came up from the pharmacy, so she held the patient's hand. They spoke softly until the medicine finally came. With it came relief, and the patient finally fell asleep. *"Doc was still holding her hand,"* said the nurse proudly.

Dr. Prieto was a busy man. He ran a big department in one of the largest urban public hospitals in the country. But for the rest of the day, he considered it his number one priority to find the resident who had done something good. He would wait until he could seemingly run into his target coincidentally. It was always when they were within earshot of at least three other residents. Only then would he start to tell the story. *"I heard what you did last night,"* he would say. We would all flinch.

But then Dr. Prieto would start to tell the story of how good it was what they had done. He would describe the acts of excellence in granular detail. He would embellish the story. He would exaggerate with magical fiction as only a Mexican poet could. He painted a detailed and complete picture of the excellence that was and the excellence that could be. *"My residents make me so proud,"* he would say, and we would all grow a little taller. We would all try to be just a little better and more noble. We all wanted to be the doctors he would praise. His residents are my age now. Most of us have engaged intentionally in lifelong careers of service to and with communities of greatest need.

Assess and Affirm Each Person's Identity

The first task in assessing and affirming a person is to ask about their self-described identity. How do they describe themselves, name themselves, or define themselves? The world is a big place, and humanity is incredibly diverse. The range of identities we knew growing up is much narrower than what our diverse patients will bring.

We can take a brief cultural history of every patient. Do not assume that someone is African American because they look or sound Black to you. Ask in a nonthreatening way. It often follows naturally from a family history. *"Are there any medical problems that run in your family? Your parents? Your grandparents? Did their culture or religion affect how they approached their own health care? How is that for you?"* What will quickly be uncovered is the "within-group" heterogeneity of people perceived to be of one race.

Latine individuals will often identify themselves culturally with their nation of origin. The lumping of "Hispanics" doesn't seem to fit. There are substantial differences between our Guatemalan and Argentinian patients. Our Mexican patients who grew up on the border in Ciudad Juárez near El Paso are not culturally the same as Mexican citizens from a rural state. In Chiapas, as many as a third of rural villagers speak Mayan dialects.

People seen as Black in America have tremendous within-group heterogeneity as well. This includes nations of origin (e.g., Nigerian or Ghanaian, Jamaican or Brazilian). Some may be related to generations of enslaved Africans who were brought to America unwillingly. Understanding how many generations have passed since immigration is one factor that affects a patient's level of acculturation. Other factors will influence culture as well, such as geographical roots in the South versus the North or growing up in a rural versus an urban community. Each generation has also had different experiences of racism.

Culture may or may not have religious elements. Some people approach their health through a spiritual lens. For example, many African Methodist Episcopal (AME) churches have health ministries or a parish nurse. Physical health and spiritual health are blended into the same worship service. In contrast, many majority-white churches hold a more reductionistic frame, in which body, mind, and soul are treated quite separately.

Gender is a core element of identity. Most men of my generation grew up with a binary understanding of sex and gender. Babies were born as boys or girls. Full stop. What we now term as "sex assigned at birth" was assumed to be the gender identity individuals would carry for life. Many cultures affirm this tradition with rituals such as "gender-reveal parties" and pink or blue balloons on the mailbox ("It's a boy!"). If that's all we ever learn, we are stuck in our binary gender rigidity.

So we now teach our medical students about the "Gender Unicorn" or the "Genderbread" person. We teach nuances of gender identity, gender expression, and sex assigned at birth. We differentiate sexual organs from sexual attractions and sexuality. We help our students accept and affirm gender-free and non-binary and trans and queer and questioning persons. And in this process, some of us learn to see ourselves in more nuanced ways. We grow and heal from our own rigidities. It's essential to my profession, but it's also a gift to my personal growth. White, cisgender guy healing.

Assess and Affirm Their Context

Family

In primary care practice, I sometimes had to give my patient a diagnosis of cancer. I would then facilitate a conversation in which both family and patient could say the word "cancer" out loud to each other. That would begin an ongoing discussion about what might come next. I would help them with the "what-if" and the "what-then" conversations. We might eventually talk about how they would want the dying process to play out. Sometimes people made different choices. I would ask, *"What would you like to know? With whom would you like me to speak?"* One man might say, *"Help me talk with my wife,"* while another says, *"Don't tell my kids."*

Sometimes family meant just a spouse and two kids. In southern culture and Latine culture, large extended families might be involved. Modern families are very different from the *Leave It to Beaver* nuclear family of the 1950s. Parents may be a single mom or two dads or two people who don't identify by gender. Kids might be being raised by a grandparent, because mom is in rehab or on the streets. With the gap in affordable housing, one household may be a trailer with mom, three kids, a grandparent, and a sister with her two kids. Or maybe there's no home at all. A single parent and one child are living in their car. We won't know if we don't ask.

Neighborhood and Social Determinants

Where you live affects your health outcomes. Neighborhoods can have great challenges, such as crime and no grocery stores. At the same time, they can have great strengths such as extended family and culture. In rural areas, transportation barriers are obvious. A clinic might be 30 miles away. In the urban environment, a clinic may be a half-mile away. But it still might mean a 45-minute bus ride with two transfers.

Poor neighborhoods can get a little frisky at night, sometimes violent. The Pilsen/Little Village neighborhood of Chicago is now the setting for many episodes of the police drama *Chicago PD*. When I drove, I could take our old car and park near the clinic. I learned to put a bicycle chain and padlock on my hood to avoid having the battery stolen on cold nights.

When I rode Chicago's L, I would get off the train at the North Lawndale stop and walk a half-mile or so to the clinic. In the daytime, this was no big deal. When I had evening clinics, it was another story. I would get to the L station at night, well after dark. I remember standing on the platform one evening as feuding gang members chased each other with guns. I stood behind a steel pillar, trying desperately to make myself invisible. For me, it was just a story to tell after the fact. For my patients, it's where young families were raising their kids. They survived crime and poverty with incredible faith and resiliency and family connectedness.

Neighborhood context has a very specific flavor when it comes to policing. Sometimes the police protect you, and sometimes the police abuse or incarcerate you. White people's advice to "call the cops" is not helpful. Drugs and gangs and shootings? Call the police! You mean the police that protect *your* neighborhood? The ones who almost shot my cousin last year? The cops who still treat all of us like criminals and all white people as victims? What world are you living in? *(Call the cops, my ass!)*

Neighborhood context can be even more complex for migrant farmworkers and their families.[2] My colleagues in Immokalee deal every day with toxic stress levels in children of migrant families. Kids see other children's parents taken away by *la Migra* (immigration). They see the resiliency these families demonstrate every day in overcoming challenges. Dr. Javier Rosado even wrote a children's book[3] to help children grieve and process the experience of frequently moving away from new friends.

Context matters. Poor neighborhoods in Chicago could be gritty and rough. Buildings that allowed immigrants were sometimes worst of all. In the 1980s, Chicago had a problem with rats. Not cute little lab rats. In Chicago, the rats had earned the title "super-rats." They looked like cats or possums scurrying through the alleys. They had evolved jaws and teeth that could chew through concrete walls, especially in public housing. They had developed resistance to all the traditional rat poisons.

So when the rats infested a building with immigrant families and young children, fathers would take matters into their own hands. One misty night in autumn, I swear I saw a Mexican man holding rebar like a sword. He was like a 20th-century Don Quixote, taking on a Chicago super-rat that was climbing out of the dumpster behind his apartment.

Lucita's father had tried all the usual strategies. Rat traps. Traditional rat poison. Baseball bat. He lived in a small apartment with a pregnant wife and three little children. He decided to make a super-poison for the super-rats. He had done some farming in Mexico and knew something about pesticides. The poisons he chose were organophosphate insecticides, available at any hardware store. They are deadly when ingested, like chemical warfare nerve agents. What he didn't know was that they can also be absorbed through the skin.

A decade later in Florida, there would be a mass poisoning of over 40 farmworkers with these very chemicals. In a field near Ruskin, Florida, dozens were poisoned from the wet insecticide sprayed on rows of lettuce. Because the growers ignored the legally required reentry times, the workers entered the field while the leaves were still wet. They began tying up the lettuce leaves to keep them off the ground. The poison was transferred from wet leaves onto exposed skin. From there, it passed into their bloodstream.

At first, only a few collapsed. No one knew what was happening, so they were sent to the hospital. They were vomiting and sweating and salivating. Some had diarrhea. Even their eyes were tearing, as if every faucet in their body had been turned on.

Fairly quickly, the emergency doctors diagnosed the problem but had limited experience. They gave the usual doses of atropine, and it barely touched the symptoms. In these cases, it takes large doses to overcome the poison's cholinergic release. Soon, more cases arrived, and they were running out of atropine. By the time a dozen patients had shown up, nurses began asking where they had come from. How many more workers were still in the field? They declared a mass casualty event. A med-evac helicopter was sent to the field to get the workers away from the wet lettuce that was poisoning them. They had to do battlefield triage.

At three years old, Lucita didn't know about any of this. She didn't know about the super-rats. She didn't know about the teaspoons of liquid poison her loving father had spread around the apartment in small trays. Lucita was in her exploring phase and stumbled over one of the trays. It splashed on her, and she tried to clean up the mess. She spread the liquid around the floor with paper towels. She held it to her nose to smell it. It smelled interesting, so she tasted it.

She got sick right away, with vomiting and diarrhea. By the time she got to the hospital, she was having prolonged seizures. She was shaking and turning blue. Emergency doctors worked on her for a few hours and then sent her upstairs. She came to the pediatric intensive care unit, the PICU, where I was a fourth-year student on call. They had sedated her and put a breathing tube into her windpipe. She had IVs and a nasogastric suction tube and urine catheter. There were tubes and tape everywhere covering her little body. The ventilator was loudly pumping air. Alarms were constantly beeping. Sedated and comatose, Lucita was calm and still. She looked like death. But angelic. Angelic, comatose death.

She looked that way for the remaining two weeks of my rotation. I came in each morning, hoping she would stir, or wake up, or move a finger. Nothing. We did lab tests. I learned to manage ventilator settings and IV fluids in a small child. I checked on her at night when I was on call and in the mornings when we made rounds. Still angelic. Still comatose. I could see Death coming, and I resigned myself to it. I finished the rotation, still imagining a hopeless outcome.

The following rotation put me on the general pediatric wards. Kids with dehydration or pneumonia might need hospitalization, but they would recover very quickly. Kids are incredibly resilient. They look sicker than death one day, and three days later, they are running and playing. We also had kids with chronic illnesses like sickle cell anemia. Leukemias were the worst. We weren't very good at curing leukemia yet, but we treated the hell out of it. Aggressive chemotherapies knocked kids down and made their hair fall out and made them vomit. Children endured painful procedures that required anesthesia, like bone marrow aspirations. Big-bore needles were jammed into a hip bone.

Maurice was one of my favorite kids. He was an ebony-skinned child with a huge infectious smile that had just a twinkle of mischief. He was a tough kid, too. He had endured sickness and pain that would have broken the spirit of most adults. I remember when they wheeled him down to the operating room one day to have yet another bone marrow aspiration. Maurice didn't want to do it. *"I'm sorry, Maurice,"* I said as I helped him onto the gurney.

The aides took him downstairs and lifted him gently onto the operating room table. He gave them a look like something was up. The anesthesiologist leaned in to put a mask over his face, and Maurice timed his punch perfectly. *Bam!* A roundhouse punch to the side of the anesthesiologist's jaw sent him reeling. When I heard the story, I grinned and almost shouted. *"Yessss!!!"* Maurice was still fighting.

A few days later, I was walking down the hall past the pediatric nursing station. My scrubs were wrinkled from a nearly sleepless night on-call. A little girl came running down the hall from behind me. I turned and looked. She had a big smile, and for a moment I thought maybe I had seen her before. I turned to a nurse who was coming out of another patient's room. *"Who is that little girl?"* I asked, as the girl ran past me.

The nurse's face broke into a big smile, and she grabbed my arm for emphasis. *"That's Lucita!"* she said. I thought of Lucita comatose, on a ventilator. *"Not . . . ?"* I stammered, pointing back toward the PICU. *"Lucita with the rat poison? Lucita in a coma on the ventilator? That Lucita?"*

"Yes!!!" the nurse said with eyes wide open in wonder and joy.

"Haaaaa!!!" I cheered and gave her a high-five. We both turned around just in time to see Lucita running and jumping up into her Papi's outstretched arms. He and his little girl were grinning and hugging in a beautiful embrace of father–daughter love. I turned to share the moment with the nurse, but she was gone. She was

changing a dressing for a child burned in a fire from an old space heater in a rundown three-flat apartment.

A psychologist in our program later told me, *"Celebrate your victories. They don't come very often. Find time to grieve your losses, but you have to make time to celebrate your victories."* Victories. I wish I had more.

Assess and Affirm Health-Relevant Relationships

People are important. Relationships matter. Our patients want to involve others in their health care, so we must ask these questions:

- Who is important in this person's life?
- What roles do they play in helping this person make health decisions?
- How would this person want you to involve these important people?

When we were designing a new clinic building for one of our facilities that served farmworkers, the immediate feedback from our team was that we needed larger exam rooms. It was not OK in that cultural setting to say, *"The rest of you can stay in the waiting room."* Visits included mothers with two or three kids but also their sisters or *abuelas* or *tias* or husbands. It was a happy chaos. *Familismo* meant that decisions were made by families, not by individuals.

The US health care system is built on an assumption of individuality and personal privacy. It challenges us when patients have a more family-based decision-making process. One health care system that has reorganized itself to be responsive to culture is the South Central Healthcare Foundation in Anchorage, Alaska. When Alaska Native people took over the governing board, they decided to shift from an individual-based medical record to a family-based medical record. It just made more sense in the Alaskan Native culture. They have since made other changes, including adding mental health specialists and Alaska Native healers to their primary care teams. They have dramatically improved both health outcomes and patient satisfaction.

In the public health department, I currently see refugees from many parts of the world. In this context, an Afghan husband and wife often come together into the exam room. The preference will be for a female practitioner to examine the wife and only in the presence of the husband. This is both religious and cultural. But these preferences may be different for different families, even from the same country. I have to ask.

Assess and Affirm Communication Style and Preferences

Different people communicate differently. Some differences in communication style are individual, and some are cultural. Some are gender-normed. Even the pacing of our speech can have cultural dynamics. My late friend Dr. Roberto Dansie was a cultural guru, grandson of a curandera. Shortly before he died, we had a long and precious conversation, mostly about this book.

He once told me of a series of conversations he had had with a Native American tribal elder, of whom he was asking many questions to gain wisdom. At some point, Dr. Dansie became frustrated. He asked the elder, *"Why have you not yet answered any of my questions?"* The elder answered, *"You never gave us time to answer, before you asked another question."* The pace of speech and questioning was an American pace. The cultural norm of the tribal leaders was to be thoughtful. They would allow many seconds or even minutes of silence after a question before giving an answer. In the end, that was the first lesson in wisdom they gave him.

Language is also a critical factor. A patient may seem to speak fairly good English, but their preferred language might be Spanish or Swahili. Do I use English for my own convenience, or do I take the extra step of finding an interpreter? A routine visit takes twice as long speaking in Urdu through a telephone interpreter. What would I want if I were sick in a foreign country?

Spanish is not just one language either. One of my colleagues said she had to unlearn some of her Puerto Rican Spanish to help her Mexican patients. In *How the Garcia Girls Lost Their Accents*, author Julia Alvarez describes the formal Castellano Spanish of a priest from Spain, the educated Español of her parents, and what her family called "the bad Spanish" of the rural *campesinas*.[4] Across Latin America, there are at least seven different words or phrases used to describe a hangover. A student said he used the word *bicho* to describe insect bites when he was at dinner with his fiancée's parents for the first time. In his background, *bicho* simply meant little biting insects. In his fiancé's parents' culture, the word could also be a euphemism for *penis*. Oops.

Assess and Affirm Health Knowledge and Health Beliefs

Before we give health advice or try to change someone's health behaviors, we need to know where they are coming from. Their beliefs and understanding may not come from our Western medical model but from their own culture. If we don't know, we have to learn. And to learn, we must ask. If you've never heard of *empacho* or *susto*, you'll never make the diagnosis.

"The spirit catches you and you fall down."[5] That was how a Hmong family understood their child's seizures. They were a special gift, a unique connection to the spiritual world. To doctors, seizures are something to be prevented with medicines. How do we reconcile such differences?

Sometimes we misunderstand each other's language. "I can't have *high* blood [hypertension]; I've had *low* blood [anemia] all my life." Some patients express misunderstandings—*"It couldn't be an STI. . . . She only has sex with other women."* Sometimes patients have to teach me their language. A man comes to the clinic and says, *"I got a haircut."* I'm thinking he's been to the barber shop, so I say, *"That's nice, but how can I help you?"* A nurse pulls me aside and whispers. *"In this neighborhood, coming to the doctor with 'a haircut' means he has a sore on his penis. It could be syphilis."* Wait, what???

It gets even more interesting across culture and language gaps. As a medical student doing a rotation in rural Haiti, I was helped by an American nurse who had spent decades in-country. She was interpreting for me as I interviewed a patient. Soon it became obvious that she was helping me a little too much. *"He says he has tuberculosis and needs medicine,"* she said. I looked at her skeptically. *"Is that really what he said?"* She admitted that it wasn't.

She was just trying to help me, but I demanded that next time she translate exactly what the patient was saying, word for word. The next patient began to tell his story. *"My bones are dead and my blood is cold and there is a fire burning deep inside my belly."* I looked at her, at a loss for what to ask next. *"Maybe we should just go back to the way you were translating before,"* I said meekly. She nodded and winked.

Sometimes people have learned various cultural practices to assist in healing. As a third-year medical student, I once examined a patient from Poland. The patient spoke little English, and I had no interpreter. He had a cough and a fever. I began to think he might have pneumonia. Then I lifted his shirt to listen to his lungs. I saw rows of large round red marks in a geometric pattern all across his back and chest. I asked the patient, and he gave me the Polish word for it. I didn't speak Polish. I still had no clue. *Giant squid tentacle suckers* became the intrusive thought in my brain, but I was pretty sure that wasn't a Chicago thing.

I know now that it was cupping. The practice is common in various countries and even among American athletes. It involves the use of smooth rounded glass jars. A flaming cotton ball is passed briefly into the jar to heat up the air but not the glass. The glass is then placed on the skin. The cooling of the air inside creates a vacuum or suction that adheres the glass tightly to the skin, which rises into the jar. The skin reddens and sometimes bruises a little. It leaves a temporary, distinct mark. Not unlike a giant sucking squid, I would say in my own defense.

Assess and Affirm Health Decision-Making and Health-Seeking Behaviors

In Mexican American farmworker culture, certain problems might lead you straight to a Western medical doctor. Other problems might require a *curandera* or *espiritualista* or even a *bruja*. In Mexico, a pharmacy might have one section for prescribed Western medicines, another with bags of traditional herbal remedies, and a third for Tarot cards, candles, and religious amulets.

Other health-seeking behaviors are tied to circumstances. Because of weather and seasonal crops, a farmworker may only get 90 to 120 days of work each year. They only get paid on the days they work. When we see diabetes dangerously out of control or an infection draining pus and spreading, it is easy for health professionals to become judgmental. *"Why didn't you come in sooner?"* we ask. But for that individual, the decision was perfectly reasonable. They were sacrificing their own health to keep working and support their family.

In low-income settings, I learned the phrase, *"Are you ten dollars sick?"* In Groveland, it might mean paying someone gas money to drive you to the clinic. In inner-city Chicago or Atlanta,

10 dollars (or now $20) might represent the copay on your health insurance. It could be the minimum fee on a community clinic's sliding fee scale. When you're scraping just to pay rent or to put food on the table, spending 10 bucks on yourself is too much.

When patients come late to a clinic visit or show up when they weren't scheduled, I try to imagine the complexities and challenges in their lives. In the community health centers, we often debated what to do with people who came late to appointments. Privileged clinicians would often take a hardline position. Every patient needed an appointment. If they showed up more than 15 minutes late, they would have to reschedule. Others of us would take the opposite position. *"Why do we have appointments at all?"* Giving a farmworker an appointment for a specific date three months from today was an absurdity. Ultimately, we landed on a compromise. We would maintain an appointment system for those patients who preferred it. Meanwhile, we would staff a walk-in clinician for those patients who came late or with no appointment.

We also learned to be humble about when our patients did and did not need to come to the clinic. We used to write prescriptions only for three months of blood pressure medicine to make sure that the patients came back for follow-up. When we shifted to writing one-year refillable prescriptions, the level of blood pressure control among our patients dramatically improved. It was a simple policy change, but it potentially prevented some strokes, heart attacks, and kidney failure.

I've seen many physicians over the years become intensely frustrated when their patients showed up with preventable, late complications of diseases. We offered screening tests or medicines that could prevent a bad outcome, but our patients might demur. Or they might listen to our advice, nod and smile, and then walk out the door and never fill the prescription.

The psychology of chronic poverty is quite complex. To understand seemingly self-defeating health behaviors, there are two critical concepts. The first is time-discounting. Time-discounting refers to how people value potential future payoffs against current costs. For a well-educated professional, investing in a 401(k) plan makes perfect sense. My immediate needs are well-taken care of. I can imagine a future in which my payoff will be a secure retirement. For someone living paycheck to paycheck, the calculus is far different.

These economic realities translate into a mindset that affects health care decisions as well. We often use a "cardiac risk calculator" to assess the probability of a person having a heart attack in the next ten years. For a 10-year cardiac risk greater than 10 percent, almost every doc in America would recommend a daily cholesterol-lowering statin. I take one myself.

Imagine that the doctor says that you have a 10 percent chance of having a heart attack sometime in the next 10 years. If you take this medicine that costs $20 a month, the risk might be reduced by as much as half. But what if you only get paid on the days when you work? What if you have a spouse and three kids, and it's a struggle just to get by? You will spend money on health care when your kids are sick but not for a medicine that *might* help you 10 years from now. It would make no sense. Today's worries are enough for today.

A second psychological frame of poverty is locus of control, measured on a continuum from internal to external. Internal locus of control is explained best by Dr. Seuss.

> You have brains in your head, and feet in your shoes;
> You can steer yourself in any direction you choose!
> You're on your own. And you know what you know.
> And YOU are the one who'll decide where to go.[6]

Physicians skew way toward this internal end of this locus of control scale. I might think, *"If I eat lots of broccoli, and exercise properly, and meditate, and buy all the right kinds of insurance, then I will live a healthy and happy life. At some time in the future, at a moment of my own choosing, I will die peacefully in my sleep."* This is a wildly unrealistic form of magical thinking. It is seen mostly among individuals of social, economic, and educational privilege.

At the opposite end of the spectrum is external locus of control. We might see this as fatalism in our low-income patients. We see them just passively accepting whatever life throws at them. Among urban youth, it may be expressed as *"I don't expect to live past 20 anyway."* Or, they might say, *"If that bullet has your name on it."* In the older generation, the expression might be *"if God wills . . ."* or *"What're ya gonna do?"* or the classic, *"Stuff happens."*

There is one particularly malignant form of external locus of control. It's when faith is placed in a powerful external authority such as a physician. These patients actually do the worst, because diabetes requires self-management or self-efficacy. The patient who says, *"Whatever you say, doc—you're in charge"* is putting themselves in great danger. These words are seductive to the physician and completely disempowering to the patient. To successfully manage diabetes, we must become less, and the patient must become more. We need healing ourselves to help others heal.

Here's the reality for our patients. External locus of control, whether fatalism, faith in God, passive acceptance, or Zen-like detachment, makes absolutely perfect sense in their lived experience. The landlord really won't fix the moldy drywall that is making their child's asthma worse. They really can't afford health insurance, but nurses scold them when they end up in the emergency room. The job market and career paths in a poor neighborhood are nonexistent. Passive acceptance is a strategy for keeping your sanity. And even when circumstances change, this can become generational wisdom.

The serenity prayer says,

> God, grant me the serenity to accept the things I cannot change,
> courage to change the things I can,
> and wisdom to know the difference.[7]

But the list of things I can and cannot change is very different for a white guy with education and professional status and a six-figure salary than it is for a family living in a run-down trailer near Stuckey Still. Part of our healing as take-charge physicians is to understand with compassion the health decisions poor people make.

Here's how a community organizer illustrated the psychology of "learned helplessness." Put a bass that likes to eat minnows in a fish tank. Then put a sealed glass jar with minnows into the tank. The bass will try to eat the minnows. Bonk. His nose bounces off the glass jar. *(Do bass have noses?)* Try again. Bonk. Nose hurts. One more time. Bonk. Still hungry. Nose really hurts. *"Screw it. Those minnows are unattainable."*

Now pour the water and minnows from the jar into the tank, so the minnows are now free-swimming. They don't stand a chance! Except the bass doesn't even try to eat the minnows. All he can think is that *"every time I try to eat one of those damned minnows, I bonk my nose. It hurts."* So even in settings where some structural barriers have been lifted, the serenity prayer is in play. Even where vocational paths have been opened or where health care is now accessible, my patients have learned to *"accept the things I cannot change."* At the end of the day, we're all different. Sometimes those differences frustrate us. Sometimes they inspire us.

Assess. Affirm. Differences.

FOR FURTHER READING

Hughes L. *The Ways of White Folks*.

Kobabe M. *Gender Queer: A Memoir*.

Lara-Cooper K, Lara WJ. *Ka'm-t'em: A Journey Toward Healing*.

Madaras L, Stonington S, Seda CH, Garcia D, Zuroweste E. Social distance and mobility—a 39-year-old pregnant migrant farmworker. *N Engl J Med*. 2019;380(12):1093–1096.

Rosado J. *After the Harvest: A Story About Saying Goodbye*.

11.

Show Sensitivity

Sensitivity means a willingness to learn about the history and lives of our patients. I became a better doctor in Groveland, Florida, after I had made at least a dozen house calls. I visited small homes on dirt roads in poor neighborhoods. I saw my patients' living conditions. I understood better their resources and challenges. I realized that much of the advice I was giving in my exam room was of no earthly value in my patients' lived reality. I needed to learn not only about culture but also about day-to-day life. Some of it was driven by local history.

Groveland, Florida, had a terrible history of racial oppression. That history was still driving Black-white relations, job opportunities, wealth inequality, and police interactions. When I read the *Devil in the Grove* years later, I recognized some of the family names as former patients. I may have taken care of family relatives of the woman who, decades ago, had accused young Black men of her rape. And I almost certainly had taken care of some of the relatives of the young men who had been falsely accused. They had been threatened by a lynch mob. Two were killed by a local sheriff. I had no idea.

You can't expect to know everything about the culture of every patient you ever care for, but it is a failure not to try. I have spent a good chunk of my career embedded in predominantly African American work settings, and I have learned a ton. But I learn new stuff every day. I am reminded constantly of how much more I have to learn across many cultures. For example, I worked six years with predominantly Latine farmworker families. I still take students on a spring break trip to Immokalee, Florida, every year for an immersion experience in farmworker health. My Spanish is still not fluent. My cultural fluency is shallow. I have only scratched the surface. I must keep learning every day.

I teach a session to our young medical students about farmworker health, from occupational injuries to social medicine. I show video recordings of farmworkers who can teach from their own lived experience. I ask each student to lift a 32-pound bucket of tomatoes up over their head as if they were passing it up to workers on a truck. I get the strongest, most athletic student in the room to hoist 80 pounds of grapefruits in the canvas shoulder bag that farmworkers use. I ask them to run around the lecture room. I ask them to climb a ladder and climb back down without hurting themselves. And then I ask the students, *"What do you think it would be like to do this for eight or nine hours straight in the Florida sun and heat?"*

I teach them a little bit about Cesar Chavez and Dolores Huerta and the farmworker movement. I hold up a short hoe and ask them to consider why Cesar Chavez called it *el brazo del diablo*, the arm of the devil. I ask them why his grandson would place it on the casket at his funeral. Cesar Chavez had fought a years-long battle to end the practice of using short hoes in "stoop labor." Workers had to bend or stoop to weed between the vegetables with the short-handled hoe. It's hard on the spine and the knees.

A long-handled hoe would have added minimal cost for the growers. Why did they fight it so bitterly? Some argue that it was a throwback to the days of slavery. Overseers on horseback could see if a person was working, because standing up meant not working. Others argue that it was just to keep the union organizers from having any victory at all. When it was banned as "an unsafe hand tool" in California in 1975,[1] some growers made their workers pull weeds by hand. Still stooping.

When I teach students about the complexities of race-ethnicity and poverty and health, I often tell a story of one of my patients. I start with the question, *"What killed Guadalupe Benitez?"* Señora Benitez (not her real name) was a short, overweight 53-year-old diabetic woman. She lived in a trailer behind a frozen-dead orange grove with her farmworker husband. She came to the farmworker clinic irregularly because they had no car. They had to ask a neighbor to drive them the 12 miles to the clinic. They came together and enjoyed their clinic visits because the Spanish-speaking staff treated them warmly. They had no children. Any other family was in Mexico. They had not formed any ties to the Mexican American community here. Her diabetes was never well controlled. She took her medicine when she could afford it, praised her doctors, and believed that enduring suffering was a sign of faith.

One day, Señora Benitez was heating water on a propane stove to take a bath. While carrying the hot water to the bathtub, she spilled some on her leg. She suffered second- and third-degree burns. Her first instinct was to put some lard or butter on the wound and perhaps some herbs. After several days, however, it was obvious that the wound was becoming infected. Reluctantly, she came with her husband to the migrant clinic. The clinic doctors recommended daily Silvadene dressings, oral antibiotics, and perhaps whirlpool therapy at the local hospital. Señora Benitez declined our hospital-based services. She could not afford any of them. She agreed to change the dressings twice a day, to take the antibiotics, and to return to the clinic in 48 hours.

Five days later, when Señora Benitez had still not returned to the clinic, a nurse drove the dirt roads out to her trailer. Señora Benitez explained that they had no money to pay for gas for someone to bring them to the clinic. The crew chiefs were not hiring her husband to pick oranges this year because of his age. By now, the wound was badly infected. The dressing had been changed only twice. She had only taken two days of antibiotics. There was necrotic (dead) tissue in the wound. Red streaks ran up the leg, and she had a low-grade fever. Two toes were beginning to turn black. She had gangrene.

Señora Benitez was admitted to the hospital, and a surgical consult was obtained. There was only one general surgeon in the community, a wanna-be vascular surgeon. He ordered an arteriogram of the leg with dye that could be toxic to a diabetic kidney. He also changed my antibiotic orders to include a kidney-toxic antibiotic. He then tried to do an arterial bypass operation. When the patient's blood pressure bottomed out, he had to convert to a below-knee amputation.

With the combined insults of IV contrast material, antibiotic, and hypotension, Señora Benitez's kidneys shut down. She was placed on dialysis. Administrators at the small tax-district hospital began grumbling about the size of her mounting hospital bill. They asked social workers to help her apply for Medicaid and Social Security disability, but caseworkers said she was not totally disabled. This five-foot-two, non-English-speaking, fourth-grade-educated, one-legged, dialysis-dependent, and diabetic Mexican American farmworker's wife was not "totally disabled," they said, because maybe she could still do a sedentary desk job like a receptionist.

At the funeral two weeks later, they laid Señora Benitez in the ground. Her husband turned from the grave and wandered toward the road. He started to walk back to his trailer, waving off all offers of help. He seemed lost as a child and all alone. We never saw him again.

So, what killed Guadalupe Benitez? The clinical answer is that she died of kidney failure and wound infections. These were driven by uncontrolled diabetes. Kidney-toxic medications added insult to injury.

But what *really* killed Guadalupe Benitez? Many medical students start with her lack of education. Other students blame her health literacy. Her highest educational attainment was completing the fourth grade in a rural Mexican school. Some blame the patient herself for delays in seeking care.

However, these answers do not address the root causes. *What really killed Guadalupe Benitez?* Some students try a glib answer. "Poverty," they say, as if the conversation is over. And maybe they're not wrong. Farmworkers are indeed poor. The Benitez family was poorer than most. If she had not lived in a trailer with no hot water heater, she never would have been burned. If she had money or health insurance, she would have had better access to health care. If she could have afforded a car, she would have had transportation to the clinic. Many of our older patients faced similar challenges. A third of Medicare beneficiaries report at least one major health-related resource barrier, such as housing, transportation, basic utilities, or safety.[2]

But Señora Benitez had no health insurance. No matter how poor she and her husband might have been, they would not have qualified for Medicaid. Even if she had become permanently and totally disabled, the immigration laws would have thrown up new barriers.

At a deeper level, poverty goes hand-in-hand with powerlessness. What political power does a disabled, low-income, Spanish-speaking immigrant farmworker have in Florida? Efforts to organize farm labor on the East Coast have had only a little success. Florida is not California.

Powerlessness may be reinforced by the religious or cultural belief that to endure suffering is pure and good. Señora Benitez believed that it was a blessing to share in the suffering of Christ. She sought to follow the example of the Virgin Mary. Mary had appeared to rural Mexicans as her namesake, the Virgin Guadalupe. Such *Marianismo* may allow powerless people to be at peace with their circumstances. It may also reflect the reality of their lives. Sadly, it is also associated with poor diabetes outcomes.

Señora Benitez also had her own sense of dignity and self-sufficiency. She believed that doctors were best seen for serious medical conditions. Other illnesses and minor injuries like burns could best be treated with home remedies. Putting butter and healing herbs on the burn injury made perfect sense in treating her wound. She thought she could never afford the silver-based cream we recommended.

Meanwhile, the first programs to be cut when clinics faced financial difficulties were transportation, outreach workers, and diabetes educators. On the positive side, at least there was a migrant health center within a few miles of this patient's trailer. By all accounts, the patient enjoyed coming for office visits. Señora Benitez genuinely enjoyed her social interactions with our fluently bilingual Mexican American staff. Still, our system consistently fails to produce physicians who speak the diverse languages of the American people. As a result, patients may be stuck with doctors like me who speak "clinic Spanish" or use phone interpreters.

There is a psychosocial element that most students miss. Why was this couple living in a trailer on the back side of an orange grove with no family? Why no association with a church (Catholic or Pentecostal)? Why were there no extended family or social connections to the local Latine community? Our patient's husband was profoundly depressed. He had isolated the couple over many years. In addition to our failure to address Señora Benitez's social isolation, we had also failed to engage her husband in primary care, or to assess his emotional health.

This story illustrates the difference between equal access and health equity. The root causes of bad health outcomes are social determinants. Neither health illiteracy nor personal responsibility is sufficient to explain excess suffering and death in communities of color. If we seek health and social justice, we have to do better. Even if we just want to eliminate variation in outcomes, we have to do better. We can't just give everyone the same majority-culture, English-language, historically white system of health care. Not if we expect to achieve optimal and equitable outcomes. Equality is giving everyone a pair of shoes; equity is giving everyone a pair of shoes *that fits*.

Cultural sensitivity requires us to develop an awareness of cultural values, beliefs, or perceptions that might influence a patient's health care. Shallow cultural sensitivity relates to observable, "superficial" characteristics such as language, music, food, and clothing. Deep sensitivity includes the core social, historical, environmental, and psychological forces that influence health behaviors in a culture.[3] Sensitivity also means knowing people's religious beliefs and practices. If you're planning a meal for a conference with a thousand attendees, you don't choose pork.

We must be especially sensitive to behaviors that might cause offence. These can lead to a breakdown in trust and communication between patient and clinician. You learn that maybe patting an Asian child on top of the head is a bad thing. Complimenting a beautiful Latine baby without touching it could be an expression not just of admiration but of envy. It could lead to *mal de ojo* (evil eye). But a red string bracelet on the wrist offers some protection. Meanwhile, around the world, both the thumbs up sign and the OK sign are quite vulgar in certain cultures.

When Saddam Hussein's statue was pulled down after his overthrow in Iraq, the crowd took off their shoes to slap the head of the statue. In many Muslim settings, showing another person the bottom of your shoe is considered the harshest of insults. When

President George Bush visited that same country, a protester took his shoe off and threw it at the president.

What if I am sitting in front of a room of students and spontaneously cross my legs, unintentionally showing the bottom of my shoe? It may mean nothing to 49 of the 50 students. But one student might have an instinctive gut reaction to feel insulted. They are then distracted by an inner dialogue about whether I meant it that way or if they are just being overly sensitive. Either way, it's both an offense and a distraction. The following box lists a few other examples of behaviors that may cause offense in various cultures.

CULTURAL SENSITIVITY:
BEHAVIORS THAT MAY CAUSE CULTURAL OFFENSE

Calling a patient by first name instead of title and surname

Touching a patient without asking permission

Making (or expecting the patient to make) direct eye contact

Getting right to business (i.e., taking a medical history) before establishing a personal connection

Taking a blood or urine sample

Patting a child on the head

Crossing one's legs; showing the bottom of one's shoes

Examining a patient of the opposite gender

Making American hand gestures ("Okay" sign, or thumbs-up gestures)

Asking a spouse to wait in the waiting room

Limiting visiting hours in the hospital

Shaking hands (right after my colleague has completed their ceremonial washing)

Treating everyone the same in a setting that respects elders

Using a medical registration form that offers only male or female checkboxes for identifying gender

Serving pork (or beef) to all attendees at a conference

Assuming that a male physician is no different than a female physician performing a GYN exam or delivering a baby

Acting as if we live in a postracial world. Underestimating the impact of everyday racial micro- and macroaggressions on our colleagues of color.

Saying, "Why didn't you just call the police?"

Lena Williams spends way more time on the issue of hair than I expected in her book about the *Everyday Interactions That Anger, Annoy, and Divide the Races*.[4] The act of a white woman with long blonde hair casually flipping her hair in an elevator provokes a visceral reaction from an African American woman. *Why?*

To understand, we must remember the history of idealizing white women's hair, especially blonde hair. This went along with the denigrating of Black hair. This is also about Barbie dolls. It's about how young Black children are acculturated to see white dolls with long straight blonde hair as the pretty ones. There is a painful history of African American women using hot irons and chemicals to straighten their hair, just to meet white people norms of beauty. To my white friends, a quick reminder about this sensitivity. No, it is not ever okay to reach out and touch an African American woman's hair. Just don't. Ever.

It's not just beauty or self-image. In business and in professional circles, many traditional African American hairstyles are considered unprofessional. To this day, there are young Black men who are asked to cut braids to meet a white teacher's standards of "appropriate" hair and dress. In the health care setting, white-majority institutions may establish norms of "professional" hairstyles. For a long time, this did not include Afros or weaves or long braids.

Think of the absurdity of having to fight for such basic rights as being able to wear your hair in a way that fits your culture or style. According to the CROWN Coalition, Black women are 1.5 times more likely to be sent home from the workplace because of their hair. Among Black teens who reported discrimination based on hairstyle, most say it started by the age of 12.[5]

Apparently, we need federal legislation just to keep employers from white-norming the hairstyles they consider "professional." The CROWN Act is an acronym for Creating a Respectful and Open World for Natural Hair. The House of Representatives passed it in 2022, but Republicans in the Senate blocked it.[6] Only 19 of 50 states have passed similar legislation. How hard do we have to fight for simple freedoms? How exhausting is that?

Businesses and health professions are starting from 1950s white cisgender norms. Individuals who have certain hairstyles, tattoos, or piercings may be deemed unprofessional. Really? What does pink hair, a nose ring, or a facial tattoo have to do with professionalism in the medical environment? The more our staff look like the patients they serve, the more welcoming our practices will be to our 21st-century diverse communities. I still look and dress like an old white guy. It's who I am. I count on my younger teammates to be fully themselves. They help make it clear that our practice is open to all patients. We need both patients and staff to be fully themselves.

One of the most important areas in which we can learn how others experience us is in the various ways in which we unintentionally hurt people's feelings. Some of this comes from implicit bias and some from not knowing where people's tender spots are. But we can learn, and we can do better.

A British survey came to a blunt conclusion. "Racist microaggressions and unfair treatment are still the norm for Black professionals in the workplace."[7] Dr. Derald Wing Sue has been a leader among researchers in defining microaggressions.[8] He says that the term refers to "subtle, stunning, often automatic, and non-verbal exchanges which are 'put downs.'"[9] He describes their ubiquity as "toxic rain: here, there, and everywhere."[10] They cause "death by a thousand cuts."[11]

Sue describes different types of microaggressions. Microassaults include racial epithets, hate symbols, or mistreating a person based on their race or gender. In my region, the display of Confederate flags outside storefronts and homes is more flagrant the farther I drive from the progressive island of Tallahassee. Some people fly the flag as a symbol of southern pride. For others, it's a *F***-You* flag of defiance. For some, it is a teenager's *"You can't tell me what to do or how to think"* sneer. In the North, it would be a "Don't tread on me" flag.

But the history of this flag is that it was flown in support of the whole system of southern apartheid. It was the flag of Jim Crow and a reaction to post-emancipation reconstruction. Its display increased dramatically after the *Brown v. Board of Education* decision that forced schools to desegregate. To a person who grew up African American in the South, it is a clear warning that you are in hostile territory. You may come into this business, but you had better be submissive. Show that you understand who's in control. *"Yessir. Yes, boss."*

I had a colleague who grew up in China. He moved his entire family from Indiana to Tallahassee to work with me on the computer modeling of racial disparities. He described driving with his family down to the coast of the Apalachee Bay, Florida's "forgotten coast." He said they thought about stopping for lunch until they saw Confederate flags outside of many businesses. He wasn't sure it would be safe for his Asian family to enter the restaurants.

Sue describes microinsults as *"subtle snubs, [that] clearly convey a hidden insulting message."* For Black students at elite institutions, they may be asked, "How did you get here?" Or to a third-generation Latino from El Paso, *"Your English is very good."* Microinvalidations occur when we gaslight people's lived experience. An example might be a white employer telling a prospective candidate of color, *"I believe the most qualified person should get the job, regardless of race."* As if racism didn't even exist.

A 2022 BuzzFeed article was titled "Latine People Are Sharing the 'Unwritten Rules' They Follow That Other People Are Clueless About."[12] Many of these "rules" developed as defense mechanisms to stave off constant microaggressions. Examples included the following:

- "Making sure our kids are always clean, have nice clothes, and neat hair . . . we don't want anyone thinking of our kids as 'dirty Mexicans.'"
- "I ALWAYS make sure to have my receipt in my hand when leaving a store."
- "Don't speak Spanish around non-Spanish speakers. They get offended and think I'm talking about them."

African Americans and other people of color in the United States adopt similar survival tactics. A recent California survey reported its results with the title, *Black Patients Dress Up and Modify Speech to Reduce Bias.*[13]

Growing up white and male, there are a thousand ways in which I can unintentionally give offense. I remember serving on the Admissions Committee for the Morehouse School of Medicine. One of my respected colleagues was presenting a candidate and mentioned a letter of recommendation. *"He describes the student as 'articulate,' which I hate,"* she said, *"but otherwise it's a really strong letter."* I did an internal double-take.

What was offensive about being called "articulate"? I thought about the letters I had written for students over the years. "Articulate" was a word I would mostly have written for students of color, wanting to make sure that admissions committees would not stereotype them as inarticulate. But I had never thought to use the word for white students, because, well, um. . . . And there it is. My implicit bias was revealed. Apparently, it was a common enough pattern for a historically Black medical school admissions committee to notice it. They experienced it as an insult. Sensitivity means listening to others reflect back to us how we are coming across.

Environmental invalidations are macro-level or systemic microaggressions. What if all the buildings in a university are named for white men? What if all the pictures on the walls have only token persons of color? Institutional invalidation is demonstrated by systematically underfunding public schools in Black neighborhoods. Then we blame Black community dysfunction for the high dropout rates. It also includes environmental issues such as the placement of landfills or industrial zones mostly in communities of color. The overabundance of liquor stores and fast-food outlets in poor neighborhoods is one more example.

Sue also captures why microaggressions can be such a thorn in the flesh. He calls it attributional ambiguity, that is, "the Catch-22 of Responding to Microaggressions":

> *Did what I think happened, really happen? Was this a deliberate act or an unintentional slight? How should I respond?*

For researchers, the Racial MicroAggression Scale (RMAS) measures "the racial indignities, slights, mistreatment, or offenses that people of color may face on a recurrent or consistent basis."[14] In addition to pathologizing cultural communication styles, denying individual racism, or invoking the myth of meritocracy, the RMAS includes "five items . . . of invisibility [such as] being dismissed, devalued, ignored, and delegitimized by others because of one's race." The scale correlates with measures of psychological stress.

Microaggressions are real. Microaggressions hurt. Microaggressions are exhausting. Education scholar William Smith has used the term "racial battle fatigue." It's the cumulative weight that Black students and faculty carry at predominantly white universities.[15] Women similarly experience both micro- and macroaggressions. The *Washington Post* published an article on "Rude Comments and Bottom Slaps: The Things Female Doctors Put Up With."[16]

Being sensitive to people's tender spots is essential to working effectively in a diverse, multigendered world. An LGBTQ-friendly provider network lists seven common microaggressions faced by trans people.[17] They include the following:

1. Asking for a "real" name or "preferred" pronouns
2. Using words like "regular" or "normal" as synonyms for heterosexual or cisgender
3. Showing intrusive curiosity or expressing assumptions about sex and bodies
4. Focusing on gender and sexuality when that's not an issue in treatment
5. Expressing cisnormative assumptions about trans people's goals for transition
6. Expressing assumptions about trans narratives
7. Assuming who someone dates (gender and sexuality are separate)

Additional insults that trans people often receive include abusive descriptions, "deadnaming" (the use of birth name without consent), and misgendering (saying "he" instead of "she" or "they").[18] Describing microaggressions experienced by LGBTQ persons "all the time," Kelsey Borresen reminds us that "it hurts whether they meant to do it or not."[19]

One additional group of people who face the challenges of stigma and marginalization are those who face mental health challenges. This group is not defined by demographics. Indeed, it may include any or all of us at different moments in our lives. Mental health is health. The late Rosalynn Carter advocated for equity in mental health treatment for decades, with a specific goal of reducing stigma. In 2007, she said this in a newspaper interview, "Stigma is the main thing. It hurts people so bad. It embarrasses them. Humiliates them. It leads to discrimination. . . . We have come a long way, but we have a long way to go."[20]

Barber et al. described three distinct forms of mental health microaggressions: (1) shaming and stereotypes about mental illness, (2) invalidating people's experience, and (3) blaming people with mental illness for their condition.[21] They list examples of what *not* to say to a friend or family member (or even to ourselves) when dealing with mental illness.

At the end of the day, sensitivity means actively seeking to understand each of our patients and our colleagues in their deepest core of individuality. This includes their social, cultural, family, relational, religious, economic, and even political context. It means trying to understand and to empathize. It means especially trying not to hurt people or to gaslight their experience. It doesn't matter whether they are different from me or I am different from them.

It matters that I seek to learn and to understand.

It matters that I care.

FOR FURTHER READING

Anzaldúa G. *Borderlands/La Frontera: The New Mestiza*, 5th Edition.

Fong TP. *The Contemporary Asian American Experience: Beyond the Model Minority*, 3rd Edition.

Lake I. *Embracing Identities: A Journey Through LGBTQ+ Experience*.

Sue DW, Capodilupo CM, Torino GC, et al. Racial microaggressions in everyday life: implications for clinical practice. *Am Psychol.* 2007;62(4):271–286.

Williams L. *It's the Little Things: Everyday Interactions That Anger, Annoy, and Divide the Races*.

12.

Nurture Self-Awareness and Humility

The flip side of being sensitive to others is becoming self-aware of my own history and culture. That means sifting through some of my own cultural baggage. My norms are not the world's norms. Multicultural experiences, especially ones that take us outside our comfort zone, are good and necessary. From them, we gain perspective.

Self-awareness is hard. We think that what we grew up with is normal. My friend, the senior Dr. Lonnie Fuller, grew up in Philadelphia. After he moved to Galveston, Texas, he said that it took him *two years* before he realized that in Texas, *he* was the one with the accent.

When our NCPC team at Morehouse School of Medicine was asked to lead cultural workshops, we were often asked to teach about specific minority ethnic groups. We were asked to teach on Hispanic or African American culture. But we were never once asked to teach on "White culture," "Anglo culture," or "doctor culture." The groups requesting the training were unconsciously saying that cultural differences represent "other people" being different. In relational terms, *"I'm normal and they're not."*

Humility is essential. There were moments in my past when I thought I truly understood. Then I found deeper levels of knowing. My head knowledge has not always transformed into heart knowledge. There are lessons of racial history that I have only recently learned. My journey in becoming an ally to LGBTQ friends and colleagues is decades behind my allyship on race and ethnicity. But I also know the joy of learning, the thrill of discovery, and the self-awareness of healing that has begun. With humility, I embrace a lifelong journey of growth.

Humility is earned every day. We all have moments when we are oblivious. I once read an exchange of letters to the editor in a women's magazine, about women's preference for female gynecologists. The magazine had published a letter from a male OB/GYN, who listed his credentials and decades of experience. He had delivered babies and provided care to thousands of women. The following month, another letter was published, this one from his wife. *"I love my husband dearly,"* she said. *"He is a kind and excellent physician. But he still doesn't get it."*

Self-awareness is the flip side of sensitivity. If my patient and I are experiencing a cultural gap or divide, I need to remember that neither of us is the "other." We're just different. Growing up as a white, cisgender, Protestant male, I grew up in the cocoon of majority norms. By definition, I have cultural blinders. Women and persons of color and LGBTQ individuals have all in some ways known what it is to be minoritized. They have almost always had to negotiate with majority culture to find their path. White guys can be oblivious.

Sometimes I notice a difference in the way my patients interact with me. I say to myself, *"that's different,"* often unconsciously. My little lizard brain, working deep down in the zone of instinct, pulls back a little. It's trying to understand if this person is odd or if they don't like me. And then the other person notices that I am pulling back. Once again, they are the one who is made to feel different.

If I am tired and people behind me in a grocery line are speaking loudly in another language, I become irritated. It happens especially with a language that seems harsh to my ears. It's not mean, it just is. We need to be self-aware of how those unconscious instinctive responses can be triggered. They are triggered not because others are different but because we are different from one another. No judgment. Self-awareness is a first step to growth. Honesty is the first step toward healing.

My own self-awareness has come slowly. My wife and I did a five-week elective rotation in a rural area of Haiti during our final year of medical school. We spent months preparing. We studied the Haitian Creole language with cassette tapes. We read books to immerse ourselves in the culture. Our experience was deep and transformational in many ways. Two moments are specifically relevant to conversations about race, culture, and self-awareness.

The first moment came after a few weeks in-country. We had been working hard in the clinic and hospital for days. One Saturday, some of the American doctors decided to go to the coast and go snorkeling. They had hired a local fisherman to carry us out to the reef in his small, handmade wooden sailboat. We dressed in full-on tourist gear, with swimsuits and hats, sunglasses and sunscreen.

When we arrived at the beach, waiting for the boat, a small crowd began to gather. Not a small number of people but a large number of small people. The Haitian children were playing a game the missionaries called, "Let's go stare at the Blancs" [whites]. I had never really been self-aware of my race. Here, the Haitian children had normal skin. We were the ones who looked different. We were "the other."

When Haitians wanted to tease the white Americans, the imitations would always involve a hat, a pair of sunglasses, and a wristwatch. With much animation and laughter, our Haitian friends would act as if they were very busy and very important. They would pace back and forth, constantly looking at or tapping their watch, much like the white rabbit in *Alice in Wonderland.* "I'm late, I'm late, for a very important date!"

"We're not all like that," we would say. And the Haitians would just look at each other and laugh. We had told the best joke of the day!

The second moment of nascent self-awareness came when we returned home to Chicago. We had done intense preparation for going to Haiti, but we had done nothing to prepare for our return to the United States. In Haiti, we had seen soul-crushing poverty, matched only by people's unbelievable strength and joy and resilience. We had seen children with bloated-belly starvation (kwashiorkor) and red-haired malnutrition (marasmus). Kids routinely dug through our garbage for scraps of food. They had to outcompete the stray dogs who were also starving. It broke our hearts.

The first day we were back home, I went to a US supermarket. I found myself walking down the pet food aisle. And it hit me like a ton of bricks. *These people have a whole aisle for dog food! These people are nuts!* And it took a minute for the obvious insight to hit me. *These are my people!* It was the first time I had ever been blessed to see my own culture from outside myself. It was my first glimmer of self-awareness.

The parallels were there for health care as well. In Haiti, I saw a man obviously afflicted with tuberculosis. He was nothing but skin and bones, coughing up blood and having night sweats. His lungs were a mess when I listened with my stethoscope. But in the United States, we would need to see a chest x-ray (now a CT scan). The Haitian doctor looked at me as if to say, *"Don't you believe your ears? That's why we have stethoscopes."* An x-ray would cost a dollar. A month of medicine would cost a dollar. The patient only had a dollar. The patient wisely used his money for the medicine. I couldn't help myself. I pulled out a dollar bill to pay for the x-ray.

It wasn't for him; it was for me. I needed to see it. I needed to know that I could believe my own ears. My ears were right. The man had pulmonary TB.

These days, doctors in training think they need an echocardiogram just to diagnose a heart murmur. A patient can't get out of the emergency department without going through the ER tunnel (the CT scanner). I find myself an outsider. I look at how we practice medicine in America, with such an abundance of resources producing such mediocre outcomes. I often ask the question—*Do we need that test? Will it change the diagnosis? Will it help us make a different treatment decision?* My own internist looked at me oddly when I asked similar questions about getting a cardiac MRI for my cardiomyopathy. *"What decision will it help us make?"* I asked. He said only half in jest, *"You can't think like that. It will get you in trouble. This is American health care."*

We must become self-aware of our own cultural norms, values, and "hot-button" issues. Once we have taken our own self-inventory, we can understand what drives our responses to others. When we know the personal filters through which we view the world, we can begin to appreciate the filters through which others view us.

Even our technologies pick up our biases. When artificial intelligence learns from huge volumes of human content across the internet, it "learns" our biases about race and gender. By asking ChatGPT to take on the persona of a journalist or a Republican or even just "a man," the software sometimes produces incredibly toxic stereotypes. One expert said, "GPT-4 was deeply racist before the company's 'red team' muzzled it."[1]

In a visual experiment, an AI program was asked to produce an image of a Black doctor caring for white children in Africa. It couldn't do it. On repeated attempts, it produced images of white doctors caring for Black children or even Black doctors caring for

Black children. Somehow sensing that it was failing, the program even produced images of giraffes and zebras to see if it was getting any closer. Its biases couldn't be undone. Lacking self-awareness, it failed.

Sometimes we have to look in the mirror to see ourselves. One of my character traits is that I'm a chameleon. I am constantly and often unconsciously expending energy to be less white or less Anglo. At other times, I struggle just to fit in with the glaring brightness of my own white-world. I know who I am. I'm not Black. Even when generous colleagues of color wink and say they count me as one of them, I know I'm really not. If I ever acted like I really thought I could be Black, they would stop saying such things. I'm not Latine, even when people call me Jorge. I'm a white Anglo cisgender straight guy. By virtue of personality and early childhood dysfunction, I developed the ability to instantly read the temperature in the room. I can subconsciously shift my tone and temperament and language to "fit in."

I fully own that I'm a white male chameleon, able at times to be a little less white but never truly Brown or Black or gender-free. And I'm okay with that. *"Hi, I'm George. I'm a chameleon. A shapeshifter."* For much of my life, it's been my superpower. It has allowed me to mix freely and to learn from many people in a non-white world. On a good day, I can even sometimes see white-world (as in a mirror dimly) through their eyes. But this strength is often just the other edge of the sword of my personal weakness, a blurring of personal boundaries and sense of self.

Porter Braswell describes the skills he learned growing up Black in a white suburb. "Code-switching may be a survival strategy but 'culture coding' can be a superpower."[2] He says, "Being able to speak multiple languages or dialects, understanding different codes of behavior and expression, feeling authentically connected to a range of styles and art—all of these abilities amount to an incredible social and cultural versatility that we should celebrate in our society." This is like the power of having a rich diversity of people on a team.

The danger comes when white people think we can do it all ourselves. There's a fine line between this culture-coding superpower and cultural appropriation. Too often, white Anglo people like me steal the power or beauty of other people's culture and make its benefits our own. It's complicated.

Racial self-awareness is even more complicated because we want to believe that we are not white. We're just normal. Michael Eric Dyson says, "Being white means never having to say you're white." He goes on to say that even white allies, "who know that whiteness is privilege and power . . . also know that whiteness for the most part remains invisible to many white folk."[3] But other folks see it in us. A collection of stories by Langston Hughes is titled *The Ways of White Folks*.[4] Dyson says it this way: "Black folk have had to know white culture inside out. We know what coffee you like, what mood you're in, whether you'll be nasty or nice to us on the subway. . . . We know the fear you feel when we get on the elevator."[5]

I remember getting my feelings hurt when a friend told me that I couldn't come to see him during our summer vacation. His father wouldn't tolerate him having a white friend come to visit. I was oblivious to all the times when I had hurt his feelings, but I felt this sting very sharply. Three of us hung out because we didn't fit in with the rich kids. All three of us got admitted to Harvard together. They would graduate and I would transfer out. I guess I never quite fit in there either.

As a teen, I began to be aware of racial injustice, but I was oblivious to issues of gender or sexuality. I was immersed for most of those years in an all-boys rich-world white-male cisgender prep school. I soaked up and internalized a profound homophobia that makes me want to weep as I reflect on it. I had zero awareness.

What was it like to be a gay teen living in a prep-school dormitory in that gay-bashing, queer-hating world? Verbal and physical bullying were directed at teen boys who exhibited any hint of effeminate behavior. Wear a pink shirt? Taunts and abuse. Express weakness or a tender emotion? Get bullied back into "manhood." Get naked with other guys in the shower after a soccer match? Maintain an appropriate homophobic distance. Snap towels at each other and use gay slurs. I still get guilt-shudders.

Guilt is not a bad thing if it leads to insight and *repentance*. It's an old-fashioned word of remorse driving a sincere desire to change. It implies a willingness to learn and grow and make amends. We have to get past the kind of guilt that only fortifies defensive walls around our tender selves. Instead, we can embrace guilt as a motivator to grow and change and cleanse ourselves. We can find redemption in becoming something better, because we have grown through and grown out of a bad place.

For me and the boys I grew up with, our sense of gender was equally warped. It was a male prep school. Nearly all of my teachers were men. The school only began accepting female students in my junior year of high school. It unmasked my complete and profound social awkwardness and boy–girl doofiness. I didn't have sisters. The last female friends I had had were in sixth-grade public school. I had been completely immersed in teenage boy culture, reinforced by white male elitist-school teacher culture.

What helped was meeting Cindy. She became my best friend in college and then somehow my girlfriend and then my wife. We hung out together. We studied together. She made me laugh, and I could make her laugh. She says I helped her make it through Calculus. She helped me make it through college and then through life. She helped me to accept being me. She taught me how to love and how to be loved. She is my treasure.

Cindy was (and is) gently but persistently assertive in being treated as an equal. She stood up to her parents when she needed to. As a preacher's kid, she could peek behind the curtain to see the church in all its glorious imperfections. When the time came, I didn't ask her minister father's permission to marry her. She had taught me that it wasn't his decision to make.

We've been married more than 45 years now, through medical school together and raising kids and becoming grandparents. I hope she keeps loving me forever. When I walked our daughter down the aisle (actually a sandy beach boardwalk), the preacher asked, *"Who gives this woman in marriage?"* Instinctively I said, *"Her heart is her own to give, but she does so with our blessing."* I learned that from Cindy. I'm still learning.

When do we learn race and gender categories? Child psychologists tell us that categorization is universal. Assigning meaning (and bias) to those categories comes from cultural and family learning. For example, infants as young as three months old can differentiate facial features in a way that adults would categorize as racial. These infants will preferentially turn toward faces that are more similar to the faces of their primary caregivers. Over the early years of development, these facial preferences (which adults would see as racial characteristics) develop further. They are then influenced by the frequency of exposure to family and friends and caregivers.

Waxman then asks the key question: "When do infants' visual categories become infused with racial bias?"[6] The short answer appears to be preschool. By age five, children are demonstrating preferences for which kids they would prefer to play with. They judge which children are more attractive and which are more likely to misbehave. They begin to generalize these preferences or biases to other children of the same racial, ethnic, or gender groups. They learn it from us.

When my son was in those early preschool years, he had a conversation with his caregiver. Ms. Powell is an African American woman whom our kids still love deeply. Those relationships are complicated, but at that age, the exchanges are pure and sweet and honest. One day, our child's caregiver referred to herself as Black. *"Ms. Joyce, you're not Black,"* my son asserted confidently. He held his arm up alongside hers. *"Your skin is dark brown and mine is light brown. See?"* She smiled and told us that story proudly. She chose not to mention that her day-to-day reality in our community never allowed herself to forget that, in America, she was indeed Black.

Just a few years later, when Dan was seven, a colleague from Jamaica planned a visit. He wanted to attend the 1996 Summer Olympics in Atlanta on his way home from an international HIV conference. I had spent time with him as an external examiner at the University of West Indies, and we had stayed in touch over the years. He asked to stay with us in our home for a few days. *"Is he a Black doctor or a white doctor?"* Dan asked. *Omigosh,* I thought. *Where does he get this racist stuff at this age?*

"Why do you ask?" I probed gently.

"Because the Black doctors are the best doctors," he said confidently. *"They're the doctors who teach other doctors!"* I smiled.

Who were the other doctors he knew? They were my colleagues and friends from Morehouse. He knew Dr. Harry Strothers, my friend and fellow workaholic. He also knew my chairman and friend, Dr. Lonnie Fuller. He was the cool old guy who had taken us to play with his radio-controlled cars and helped us launch the sailing dinghy I built. Dr. Fuller built incredible model planes and boats and cars in a tricked-out workshop. Dan was charmed.

Dan had also met Dr. Louis Sullivan, former HHS secretary and then president of Morehouse School of Medicine. He saw how everyone treated him with the highest respect and deference. Dan had formed his racial categories. They were built on his experience knowing Black doctors as the ones who teach other doctors. Sure, it was a form of racial bias. But it was an antiracist bias. I decided I would let him keep this one for a little while longer.

Self-awareness requires humility. Humility means recognizing that none of us ever fully attains cultural competence. Instead, we make the commitment to a lifetime of learning, of peeling back layers of the onion of our own perceptions and biases. We become quick to apologize and to accept responsibility for cultural missteps. We embrace the adventure of learning from others' own lived experience.

My inadequate Spanish skills have led to many humbling experiences. There was a Mexican woman who spoke no English in the South Lawndale clinic in Chicago. Our staff were fluently bilingual, but they were super-busy. Our access to interpreters was quite limited. The woman came to me early in her first pregnancy. By the time I was ready to leave Chicago, I had provided all her prenatal care and delivered her two healthy babies. All with very stumbling Spanish. When I told her I was leaving, she wanted to tell me what I had meant to her. She started out hesitantly.

"Tengo el amor del Señor en mi corazon," she said. I misunderstood immediately. I did not know that *el Señor* was a way to say "the Lord" in Spanish. I just thought it meant Mister. I also did not remember that she had an evangelical faith in her Lord, Jesus.

"Perhaps you also have el amor del Señor en tu corazon?"

Wait . . . I was translating again in my head. *You have love in your heart, and you want to know if I have the same love in my heart?* I started to back up unconsciously. I looked at her strangely, and she realized what I was thinking.

"Aieee, no!" she cried out. *"El amor de Jesus,"* she said. I was embarrassed and apologized profusely. *"Si, tengo el amor de Jesus en mi corazon,"* I said. *"I do indeed have the love of Jesus in my heart."* And I really needed it in that moment and in many moments since.

We have to be humble also because our subconscious denial will make us completely oblivious to many of our flaws. Denial is not stomping our foot and saying that *"I'm not a racist!"* Denial is a subconscious or unconscious defense mechanism. It can make me blissfully unaware of my own implicit bias, or stereotyping, or racist thoughts, or white privilege. I have personal experience of how stubborn denial can be.

In my house is a deacon's bench. It was my grandfather's bench, handed down to me by my mother, with a story attached. This bench was in the workers' waiting room in my grandfather's orthopedic surgery practice. I accepted the story for years without a thought. I loved my grandfather Staben. He was awesome, a kind and gentle and dignified man.

Once I asked for more details. My mother explained, *"It was for the workers to sit on in the workers' waiting room. They would come in all dusty. The doctors didn't want all the other patients to get dirty."* Now you would think that my antennae would have perked up at the sound of *"the workers' waiting room."* Especially after caring for thousands of Black patients, some of whom had escaped from the segregated Jim Crow South.

It wasn't until I was speaking with a progressive lawyer in small town Central Florida that the bell finally rang in my brain. He was speaking about one of the older physicians in town. He said, *"I used to aggravate him by seeing him as a patient and sitting in the colored waiting room."* The gears turned. The shoe finally dropped. Colored waiting room. *The workers' waiting room.*

My beloved grandfather, practicing orthopedics in the 1940s and 1950s in Springfield, Illinois, the city where Abraham Lincoln practiced law, had two waiting rooms. My grandfather enforced segregation in his medical practice. The good news is that he cared for Black patients. The bad news is that he had a *"colored waiting room."* And I was more than 30 years old before that seemingly obvious conclusion even danced close to my conscious thought.

Denial is a powerful thing. To her dying day, my mother would not believe that this could be true about her father. She adored and hero-worshipped him. She saw the world through a generous, rose-tinted set of glasses. But mom was in denial. I was in denial.

Grandfather Staben was not perfect. He was a product of his day. I like to believe that he provided compassionate care to all his patients. But he enforced racial segregation in his practice. He had a colored waiting room. I love my mother, and I love my grandfather. But none of us is perfect. I was oblivious.

Denial is also a defense mechanism. It prevents us from seeing the privilege we enjoy or the pain that we inflict. And as any drug addiction counselor will tell you, denial is rigid and strong, but brittle. It resists obvious evidence or truth until it begins to crack. And when it cracks, it can crash down with spectacular force. It's scary to feel it begin to give way. To feel that first crack I think is the source of the anger and defensiveness Robin DeAngelo has described as "White Fragility."[7] In the prologue to *Invisible Man*, Ralph Ellison describes the dangers inherent in breaking through my denial as being akin to waking a sleepwalker: "I remember that I am invisible and walk softly so as not to awaken the sleeping ones. Sometimes it is best not to awaken them; there are few things in the world as dangerous as sleepwalkers."[8]

Sleepwalkers are the un-woke. Sleepwalkers are straight white folks in denial. Sleepwalkers are dangerous. But I too have pockets of denial.

I can't bear to think of myself as a racist, because most of my self-esteem is built on my self-image as one of the good guys. Me a racist? I can't bear the thought. Just like all the patients I've ever confronted about their drinking or drug abuse. *"I'm not an alcoholic. I'm not an addict. Why would you say such a thing?"*

Denial still holds me back. How is it that I can be quick to acknowledge rampant discrimination and disadvantage experienced by people of color, but I find it so doggone hard to acknowledge that every day, in thousands of ways, I am advantaged? I enjoy the very white male privilege I would hope to overturn. I am, at the same time, that rich white kid that I resented and that rich white man that I became, even as I am forever the janitor who cleaned rich kids' toilets.

The very power of denial is that we are completely unaware. For example, white people get a greater placebo effect when a useless cream is applied to a skin rash by a white or Asian male physician than when it is applied by a Black or female physician. It's all happening at a subconscious, neuro-immunologic level. That's how insidious implicit bias can be.[9]

We saw this denial whenever we did workshops on cultural and racial competence. Dr. Kofi Kondwani and I (and sometimes a Latina colleague) provided a series of trainings to virtually all of the staff of the Alabama Department of Public Health. Their leaders had made participation mandatory. Most participants were polite but cautious. African American participants were more enthusiastic (*"they really need this,"* they would whisper, looking over their shoulders). In those sessions, we heard all of the typical responses catalogued by Robin DiAngelo:

- I don't see color. I just treat everyone the same.
- I don't care if you're Black, white, green, or purple polka-dot.

The common theme to all these responses is how important it was for white participants to protect their walls of denial. To acknowledge being a racist or benefiting from white privilege would conflict with their core self-image of being a good person who *"just treats everyone the same."* When their own testimony seemed insufficient, they would play the ultimate power card, the MLK card. *"Didn't Martin Luther King say that we shouldn't judge people by the color of their skin but by the content of their character?"* Apparently, this is the one quote by MLK that white Americans can quote nearly verbatim, but most of us still miss the context. The actual quote is this: "I have a dream that my four little children will one day live in a nation where they will not be judged by the color of their skin but by the content of their character."

White folks like me want to jump ahead of the hard work of breaking through our walls of denial. We want to skip engaging in the hard work of self-examination and truth and reconciliation. We want to leap ahead to a postracial world, where there is no racism and the color of our skin really doesn't matter. Dr. King suffered no such illusions. He knew it wasn't our reality. It was a *one-day-in-the-future* dream. We might achieve it, one day. But only if we were willing to do the hard work. In the words of Michael Eric Dyson, this is "the paradox that many of you refuse to see: to get to a point where race won't make a difference, we have to wrestle first with the difference that race makes."[10]

In my mind, I have many metaphors or ways of thinking about race in America, and none of them are adequate. I think of a dysfunctional family, of being children of an abusive parent who favors one child while abusing another. And then the children grow up and don't know how to sort it out. And their kids are a mess too. But in the context of our denial, I think the model of addiction can help. I am addicted to white privilege. I have to confront the racist stuff embedded so deeply inside myself. I am addicted to living within white-normed social structures and economic structures. And the first step in my process of recovery is to break the denial and to acknowledge that I have a problem.

"*Hi, I'm George. I'm a racist and a white-privilege addict.*" Or even, "*Hi, I'm George. I'm a White Guy. And I'm beginning to understand how and why that matters in our country.*" But hearing the cracks in my walls of denial, feeling the floor tremble beneath my feet, makes me recoil in terror. I want to feel good about myself. I want to be one of the good guys.

Another opportunity for us to engage in humble self-awareness is in the arena of gender justice. When I transferred as a resident physician to Cook County Hospital. Ms. Andrea Muñoz was our residency program coordinator. She was Dr. Prieto's right-hand person. She ran the details of our residency. She also had a fierce sense of social justice, polished by years of working in the farm-worker movement with the movement's co-leader Dolores Huerta. Ms. Muñoz waved me into her small office from the clinic hallway. She had heard me talking about one of my fellow residents. *"Did you just call her a 'sweet girl'?"*

"Um, yeah," I said, thinking that in the South, it would be a compliment. Right away I had the sense that I had said something wrong. *"She's a woman,"* she said fiercely. *"She's your colleague. Don't ever call her a girl, okay?"* Um, okay. I hadn't really thought about it that way before. Dumb, dumb, dumb! Blinders. Always getting me in trouble. And thank you, Ms. Muñoz, for making me a better person.

In some ways, gender bias is even more deeply embedded than race. Infants perceive gender differences. Even before kindergarten, they begin to put those differences into social categories they learn from their parents and caregivers. Before the baby is born, nurseries are decorated in blue or pink. At the baby shower, gifts are given that reflect our cultural definitions of what defines a boy or a girl. Is it any wonder that our brains have been programmed to see gender in such binary terms?

All this is reinforced in a thousand different ways by our cultural definitions and social structures. How we dress, what bathroom we use, what sports team we can join, what dorm room (or hospital room) we can share—these all are binary-gender coded. Even our religions, and sometimes especially our religions, reinforce these rigid binary definitions of gender. Jesus and Buddha never did, but sometimes our religions do. They reinforce a male-dominated version of gender identity. They often define very rigid family and societal roles for each gender.

Secular society does the same. *Men Are from Mars, and Women Are from Venus*, says the book title. Notice the assumptions:

(a) that there are only two choices (binary-gendering) and (b) that people of these two genders are very different psychologically in ways defined by their gender. But isn't the world so much more complicated than that?

Much of our core sense of self and our family roles are wrapped up in these gender identities. It can be scary to try to deconstruct them. Can I even imagine myself in a different gender frame? I cannot hope to be in a meaningful relationship with persons of color, an ally of gay or trans friends, or a voice for gender justice if I cannot admit to myself that I am a white, cisgender straight guy. And I have all kinds of conflicted feelings about it.

The good news is that we can overcome our own unconscious bias. We can become a more self-aware person. We can work to create more self-aware organizations. We can bring programs that reduce bias and discrimination in measurable ways.[11] We can change our teams and our institutions, but it takes time and effort. We must lead in a consistent manner over an extended period of time.

A first step is to practice organizational self-awareness. That means actively seeking to understand the culture of our own institution. After spending 25 years working in a historically Black medical school, six years working in a community-based migrant and community health center, and several years training in a large diverse urban public hospital, I came to work at Florida State University College of Medicine. This school is in the top 10 of all majority institutions in the country for medical student diversity. We have high proportions of both African American and Latine students. But I had only been at FSU for several months when I walked away from a meeting and said to no one in particular, *"Dang, this place is white!"*

I honestly didn't know what had triggered the thought. Was it the way in which all the white people arrived at the meeting with

SWAT team precision exactly on time? Or was it the way a colleague of color was teased for showing up a few minutes late? Was it the presumptuous use of first names? Was it just a head count that I had unconsciously learned from my colleagues who instinctively check every room they enter to see if they are the only person of color or woman or gay person present?

Maybe it was the discussion of minority issues in the third person (those people). Or perhaps it was the mention of racial identity only for minorities (she's a Black nurse). Could it have been the complete discounting of Tallahassee's own segregated health care history? I've spent hundreds of hours in meetings where I was the only white person. Now I was sitting in a room with mostly white people, surrounded by a community that is 30 percent African American. Later that day, an African American colleague poked her head in the door of my office. *"I heard you say that, and I almost busted out laughing!"* she said. *"I'm so glad you said it!"* And then she was gone.

One of my roles at FSU has been to serve as chair of the Council on Diversity and Inclusion. In that role, I was surrounded by people who have tremendous lived experience. They continue to teach me every day. They also describe the myriad ways in which they can feel marginalized in our own institution. I count it as a great strength of our College of Medicine that such a council existed and was empowered to take action. We had a voice with our dean and with senior leaders in our COM Executive Committee. At the same time, I grieve that our governor and Florida legislature has passed laws to make any such Diversity/Equity/Inclusion (DEI) activities illegal.

Part of me felt that we should not have this council led by a straight, cisgender, white, Anglo male. But I also didn't want to pile on with more of "the Black tax," the expectation that a small number of minority faculty will serve on every committee and mentor every minority student. Another member of the Council, herself an African American woman, helped convince me. She told me, *"You can say things in a way that the dean can hear it. Maybe because it's coming from a white man. Maybe it's the way you can say hard things in a gentle way, and then say it again in another way. You're polite and respectful, but you don't move on until they hear you."* I hope so.

Cultural competency in any setting may require decades of immersion, not just in the clinic but in the community as well. Even then, we are at best amateurs in another person's culture. A realistic goal for busy clinicians is to learn specific behaviors and habits that will allow us to be more culturally effective.

We also must continually learn ways to avoid missteps that are culturally offensive or culturally dysfunctional. We must be quick to apologize. Asking forgiveness of a patient or a nurse's aide is not taught in medical school, yet humility is an essential skill. We need humility to say, *"I'm sorry."*

No one ever fully attains cultural competence. Humility is what gives us the freedom to peel back layers of our own perceptions and biases. Tervalon argues that cultural humility is more important than cultural competence.[12] One of the quickest ways to exercise humility is to take on the role of student. Elevate our patients or other community members to the role of teacher. Each person is the world's expert on their own experience and cultural perceptions.

At the end of the day, I can no longer avoid the fact that white privilege and white denial are essential elements of my core identity. I am a white guy. And by God's grace with the patience of friends and colleagues, I am healing. I am humbled by life. I am growing and learning. I am taking baby steps toward standing for racial justice and gender equity and LGBTQ alliance. I am on a wondrous journey of growth and self-discovery.

I am, indeed, a white guy healing.

FOR FURTHER READING

Hughes L. *The Ways of White Folks.*

Lekas HM, Pahl K, Fuller Lewis C. Rethinking cultural competence: shifting to cultural humility. *Health Serv Insights.* 2020;13:1178632920970580.

Lupton RD. *Toxic Charity: How Churches & Charities Hurt Those They Help.*

Nordell J. *The End of Bias: A Beginning: The Science and Practice of Overcoming Unconscious Bias.*

Oakley B, Knafo A, Madhavan G, Wilson DS, eds. *Pathological Altruism.*

HEALING AND HOPE

13.

Inner Healing

Full disclosure—I want to change the world.

I want to heal the world. I want to heal our nation of all its racial divisions. I want to heal my state of its polarizing politics. I want to end all of its bullying of the marginalized. I want to heal my community of all its inequities and its denial. I want to heal my institution of its biases and its pride.

I want to heal it all. And deep inside, I know that my own need to be a healer, my drive to make a difference, is inextricably intertwined with my own brokenness. I also want to be healed. I need to be healed.

I came from a dysfunctional family. I was born to a broken father who was himself abused by an alcoholic and abusive father, the World War I war-hero grandfather I never knew. I was born to a mother who was our saint and our solace, our source of unconditional love and grace. But this same grace and patience that allowed her to endure decades of emotional abuse also made her the perfect enabler of my father during his "dry-drunk" rages or his occasional actual-drunk spells. She enabled his self-pity and his incessant neediness and insecurity. She submitted to his overarching need for control, even as she found in him all that there was to love.

So fair warning. I see America through the eyes of a white guy who knows a dysfunctional family when he sees one.

By now, many readers will have given me various diagnoses or at least wondered what my diagnoses might be. *From what exactly am I healing?* I have used the language of psychology to describe my own deep childhood sense of inadequacy. I am driven to somehow be enough. I have used the language of family dysfunction to describe the emotional abuse of my father and he from his father. And I have used the language of addiction to describe seeking recovery from racism and genderism, as well as my own addiction to self-sacrificing altruism. Finally, I have used the language of racial reconciliation and social justice to describe our need for societal healing in America.

There was a moment in my life when I became acutely aware of my need for healing. I had been working an exhausting schedule, on-call day and night for a full year straight with no backup. I had taken on a leadership position as medical director of our multiclinic community health center. Meanwhile I was the only physician, partnered with a wonderful nurse practitioner, caring for all the patients in a busy rural clinic. My schedule was day and night, 365 days a year, for our patients in the hospital or nursing home. I was also managing the doctors and clinical programs of two other clinics, three dental units, and a birthing center. I was becoming exhausted. I needed help. Desperately.

We finally hired a second physician for this site through the National Health Service Corps. Dr. Redd (not his real name) was well trained. He was an MD family practice physician who also had a master's degree in public health. Just like me. He could articulate a vision of community health development. Just like me. He had a positive spirit and a warm way with people, but he was a bit of an introvert. He needed time to think about what he was doing. Just like me. The only difference was that he was tall and athletic, with movie-star good looks. Not like me at all.

We worked very well together for the next year or so. He was (and still is) an impressive physician and human being. He was my partner, my backup, and my friend. I could actually take every other weekend off. I finally had some relief, and I began to think that it would all be okay. Then I got a call from the emergency department at a hospital 30 minutes away. My friend and colleague had been admitted after having had a seizure in his bathroom at home. I raced to the hospital straight from my house in blue jeans and a scruffy jacket. *"I'm Dr. Rust,"* I said as I walked into the emergency department. It wasn't my primary hospital, so no one knew me there. ER nurses looked at me skeptically.

My friend was being admitted to the hospital. A family physician whom I knew was his doctor. He pulled me aside and said, *"Let's talk."* He explained to me very calmly, but firmly, that my colleague had a drug problem. A major drug problem. Morphine and hydrocodone. He had been injecting opioids into his veins. On this day, he had shot up in a tiny vein between his toes, to hide his addiction from his wife and from all the health professionals who thought we could spot a drug addict a mile away. I had trained at Cook County Hospital at the height of a heroin crisis and worked every day with this guy and never had a clue? He was a great doc. He cared for people with the most challenging complexities compassionately and efficiently. He was my perfect doc. He was *just like me.*

It turns out he was using morphine and other drugs to come down from the incredible stress of doing what we did all day long. His wife said that sometimes in the evening he would be so exhausted he would just sit in a chair with his head slumped and his eyes glazed over. In retrospect, she realized that he was not just exhausted, he was drugged. Self-drugged.

Our state was ahead of its time in helping health professionals with addiction. What was then called the Impaired Physicians Network has now become the Professionals' Resource Network (PRN). It is a national model for dealing with professionals whose problems of alcohol or addiction or mental illness limit their effectiveness. In some divine coincidence, Dr. Kerr had been active in building the program. He knew exactly how to get Dr. Redd started. He would stay in the hospital overnight and then move immediately to a drug rehabilitation program designed for physicians. Doctors can be especially challenging to work with. We intellectualize and rationalize and take over group sessions. The answer is to put us in a group with other docs who are also dealing with drug addiction. They can be brutally honest about what it takes to recover.

When I got home from the hospital that night, I fell into bed exhausted. I woke up the next morning and tried to make sense of it. I realized that I had to go see our hospital patients. I let the nurses know that Dr. Redd would not be on-call that weekend. Or that week. Or ever? I suddenly found myself sobbing like a little child. I wept a little for my friend but mostly for myself. I was back on the burnout treadmill, and I didn't know when I could ever get off. I think I've cried like that maybe two or three times in my whole adult life.

Wait, who's the patient here? My friend is the one with the addiction. He's the one in recovery, right? But how is it that this friend with opioid addiction could be so much "just like me?" About that time, I started reading a book that helped me understand my own need for healing. *We Are Driven: The Compulsive Behaviors America Applauds*[1] was written by faith-friendly psychologists. Through personal inventories and checklists, they helped me to see explicitly the similarities between drug addiction and my more socially acceptable compulsive behaviors.

My inadequacy had been expressed over the years in what academics call the CV-deficiency syndrome. It's the compulsive need to have more professional degrees behind our names. One board certification isn't enough, so I'll get two. An MD degree isn't enough, so I'll get a master's degree in public health. I feel less-than, so I have to become more-than. I could publish scholarly papers—is 100 enough? My name became embellished by abbreviations and credentials: George Rust, MD, MPH, FAAFP, FACPM, . . . M-O-U-S-E. As a psychologist might say, we don't build walls around areas of strength.

One of the insights that came from reading this book was the notion that helping others in community service could be a form of addiction itself. Sacrificial service especially could be a form of unhealthy, compulsive behavior. Mother Teresa syndrome, they called it. *Wait, whaaaattt?* I thought that what I was doing was a faith-driven, sacrificial-service mission. It was supposed to be good and pure and noble.

The authors had me cold even with their chapter titles. "Events That Set the Cycle in Motion—Family of Origin, or Major Life Trauma." Emotional abuse, unpredictable rage, family dysfunction—check, check, check. Freshman roommate's suicide? Guilt over missing all the warning signs? Double-check. Subsequent chapters addressed those "whispers from the past." They called out my negative self-talk of inadequacy or shame. They summed it up in this chapter title—"Driven to Be More to Keep from Being Less." Ouch! Nailed it.

They described my compulsive behaviors as "addictive accomplishments." My drivenness expressed itself in being a rescuer, a martyr, and sacrificing self for others. Others have called it pathological altruism[2] that takes well-meaning behavior too far.[3]

The answer is not to just go all in on selfishness. We have to distinguish psychologically healthy, morally robust altruism from this unhealthy, self-sacrificing, ego-propping altruism.[4] Being generous and considerate of others is generally a good thing. Helping those in need is good and right. But doing so in a way that always places my own needs (and my spouse's or family's needs) second to the needs of others is not so healthy.

I can spot pathologic altruism in other people a mile away. Among dedicated colleagues, I have seen it lead to burnout, divorce, absentee parenting, and addiction. In my own life, it sometimes made me choose work or mission over parenting. I remember flying somewhere to give a speech when my wife was soon to deliver our second child. At the time, I had no thoughts of how selfish that might be. But healthy self-care is not selfish. We now start teaching our medical students about self-care from their first day of class because frankly, my generation of physicians was no darned good at it.

In community health work, I often see two variants of pathological altruism:

1. Self-sacrificing service to the point of self-destruction
2. Altruistic service that actually harms those we are intending to help (e.g., the "toxic charity" of church mission trips)

Dr. Paul Farmer was a hero to many of us in the mission of global health equity. He built a program of community health development in Haiti (*Zanmi Asante*). He then expanded the *Partners in Health* model to scale across several continents. An infectious disease specialist at Harvard, he took on the issue of multidrug-resistant tuberculosis. He then proved the value of treatment as prevention for HIV. He built out programs that relied on local strengths and talent. He trained community health workers to deliver needed care in a cost-effective and sustainable model. Clearly, this was altruism at its best and highest form. His book, *To Repair the World*,[5] inspires our students, just as Dr. Farmer inspired many of his colleagues.

A more complex and nuanced perspective is presented in Tracy Kidder's book, *Mountains Beyond Mountains*.[6] In reading it, I found myself transported to the Haitian countryside where my wife and I had had our first experience of global community health. Dr. Farmer saw beyond the beauty and the poverty to see what so many Americans fail to see—the strength and resiliency of the Haitian people. He built creatively on their capacity to engage in community-based public health work. But I also found myself profoundly saddened at a moment in the book when Dr. Farmer faces a choice between his life's work and his family roles.

How many times have I seen this happen among my most dedicated colleagues? How many children of doctors or civil rights leaders wished only that their mom or dad would have given their parenting the same passion and energy that they gave their mission? I say this not to judge, but it resonated deeply with me. By the time our second child was born, it was obvious that I was consistently choosing my work over my role as a husband and as a father.

I am blessed to have a wife who loved me enough to call me on it. At the same time, she loved me through it. My life as a migrant clinic doc was clearly not sustainable. I had to make a change to be a father but also as a matter of self-care. I had to leave the clinics. I had to find a role in which I could still make a difference but in a way that flowed from my strengths.

I needed to do what I was built for, to engage in meaningful work that was also re-energizing. I needed to care for others, but I also needed to teach and write and have boundaries. I needed to go home at a decent hour to be with my kids before bedtime. I also needed some introvert time, solitary quiet time for reading and writing and recharging. I needed to heal if I were to be able to keep healing.

Many years ago, as my insights were beginning to emerge, I gave a talk about burnout to friends at the Christian Community

Health Fellowship. It was a room full of incredibly devoted health professionals. Many of them were beginning to question the sustainability of the paths they had chosen. I talked somewhat clumsily about my newfound insights. I spoke of my need to be "Amazing-Man"—serving the poor, changing the world, being the smartest guy in the room—just to feel halfway good about myself. I felt like it was never enough. I was never enough. Of course, I enjoyed the applause at the end of my talk. Of course, I listed the speech on my CV. Of course, I still need healing.

The trouble with these compulsive, inadequacy-driven behaviors is that in and of themselves, they are good works. The world needs people willing to help meet the needs of others. Communities need people willing to serve and some willing to lead. Do I stop doing everything until I get my head on straight? Must I have pure motives and a clean bill of psychological health to continue? If so, I'm afraid that this work would come to a screeching halt all over the world. Mixed motives are the best we can hope for. A psychologist researcher at Morehouse gave me some helpful advice one day. Talking about our drivenness and passion for making a difference, he said, *"It's a powerful big dog, my friend. You need to keep it on a leash."*

And these experiences were part of my process of learning to find balance. I had to set boundaries. I had to engage in self-care. I had to practice the sometimes psychological, sometimes spiritual, discipline of knowing that I am enough. Or at least that God's grace is sufficient. I had to leave the farmworker clinics because I had made the workload and call schedule sustainable for everyone except me. I had to leave because we had two children and I wanted to be present in their lives. My wife had her own reasons to make a change, being on-call 24/7 as the only pediatrician in South Lake County. It was not sustainable.

In this process, I gained insight into my introverted personality and my need for quiet time to re-energize. I had to align my true self with the mission that I was better built to do. I found a life that balanced serving with teaching and writing. I even came to love doing research. We could ask important questions and answer them with methodologic rigor. *"What if We Were Equal?"* asked Dr. Satcher. We ran the numbers, wrote the paper, and entered into a national conversation about eliminating health disparities.

So how does this journey of healing relate to white guys seeking social justice? Who we are enables what we do. What's inside us spills out when we're bumped. If we are angry and driven, we probably aren't helping. If we are self-confident and oblivious, we probably aren't helping. If we are fragile or timid, we probably aren't helping. If we are in denial, pretending that we live in a postracial world, we probably aren't helping. In the end, if we aren't doing the hard inner work of healing, we probably aren't helping.

Ruth King talks of *Transforming Racism from the Inside Out.*[7] She speaks of moving from implicit bias, subconscious denial, and inner conflict to "wise awareness." She offers specific mindfulness techniques for moving through this process. The first few times we try it, we're going to see some ugly stuff inside ourselves. Everything in us is going to want to shut down and run away. We tell ourselves that it's not who we really are. And in one sense, we are right. These are just thoughts and feelings deep down inside us. We have the power to observe them and feel them.

We can realize that these thoughts and feelings are separate from the self who is observing them, the self who can make conscious choices about what to let go. And in detaching ourselves from the superficial icky thoughts, we find enough peace to swim deeper, where we find new and deeper, ickier thoughts and feelings. With proper grounding and calming techniques, we can find the peace and courage to stay in those moments a little longer each time.

Learning to meditate as a spiritual discipline or as a secular practice of mindfulness can teach us self-calming, self-awareness, and self-compassion. The practice allows us to dig deeper while maintaining a "third eye" self that gives distance and perspective. It's our safe-ground solid foundation for letting go. King suggests a 5-5-5 approach—meditate for five minutes a day, five days a week for five weeks until a habit or new discipline is formed.

My racing brain doesn't do well with sitting meditation or slow-motion yoga, so my own practice takes different forms. One is a combined eye movement and breathing technique before I sleep at night. A second is a walking meditation that uses a mantra cycled with my steps, in a rhythm that brings peace. My walking path is often through the beautiful tree-covered canopy of the FSU campus. My mantra comes from the Hebrew prophet Micah. It has the perfect rhythm for my pace and the perfect balance for my dysfunction: *"Do Justice, . . . Love Mercy, . . . Walk Humbly, . . . with thy God."*

My third meditation is simply to be in and of nature, especially connecting my soul with the earth's water. I often fish alone. Miles at sea, I stare endlessly at the shimmering Gulf waters. My gaze is brightened by the wondrous surprises of nature—a pod of dolphins, a sea turtle, ocean birds, or a fresh rain. I notice the sea color change as we reach deeper waters. It's my solace. When I fish with a buddy, it's a friend who seeks the same solace. He has seen and experienced horrible trauma both as a Black man and as a police officer. He also needs the healing of the salt air and sea. In these moments, we need no words to be together.

Many forms of meditation start first with simple mindfulness, a conscious awareness of sensations in the moment. For students who get stressed before exams, I sometimes recommend the 5-4-3-2-1 exercise. It can be adapted for people with varying sensory challenges. Start by looking around the room, left and right. Name five specific things that you see. Then notice four things that you can touch or feel. Notice how you feel in your seat and then how your feet are connected to the ground. Notice the feeling of your breath, in and out. Then listen. Focus on three distinct sounds that you hear. Some will be external. Perhaps the third will be the sound of your own breath. Listen to it, in and out. Then go deeper inside. With your breath, notice two things that you smell. Can you experience their scent and yet be distant from it? Now feel the inside of your mouth. Can you notice the taste of your own lips or tongue or self?

These self-calming techniques get better with practice. They aren't going to help in the moment when you've just been accused of racism or when you've experienced another microaggression. They won't save you when someone has just stepped on your last nerve. Unless you've practiced them as a discipline. Every day. When you are not stressed and when you're only a little stressed. You'll get better and better at it, until you can call up a sense of peace and third-eye distancing whenever you need it. These are what allow us not to run away or hide from racial tensions but to work through the conflict.

Resmaa Menakem describes racialized trauma as "soul wounds" that we each carry in our bodies.[8] Whether we are Black or white or other, we carry this load, albeit in different forms. He points out how such traumas are passed down through generations, sometimes through culture and sometimes through the epigenetic expression of our DNA. He offers practical thoughts and body-centered skills for healing in this space.

One of the critical insights Menakem offers is that calming techniques can be used wrongly for an outcome that does not heal: "Instead of inviting and accepting healing, they use settling in a neurotic way, to *avoid* healing . . . they flee the situation, and then partly soothe and settle their bodies with meditation, prayer, yoga, hiking, and so on."

Psychotherapist and Buddhist teacher John Welwood called this "spiritual bypassing" and "premature transcendence." He notes how we may use spiritual practices to sidestep or avoid facing unresolved emotional issues, psychological wounds, and unfinished developmental tasks.

I recognize myself in some of Menakem's insights. He observes that "some people can become extremely calm and low-key under stress. . . . They use their body-settling skills to disengage and disassociate."

How do you think I made it through childhood? When dad is yelling and mom bursts into tears, where can a little boy's mind go to hide? But I'm slowly learning to do it the hard way. On a good day, I can use my calming techniques to stay in the moment and work through the hard stuff. One day at a time.

One area of inner healing that requires self-calming and self-compassion is the discipline of self-examination. Identifying implicit biases is hard and sometimes painful but necessary work. It becomes possible only if we are kind and gentle with ourselves when we trip over our own ugly spots. In *The Inner Work of Racial Justice*, Rhonda Magee says, "We can do more harm than good if we are not able to bring kindness and compassion to it."[9]

That one's hard for me. Sometimes I burp up a racist thought or gender bias like a bad onion from yesterday's cheeseburger, and I hate myself for it. Decades of consciously working on this stuff, and I still have those dirt-nuggets buried in me. *What an idiot,* I say to myself. My inner voice can be harsh with negative self-talk. Self-compassion is often harder than feeling empathy or compassion toward others.

But with practice, I can choose to consciously observe the thought or feeling. I can examine its origins and then watch it leave my consciousness. I can remember that the self who is observing is also the self that is wanting to become better. One of my colleagues is a white Anglo sister who spends her workdays caring for migrant children. She has this to say about negative self-talk. *"Would you talk to your patient that way?"* Can we at least show ourselves the same nonjudgmental, compassionate caring that we would show to our patients or our friends? Can we choose to be therapeutic in those moments? Can we hold our own hand on a journey of self-discovery and growth, just as we would hope to do for others?

Let's do an exercise together. So much of our own core sense of self is wrapped up in our gender identity that it can be scary to deconstruct. But what if I could put aside (somewhere safe) my "sex assigned at birth" and my culture-bound gender designation. Can I engage in a journey of self-discovery beyond one gender? What are the personality traits and feelings I have that are more in the zone of masculine gender norms in our society? Which ones are more feminine? Which ones do I feel more pressure to express? Which ones do I tend to tamp down? What about me doesn't really fit any of these norms or fits both at the same time? Try to observe these thoughts and feelings in compassionate self-awareness without judgment.

Are there moments when I could relate to a sense of feeling genderqueer, or non-binary, or gender-free, or just me? Imagine that we are completely free to be ourselves. Can I imagine being a two-year-old playing on a playground with other children? Imagine relating to each other as little kids, entirely uninhibited by society's gender expectations.

Take a deep breath. Be mindful of how you are feeling. Be self-aware. Did the thought experiment make you feel free? Were you more at peace with yourself? Or did it cause your muscles to tighten, your breath to quicken, or your anxiety to emerge? Either way, notice the thoughts and feel the feelings. Observe them and notice that you have a separate self that can see the thoughts and feelings without *being* them. Take another deep breath and seek the compassionate perspective you might have if you were counseling another person who was experiencing these thoughts and feelings.

Can you see two men kissing in public and feel warmth and joy for their love? If you identify with them, do you fully accept and love yourself? Can you imagine loving a person whose outward appearance above the waist matches the woman that she is but whose genitals still match the male sex they were assigned at birth? Do you feel love and acceptance, or is there something in you that recoils? Perhaps you identify personally with this. Maybe you went through a time of inner conflict between who you are and who others thought you should be?

Be mindful and self-aware. Notice the thoughts and feelings without allowing them to define the *you* that is observing. Do you feel vaguely anxious? Where do those thoughts and feelings come from? Was homophobia or transphobia explicitly taught to you by your parents or teachers? Did it come from school bullying and peer pressure? Is it from culture or religion or politics or online social networks? Take some more deep breaths. Close your eyes. Relax your muscles. Can you let the sense of your instinctive reactions drift to one side? Look for a path toward empathy and warmth. Can you embrace people as they are and as they love?

For many of us, such exercises help us call out biases we are already struggling to overcome. They may also help us uncover new biases we were not even aware of. We call these implicit biases. Discovering these can be quite threatening to our self-image of being good people. We believe in our hearts that we are not racist or misogynistic. But maybe we are?

Peeling back layers of the onion, we come to understand that there is always another layer. The good news is that we are making progress on the journey. Each layer of the onion we peel back can turn an implicit bias into a conscious bias. Now we can work on it. We can learn more. We can actively engage in justice and allyship. That's progress.

Some of my self-compassion is to understand the connections between my current character traits and my dysfunctional history. My chameleon nature was born from early childhood, hiding from a father's unpredictable anger and hurtful words. Those were in turn born out of *his* childhood experience of his father's alcoholism and violence. My chameleon nature at times puts me in the role of being peacemaker. At other times, I seek only to blend into the wallpaper to avoid being hurt. I do need healing. We all need healing. And much of the healing I have found is in the embracing of my gift and owning my vulnerabilities. I live in recovery, one day at a time.

Leonard Cohen said, "There is a crack in everything; That's how the light gets in." Hemingway said, "The world breaks everyone, and afterward many are strong at the broken places." I tell our students that we begin to be able to help broken people when we at some level can embrace our own brokenness. This too is a gift.

I realize that I am writing all this as a white guy. For me, I have work to do that relates to my white-guy privilege and bias. Some of these approaches of inner healing may also apply to people of color, to feminine people, to gay people, and to trans or gender-queer individuals. They may or may not be helpful to people with any of the various intersections of marginalization. It is not mine to say.

We all have our stuff to deal with. It's not useful for me to tell you what *your* stuff is, but we all have stuff. And none of us is immune to internalized racism or gender rigidity or sexual bias. Some of our stuff may be our reaction to marginalization. Some of it may be in how we've grown up marginalizing others. Some of our stuff may be internalized trauma.

We may even need to seek professional help to avoid injuring ourselves further in remembering our trauma. We may have angry feelings to deal with. We may have fears or perhaps grief to process. We won't know until we look inside. We won't grow until we let go and engage in the process of becoming our better selves.

Here's an example of how we can work on our own fears. In this case, it is a fear that is both instinctive and subconscious, learned at a very early age. My wife showed me a picture of a snake the other day. I recoiled and asked her not to do that ever again. If I see a picture of a snake, the adrenaline squirts into my bloodstream. My heart starts racing and my pupils start dilating before I can even know what I've seen. And that's just a picture!

Never mind that I have held garter snakes in my hand. I know that most snakes are harmless and essential to our Florida ecosystems. I can tell the difference between an indigo snake and a water moccasin. I know which one can cause actual danger. I once was chased down a wooded path by a small water moccasin while a bunch of good old boys at the fish camp laughed. They cheered both for me and for the cottonmouth all at the same time. They just wanted to see the show. A big water moccasin once swam toward our canoe while my daughter and I paddled furiously in reverse. The point is, water moccasins are dangerous and aggressive. They are the a**holes of the snake world, but that doesn't make all snakes dangerous a**holes.

Fight-or-flight responses tend to form fast-track neural pathways in our brains. They're like my armed robbery fear track that can be triggered by loud red pickup trucks. One technique for managing these is summarized in the mnemonic RAIN: Recognize, Allow, Investigate, and Nurture.[10]

R is for "recognize." I can't deal with it, until I become self-aware of this bias. I now recognize this fight-or-flight reaction I have to snakes.

A is for "allow." The other day I fussed at my wife for showing me a picture of a snake. But today, I bring it into my consciousness. I am grounded and at peace enough to address it. I allow my mind to call up the image of a snake, with all of its attendant thoughts and fears.

I is for "investigate." A dangerous snake once chased me. I call up that memory. I notice my feeling of fear. I notice how my pulse, even now, has quickened. I remember learning from a young age that my father was deathly afraid of snakes. My brain now is hard-wired to think that snakes are dangerous and scary. None of this is occurring at a conscious level, until I bring it forward.

In the original version of RAIN, N was for "non-identification." That seems a bit abstract, but it's a way of noticing that I can have two selves in this moment. I can certainly have a self that is feeling scared of snakes. But I can also have a self that is sitting quietly and observing this fear. It doesn't matter that the fears are irrational. They are real. Still, I can distance myself. I am not the fear, I am me. As Magee suggests, "Now allow these thoughts, sensations, and emotions to drift away, to fall into the earth. Let them go."

In other versions of RAIN, N is for "nurturing." I can feel compassion for the little boy of my past and for the frightened man of my present. I can speak self-affirmations of love and comfort to this fearful child-man. I can hug myself (when no one's looking). My heart still races when I see a snake, but now I am okay with it. I can calm myself. I can see my neural pathways of bias or fear and choose not to ride them. I can use my learning to decide what is the appropriate response. If it's an indigo snake, I smile. If it's a water moccasin, I pick up a big stick and slowly back away.

It's not enough, though, to do the inner work just for my own peace of mind. I need to do it to have relational healing as well. Here are two sides of the coin of disciplined self-growth. On one side of the coin, the 12-step approach asks us to make "a searching and fearless moral inventory of ourselves." We are to "admit to our Higher Power, to ourselves, and to another human being the exact nature of our wrongs, and to ask that these defects of character or shortcomings be removed." That's hard work. It takes a lifetime. Some of this language seems pretty blunt and harsh. It is written for clarity and to leave no room for denial or rationalizations, in the context of addiction.

But even as I am rigorously taking moral inventory, I must not be tearing myself apart. We do this by engaging in self-compassion, differentiating self from thoughts and cultivating an awareness of our emerging better self. Minoritized communities don't need white (or male or cisgender) guilt and shame. Notice it. Deal with it. Let it fall away. We can't lay it on others and expect their forgiveness. We can't expect others to make us comfortable in our own skin. This is our work to do.

Grow in your self-awareness. Face the truth. Feel those feelings. But also be grounded in your compassionate self, the self that can observe these feelings but not *be* these feelings. Stay grounded and at peace, focusing on the self that is seeking to understand and grow. This is the self that can examine and even regret, but the self that can also be therapeutically compassionate. The centered self can also discern (in consultation with others) how best to make amends. This is the self that can both grow and let go.

The inner work of healing doesn't have to assume pathology. None of us has yet achieved cosmic perfection. Most of us have unresolved psychological issues. Most of us have internalized implicit biases around race or gender or sexuality or abilities. We can see our journey toward being an effective ally, or being a champion for justice and equity, as being a journey of healing toward our most positive potential. I'm doing the best I can. In fits and starts, I see progress. I'm doing a little better now than before. I have a long way to go.

In the Christian traditions, we speak of grace and unconditional love. This was at the essential center of my own healing, although I wish I could have skipped some of the acculturated religious baggage. In the Buddhist tradition, Ruth King describes a discipline and practice of "metta, a Pali word for unconditional kindness—friendliness and genuine acceptance."[11] The Dalai Lama has said that his true religion is kindness. Self-love and self-compassion are essential for creating that safe space in which we can examine ourselves. That's how we let go of that which holds us back or hurts others. Being okay with ourselves now is how we grow into being the open and loving people we want to become.

Over the years, I have learned tremendously from patients and friends who are living in recovery, whether from addiction or chronic mental illness. I have found that the people who are most successful are those who have many pillars supporting their recovery. Inner healing requires a balance of inward and outward activities, some that may be clinically therapeutic and some that are more broadly healing in their nature.

For some, medication is essential. It may provide the initial healing that allows us to attempt other modalities. Professional therapists can unlock new insights and teach us techniques to manage our runaway thoughts. Some form of regular exercise is essential, perhaps as powerful as Prozac when it comes to treating depression. Being outdoors, being in and of nature, even taking a brief walk, all help bring our spirit and our brainwaves into connection with our world. What and when we eat has a long-term impact on our metabolism, as well as our gut microbiome. These in turn affect our brain biology and our mental health.

For many of us, tapping into our creativity is a source of solace and healing and hope. Listening to music, creating music, even simple tapping or whistling or singing in the shower, can all enhance our recovery. For others, creativity may include painting or sculpting or making jewelry. Many find knitting or crocheting to be contemplative. For me, building a wood-strip canoe was pure therapy.

A daily discipline of meditation or other grounding techniques is essential. For some, this could include a spiritual component, in whatever ways we might define connecting to something beyond ourselves. It may also connect us to a spiritual community, perhaps to others who seek healing and others who seek to change the world. We all have our journeys. We all need each other.

Having a support system of people in your life is an essential pillar of healing. We need people who will love us and support us no matter what. We need people who will tell us when we need a breath mint or when we have bias. We need people who will tell us when we need to take our meds or to check in with our psychiatrist. Sometimes these can be family, but sometimes family isn't the right answer for now. Some support groups like AA are formalized. Some are just friends and fishing buddies. None of us can do it alone, not even us introverts. Perhaps especially not us.

The point is, if we are to do the hard work of inner healing, most of us need a full-on, multidimensional recovery plan. That's true whether we need healing from the daily traumas of racialized or genderized stress or from trying to heal from racial bias or from being too judgy. We need professional support, social support, friends, and fellow-recovery peers. We need music and arts and creativity and spirituality. We need disciplines of grounding and self-calming meditation. And we need to balance the practice of generous compassion and of setting boundaries.

There is no one simple fix. It takes time. Building the harmonies and synergies of all our sources of our recovery will grow and change over time. They become even more beautiful as they become both the source and the expression of our healing.

Let's do what we have the power and privilege and influence to do right here and now, starting with our zone of greatest influence—our inner selves. Let's do the hard work of inner healing first, even as we move forward to do the work of relational healing and structural healing.

FOR FURTHER READING

King R. *Mindful of Race: Transforming Racism from the Inside Out.*

Lama D, Tutu D, Abrams D. *The Book of Joy: Lasting Happiness in a Changing World.*

Magee R. *The Inner Work of Racial Justice.*

Menakem R. *My Grandmother's Hands: Racialized Trauma and the Pathway to Mending Our Hearts and Bodies.*

14.

Relational Healing
From Bystander to Ally

So how do we find relational healing in this dysfunctional family we call America, where both Black and white share centuries of ancestors borne of an abusive relationship? How do the descendants of the colonizers make things right with the descendants of America's native peoples? As a child of this dysfunction, how do I reconcile with those whom my privilege has disadvantaged?

No matter what troubles I have seen in my life, I have not experienced being the unfavored child of this dysfunctional American family. I have not been the one who bore the brunt of the abuse and then didn't get included in the inheritance and to this day gets blamed for their own poverty. Ta-Nehisi Coates says that "in America there is a strange and powerful belief that if you stab a Black person ten times, the bleeding stops and the healing begins the moment the assailant drops the knife."[1] A generation earlier, Malcolm X painted an even starker image. He said that many white people "haven't even begun to pull the knife out, much less try to heal the wound. They won't even admit that the knife is there."[2] But denial doesn't work. We all need healing.

Here's a framework for seeking relational healing. I call it CARMA.

C: Connect and Communicate
A: Accept/Admit/Acknowledge/Apologize
R: Release/Repent/Redirect/Renew
M: Make Amends/Make It Right
A: Advocate/Ally with Others

The C in CARMA Is to Connect and Communicate.

We can't achieve reconciliation in the world unless we can achieve it in our own lives, with the people closest to us. We can't do racial reconciliation in the abstract—we need to reconcile with those whom we have hurt or who have hurt us, whom we have advantaged or disadvantaged. We have to connect. We have to communicate. We need healing.

Schools, neighborhoods, and churches in America are racially and socioeconomically segregated. To have any chance of reconciliation, people in disconnected groups must connect. bell hooks wrote that "healing is an act of communion."[3]

Sometimes relationships are seriously damaged. Forced reconciliation can actually cause harm. I came to some measure of reconciliation with my father in his later years but only by first learning to set boundaries. If I get this close, we can have a conversation. If I get closer, he's going to poke my tender spots. That defined the boundaries. We would visit but stay in a motel. When he started to drink and say stupid stuff, we would head back to the motel. We protected our kids, even as we wished they could spend more time with my mom. It was a dodgy dance of dysfunction.

My brother had a rougher road. All his life, he had stood up to our father. Valiantly, he protected me and our mother at his own peril while I quietly blended into the furniture. They continued to poke at each other and hurl their grievances until the end. Each expected and needed an apology from the other, and neither was able to give it.

For that reason, I was the one who arranged for Dad to move to his first assisted living facility when Mom was hospitalized with a bleeding stomach ulcer. I was also the one whom the paramedics called at 3 AM when Dad had fallen out of bed drunk. They put him on the phone only for him to tell me, *"I'm fine. Just tell them to put me in bed."*

No Dad, you're not fine. I didn't know until then that you could get kicked out of a senior-care home for bad behavior. Yup.

As he neared the end of his life, I saw more clearly the hurt little child inside him. I could feel compassion. He lost his power to hurt me. By the time he was in his last memory-care facility, I remember how small he looked, hunched over in his wheelchair. I leaned over and kissed him on the head, something I had never done before. I felt his loneliness.

I spoke at his funeral. I painted a positive spin on my father's bitter life and even cried a bit. My brother observed wistfully that I had come to some sense of peace with our dad. *"You obviously found some way to connect,"* he said. *"I never did."*

After high school, my brother and I had drifted apart. He married, had kids, and built a career. I went off to medical school and became a bit self-righteous. We sent cards on Christmas and birthdays.

After Dad died, my brother and I sensed that the time was right to reconnect. We made plans to spend a week together camping in the Chassahowitzka Wildlife Refuge. There was moss hanging down from the branches of old-growth cypress trees, next to creeks fed by springs of crystal-clear water. We spent our daylight hours fishing from an old wooden jon boat. There was a spot in the river where we caught freshwater bream on one side of the boat and saltwater mangrove snapper on the other. It was magical.

In the evening, we would sit in camp chairs watching the fire, seeking peace with each other. My brother and I had come to very different places in our politics, especially around issues like Obamacare. Avoiding conflict, I did not want to talk about it. But my brother did. And he was persistent, even as he was respectful. *"I want to know what you think. I know you have a different view, so I want to understand why."*

I explained, in a gentle and respectful way, that I saw people suffering every day because of their lack of access to good health care. I wanted everyone to have the best care our country could offer. I saw that other countries had found solutions. I wished that we could move toward a more fair and caring system. I said all this very softly and gently, watching my brother for his reaction. This trip was all about making peace.

Then he explained his perspective, and for the first time, I really listened. He wanted to choose his own doctor and go to whatever specialist he wanted. He wanted to have a relationship with his doctor free from government intrusion. He wanted that doctor to be able to choose where and how to practice medicine, with no government limits.

Somehow that clicked for me. He had a deep emotional need for a system free of controlling authority figures. It made sense. My brother was also describing autonomy, one of the core ethical values in medicine. We could each respect each other as coming from a place of moral and ethical goodness. We could still love each other. We disagreed, but that was okay. And we will forever cancel out each other's vote.

When our mom got cancer, my brother was there for her as he had always been. He stayed at her house, managed her affairs, and spent time with her every day. Later, he would become a friendly face to all the residents of her nursing facility. Mom and Paul would have a special chocolate treat each afternoon and look at old photo albums that made her cry with fond memories. I saw the tenderness of their love for each other. I saw the intense bond they had formed in defending each other for their entire lives. And I loved them both more than ever. When Mom passed, we came together again. We both felt the healing.

In my work life, I have also had to engage in relational healing. Over the years, I have held various positions of leadership as a white guy in majority-minority organizations. Medical director, department chair, center director. I built and led diverse teams. In the Forming-Storming-Norming-Performing cycle of team dynamics, the storming part often included overtones of race and gender, of old wounds and mismatched power. We learned to work through it.

When I recently went back for a visit to Morehouse, a former colleague thanked me for the organizational culture we had created in the National Center for Primary Care. *"We could be honest, we could be ourselves, and we could talk about anything,"* he said. *"It doesn't happen by accident. It takes leadership. You have to be intentional. And you were."*

In the context of a non-white world, how do white guys connect and communicate? How do we enhance each diverse team member's sense of *belonging*? The first step is simply to get to know people who are different from you. Spend time with people of diverse race or ethnicity, or sexuality, or gender identities. Be people together. Form relationships. Learn from each other. But don't force it. Sometimes the Black kids do need to sit together in the cafeteria. It's the same for people of color working on your team. You need to let it be.

If you're the team leader or boss, recognize also that there's a power mismatch. You're their boss, not their buddy. Both of you need some boundaries. But don't be too rigid. In my experience, African American and Hispanic organizations have strong core values like *personalismo* and *familismo*, balanced by *respeto* and *dignidad*. Personal relationships are important, as is creating a sense of family among members of the work team. But even in closeness, show respect.

It's important to let each of your colleagues know your commitment to diversity in all domains. While I was writing this chapter, I got this message on LinkedIn from someone I thought was just another straight white guy.

> *Hi, George, I hadn't heard that you left Morehouse. Anyway, I started transitioning and came out as trans in July 2019 . . . I hope you are doing well.*
>
> *Alice*

It had been some years, so it took a moment to remember who this person was. I had known them before only in their male gender expression. I felt warm and good that Alice had reached out to share their transition with me. I wanted only to help them feel warmth and affirmation in return.

> *Hey Alice,*
>
> *So glad to hear from you. We are all on a journey to becoming our true and better selves, aren't we? Hope to see you again one day.*
>
> *Peace,*
>
> *George*

One thing I have learned from being embedded in minority organizations is to recognize diversities within diversities. No one person can speak for their entire group. When we did an Asian supplement to our Georgia Health Disparities report, Atlanta's Center for Pan Asian Community Services conducted surveys across 12 different language groups. Even within those groups, there were significant heterogeneities.

Mistakes are often made by majority-white institutions who consult with "the community" by seeking the input of one visible spokesperson. In our community, there is an extraordinary

African American minister and civil rights leader who has built tremendous resources to serve his community. But he has one person's point of view. He has his own organizational loyalties and a certain generational perspective.

At a point when FSU was deciding where to build a clinic, he was the main source of input from "the Black community." Unfortunately, he completely missed the concerns of another group from "the Black community." It blew up as a conflict, an unforced error on our part. Our leaders learned their lesson, and on the next go-around, they consulted with various stakeholders and came to a much more positive community partnership.

A second step, and this is crucial, is to get off your own turf. Get out of your safe space. Find a way to be with others in *their* safe spaces. The great gift of working in a farmworker clinic and an HBCU was that I was working in organizations centered in African American or Latine culture and power. I was in the minority, and the power dynamics were right. Everyone could be robust in their self-expression, fully belonging without shape-shifting to meet white norms. And they could direct me within *their* cultural values and sense of mission.

Finally, if you are a leader on diverse teams, invest in people's success. See their strength and resiliency and potential. A parting gift when I left Atlanta was a framed Morehouse T-shirt with signed notes from many of the people I had worked with. Many noted how we had supported them getting advanced degrees or promotions. Soon, even the mid-level leaders in our center had gotten a reputation for asking their team members, *"Where would you like to be in five years? How can we help you get there?"* We didn't just ask. We followed through with tangible support.

Ultimately, relational connection and a sense of real community must occur at a deeper, even spiritual level. Desmond Tutu uses the word "Ubuntu" to describe "the essence of being human . . . in community, in koinonia, in peace." Tutu offers a Xhosa saying:

"A person is a person through other persons. . . . I am because I belong."[4] That's "Ubuntu."

The First A in CARMA Is to Accept/Acknowledge/Admit/Apologize.

If you think you are part of a diverse team, it may not be enough. In a historically white institution, the organizational culture is probably way more white-normed and male-normed than you can see. Spend time at an HBCU or an African American community nonprofit. Lots of time. Go to concerts (or weddings or funerals) at a Black church or a Spanish-language mass. Accept invitations to a Passover *seder* or a Ramadan *iftar*. Go with friends to a gay club or a Pride parade. Have town-hall meetings in church basements where you are the only white guy in the room, and really listen. Leave the country and immerse yourself in another culture, not surrounded by Americans. Know that you are just toe-dipping but try to see yourself and your organizational culture as others would see you. Get outside yourself.

Begin addressing some of the ways in which white-guy norms may have left people on your team or in your organization feeling "othered." Ask the naive questions. Explore openly whether your meetings and leadership conversations have a male or female-normed pattern of communication. Have a conversation about friendliness *("Hi, just call me George")* versus respect *("They call me, Mr. Tibbs!")*. These patterns instantly communicate which cultural group is dominant in a meeting.

In a new language, right after I learn to say hello and goodbye, I try to learn *"I'm sorry."* I know I'm going to misspeak or offend or make cultural missteps. But apologies are not enough. Desmond Tutu says, "If I come into your house and steal your belongings, I cannot then go home and say, 'Well, I forgive myself, so all is right in the world.'"[5] He and his daughter describe action steps, including admitting the wrong, apologizing, and asking for forgiveness.[6] But they emphasize a step that is often neglected. "Make amends or whatever restitution or reparation is called for and needed."[7]

The challenge in a group built on white-guy-normed expectations is that people from minoritized groups will have learned to adapt. They may have survived by convincing you that you are just fine. They might even say that they like it better your way. Have Asian team members adopted Anglo names to make it easier for other people to pronounce? Do people cover their tattoos? Such is the price of surviving in the work setting. What's required is to respectfully listen and talk about differences in a safe space. It can't just be your safe space. It must be a safe space for the most marginalized people. This all takes time, often years. Don't rush it, but don't put it off either.

Michael Eric Dyson reminds us that "whiteness . . . is most effective when it makes itself invisible, when it appears neutral, human, American."[8] Overcoming this will take a very intentional process that amplifies minoritized voices. If you're a white-guy leader in this setting, you may need to do dozens of sit-down, shut-up-and-listen sessions with small groups of minoritized individuals. It will only be effective if you have earned trust over time.

You need people who will tell you how it really is for them. In this context, outspoken people and angry people and "troublemakers" are your most valuable asset. You need to listen to all the voices. And then you need to be their ally and amplify their voices when you go back into the room with your white-guy-normed team. But remember who has the power in your organization. You're putting your minoritized colleagues in danger. Don't expect them to fall on this grenade for you. They may be going along to get along, and they can't be sure that you can or will protect them.

Start with respect. Have repeated conversations about how we show respect to each other. Explore the diverse ways in which people receive being respected. Shift your meetings in the direction of respect versus superficial friendliness. Shift your communication style in the direction of more respectful listening. Make sure each person feels heard. The more the white guys have the power, the more it is that *we* are the ones who need to change.

We are living and working in a non-white, multigendered world. If Michelle Obama didn't feel that she could wear braids in the White House, how does a young African American woman handle her cultural expression in your organization? Are braids okay? Young people are fine with tattoos and nose rings and body piercings. Are you? Purple hair? Non-gendered clothing choices? How far are you willing to go to make sure that anyone on your team can be fully themselves? How do you make sure that no one is trying to be "less Black" or "more American" or "less gay"? How far are you willing to go to make sure that everyone adds value to your team precisely because of who they are?

I was getting a little preachy about this in one of our Executive Committee meetings. One of our senior leaders leaned over and whispered, *"But what if being fully themselves means they're a racist a**hole?"* So yes, there are some boundaries, some guard rails that make it safe for everyone to be fully themselves. No one has the right to make another person feel "less than" or "other." Your right to individual expression ends where your fist hits my nose, both physically and relationally.

The R in CARMA Is to Release/Repent/Redirect/Renew.

White guys, let us not underestimate the grievous violence and oppression that are at the core of our history as a people. Our land is stolen land, stolen first from American Indian nations and then again from Mexico. It began first with colonization and then slavery. Those were the horrific start but not the end. Do not minimize the subjugation of women under male control, through religion and culture and even the law. In the past, our Constitution denied women the vote and even their personhood. We continue to pass intrusive laws to control women's bodies in reproductive choices. In the 21st century, we carry forward economic inequalities across race and gender. There has been an ongoing effort to undermine the self-worth and humanity of all people of color. Trans people are being targeted with extreme prejudice.

We must not underestimate the pain and grief of it all, often caused by straight white men who have gone before us. I know that I am not those men. I know that I did not do those historic wrongs. But I live in the legacy of those wrongs. And I benefit from the racial and gender advantages passed on to me in wealth and health and education. I live in privilege. I didn't ask for it, but we are the children of that dysfunction. And denial does not lead to healing.

Liberation theologist James Cone summarized "repentance for white people" as "dying to whiteness."[9] Michael Eric Dyson devotes an entire section of his book to this challenge of "repenting of whiteness." How do I do *that*? Robin DiAngelo says it like this: "I strive to be less white, . . . to be less racially oppressive . . . more racially aware . . . interested in, and compassionate toward the racial realities of people of color."[10] Can I do that? Where do I start?

There cannot be reconciliation without truth. There cannot be redemption without justice. One of the ways we perpetuate ongoing racial injury in the United States is when we engage in denial. We gaslight those who would remind us of our history. We pretend it never happened. We turn the knife and reopen the wound. Rev. Joseph Lowery, dean of the civil rights movement, often said that "we live in the 51st state, the state of denial."[11]

On the front page of my newspaper one morning, our Tallahassee Memorial Hospital (TMH) ran an ad saying, "Caring for *you* for 75 years." If I were an older African American adult reading this, I would react with some anger. *"The hell you say!"* TMH began its history caring only for white people. They began admitting people of color only after Medicare forced the issue in 1964 by threatening to withhold funding from segregated hospitals.

Saying that TMH has been caring for "you" for 75 years says one of two things. Either TMH would like everyone to forget its segregationist history, or they only think of the white community when they think of "you." Those who were marginalized and injured by a segregated medical care system are in the category of "other."

When President Bill Clinton offered our nation's apology to survivors and families of the US Public Health Service's Tuskegee syphilis study, he told survivors, "What was done cannot be undone, but we can end the silence."[12] Deconstructing our denial is a lifelong project.

AA's Twelve Steps include the following:

- [Continue] to take personal inventory and when we are wrong promptly admit it.
- [Make] a list of all persons we have harmed and [be] willing to make amends to them all.

So how do we do that? Moses H. Cone Memorial Hospital in Greensboro, North Carolina, provides an example. In a community partnerships meeting, a senior executive publicly apologized for the fact that their hospital had offered unequal care during the era of racial segregation. Two miles away was the site of 1960s lunch counter sit-ins. But this 21st-century meeting was the first time that anyone had ever officially acknowledged the segregated history of Greensboro's health care system.

The apology was taken as sincere because there was a real commitment to making amends. The hospital offered real structural change, real dollar resources, and a real commitment to achieving the goal of equitable health outcomes. Archbishop Desmond Tutu said this: "Forgiving and being reconciled are not about . . . turning a blind eye to the wrong. True reconciliation exposes the awfulness, the abuse, the pain, the degradation, the truth . . . but in the end it is worthwhile, because there will be real healing."[13]

What do we do with the sadness we feel over the sins of past generations? Can there be generational remorse or repentance? Can we say, *"I'm sorry"* for the sins of our fathers or forebears? I say yes, for two reasons. One is that we often live in circumstances of relative privilege born of the history of our not-so-distant ancestors. We must not only apologize for their actions but for our own lack of action now. We can experience a genuine sense of repentance that leads us to make amends and to set things right.

Second, do we not feel national pride for what America has done right in the world? Do we not feel local pride when our community responds with resiliency to a natural disaster? Do our hearts not swell at the patriotic themes of the Fourth of July? Should we not then also feel national remorse over slavery and Jim Crow or the criminalization of same-gender sexuality? Family dysfunction and abuse, with all its guilt and shame, carry down over generations. Truth and reconciliation are needed. If the abusers have passed away, then the generations that follow must stand in for them to seek healing.

At times, we need to make room for the release of pent-up emotions. I described in a previous chapter how our students reacted during a resurgence of white nationalism alongside multiple police murders of unarmed Black civilians. Students of color needed to express their anger, rage, frustration, and exhaustion! Where was it safe to let all that storm of emotion out in our buttoned-down, professionalized, historically white FSU College of Medicine?

In those moments, they taught us how to release and renew. Let it be raw, and let it be real. Validate the feelings. Create safe places. Share in the anger. Absorb the anger with generosity and grace. Be silent in that sacred moment.

White guys get angry at injustice too. But we also may need to process white guilt or white shame or male insecurities. I'm often struck by how people react to Dr. Henry Louis Gates when he gives them their ancestral histories on the show *Finding Your Roots*. Sometimes African Americans are moved to tears by the stories of resiliency shown by slave ancestors. European Americans often take pride in the courage shown by ancestors who left everything to come to America.

Others find out bad things about their forebears, whether they were born out of wedlock or born of the rape ("union") of a slave by a slaveowner. Those who learn that a great-great-grandfather was an unrepentant slaveowner may react with a sense of shame. *What do we do with that?* Truth is, none of us have any control over our own ancestry, neither to take pride nor to take blame. What we must own is what we are doing now with the inheritance.

The M in CARMA Is to Make Amends/Make It Right.

Making amends is essential, if done in a constructive and community-affirming way. It must also be proportionate to the centuries of harm done. We need to start in our own little spheres of influence. It was one thing for me to identify gender differences in salaries when I was chairing a department, but saying *"I'm sorry"* wasn't going to cut it. Not until I got the institution to make salaries equal did I have any moral authority to say that we were going to treat everyone fairly. Desmond Tutu talks about white people in South Africa feeling entitled to reconciliation and forgiveness "without their having to lift so much as a little finger."[14] Does this not describe 21st-century America?

Relational healing means truth before reconciliation and justice before redemption. History must be rewritten to include the perspective of those who saw it from the painful side. The consequences must be measured. Reparations or recompense must be made, no matter how costly or how long term the price, The same principles apply to healing teams. Often I have colleagues come to me for advice on situations where the racial dynamics of their teams are going off the rails.

In one example, a highly accomplished, scary-smart, sharp-tongued, and brilliant tenured professor was unintentionally but repeatedly undermining trust and destroying confidence in a researcher they mentored. They couldn't identify with the lifelong experience of an African American scholar so often made to feel "less-than." It is critical to build competence and confidence in parallel. Don't find what's wrong with people's work until you've found 10 things that are right with it. Overpower microaggressions with microvalidations. And if you inadvertently knock someone down with your critique, apologize and work harder at building them back up.

A research team was being led by a super-smart, task-driven, young white PhD researcher. She was quickly alienating several similarly young, equally smart African American PhD colleagues. In her temperament, the white PhD was task-driven and a bit controlling. Her colleagues of color expected a collaborative process, and she was acting like their manager. They expected to be treated with respect and equality. They needed to see trustworthiness before they could trust.

In all her whiteness, she was completely missing the racial dynamics that amplified her missteps. She was assuming privilege and power. She was valuing tasks over relationships. She was focusing on her short-term objectives rather than group attainment of goals. In the words of an old African proverb, sometimes you must "go slow to go far."

Another colleague was building a unit to engage our community in research, focusing especially on minority populations. She heard me speak on community partnerships and about building trustworthiness as an institution. She asked for my help. But she had already finished hiring a team comprising almost entirely white women. *"What can I do to build trust?"* she asked. What indeed.

The Final A in CARMA Is to Advocate/Ally with Others.

In each setting, we must find a way to use our voice, to spend our privilege, and to be an ally. John Lewis said this: "A young person should be speaking out for what is fair, what is just, what is right. Speak out for those who have been left out and left behind."[15] Young or old, we must all speak out.

In his Nobel Prize acceptance speech in 1986, Holocaust survivor Eli Wiesel said, "Neutrality helps the oppressor, never the victim. Silence encourages the tormentor, never the tormented."[16] As early as 1946, Albert Einstein called racism America's "worst disease." He went on to say that racial segregation was "not a disease of colored people, but a disease of white people," adding, "I will not remain silent about it."[17]

One of the simplest yet toughest disciplines is to know when to speak up and when to shut up. If we consider speaking up as just a thin slice in a much larger sandwich of important behaviors, we'll come closer to getting it right. Here's the sandwich:

- Be Quiet/Listen
- Affirm/Echo
- *Speak*
- Affirm/Echo
- Listen/Be Quiet

In 2023, three Tennessee legislators took to the floor of their statehouse chamber to advocate for gun legislation after a mass shooting. They hadn't been allowed to speak under regular order. Two were young Black men, Representatives Justin Jones and Justin Pearson. The third was a 60-year-old white woman, Gloria Johnson. Guess who was expelled and who wasn't?

In all of the media appearances that followed, Representative Johnson could be seen encouraging and supporting her young African American colleagues, without stepping forward to take the microphone. When she was finally asked about why she was not expelled but her two colleagues were, she said simply: "I think it's pretty clear. I'm a 60-year-old White woman. And they are two young Black men."[18] An MSNBC commentator reacted spontaneously, "That's what an ally looks like."

Don Lemon says it this way: "Sometimes you're the right messenger for the moment; sometimes you have to be brave enough to be quiet and carry water for someone else whose voice deserves to be heard."[19] There is a discipline of knowing when to step up and when to step back. Here's my process:

- Hang Back to Learn and Understand Context
- Step In to Be an Ally
- "Step Up" to Engage in the Fight
- Step Back for (non-white-guy) Heroes to Shine
- Be Supportive and Available
- Step Away to Create Space for (non-white-guy) Leaders to Blossom

Sometimes being the white guy is useful. When dealing with larger and whiter institutions than Morehouse, I sometimes was given the role of white-guy liaison. I was the designated "whitesplainer" when leaders at historically white institutions were unintentionally sabotaging our partnership. For example, our research team at MSM's National Center for Primary Care had developed some positive relationships with smart folks at Georgia Tech. They had big data analytical expertise and computer assets that were different from what we had. At the same time, they truly valued our expertise in clinical medicine and our nuanced understanding of the intersections of race, health, and poverty. The potential synergies were tremendous.

But when I first met with my Georgia Tech counterpart, he started rattling off all the brilliant colleagues that could work with us. Each of them could bring a half-dozen PhD post-docs to work on our projects. *Great, right?* And authentically generous. But our young, small, underfunded historically Black medical school had nowhere near this scale of human capacity. Five full professors and their dozen grad students would overwhelm our team. They would end up dominating, no matter how noble their intentions. They would end up taking our Morehouse ideas and becoming the lead authors on "our" papers and "our" grant proposals. If we weren't careful, we would be co-opted. Again.

I pulled my Georgia Tech counterpart aside and asked if we could talk about the dynamics of a relationship between a large institution and a smaller one. He seemed open. *"There really is a cool synergy here,"* I said. *"But picture an elephant and a flamingo trying to dance. Entertaining to anyone watching, kind of dreamy for the elephant, but scary-dangerous for the flamingo."* He nodded. *"I don't want Morehouse to get stepped on while we're trying to do this dance."*

Then I told him my leprous lumberjack story, one that has framed all of my work with community partners. I was in medical school and preparing to do overseas medical work. Dr. Paul Brand, one of the world's preeminent leprosy specialists, spoke to a group of us in a workshop on community health. After decades in India, he had come home to lead the Hansen's disease (leprosy) hospital in Louisiana.

Dr. Brand described his practice of trying to shake hands with each of his patients. He wanted to give them a human touch and to make sure they knew he wasn't afraid of their disease. He wanted to erase the historic and biblical and persistent stigma of having leprosy—seeing each person not as a leper but as a person healing from leprosy. He told of a lumberjack, a mountain of muscled manhood in a flannel shirt. Dr. Brand would reach out his hand to shake, and Mr. Lumberjack would just cross his arms and shake his head. Finally, after some weeks of this interaction, Dr. Brand asked the man, *"Why won't you shake hands? You're not infectious. I'm not afraid."*

And the man replied, *"I have no feeling in my hands, but the strength is still there. When I shake hands, I sometimes don't know that I'm squeezing too hard until the other man cries."* Dr. Brand looked at us, an eager group of white American physicians-in-training. We were all full of idealistic zeal to go help the poor and make a difference in the world. He said, *"As American physicians, you have money and resources and knowledge and technology, but they are way out of proportion to that of the people you would serve. You bring great power and great strength. But without sensitivity, it can crush the people you are trying to help."*

My Georgia Tech colleague took it to heart. We talked a few more times to develop a strategy, and out of it came the NCPC Research Wizards of Methodological Magic. Every Thursday morning, the Wizards team would meet around a small table in my office. From my Morehouse team, we would have a couple of PhD researchers and maybe an emerging MD clinician-scholar. From Georgia Tech, we took on a PhD candidate and his faculty advisor. I was there as a facilitator since I knew just a bit about everyone's areas of expertise.

It worked. We tackled the question of why there were racial disparities in childhood asthma and cancer and multimorbidity. The rule was that everyone on the team participated in every project. We each could bring unique knowledge or methods and teach it to the others. We produced a bunch of peer-reviewed published papers, the coin of the realm in academic careers. Papers led to grants, which in turn funded salaries for our team.

More importantly, the work brought us into the larger national conversations about health equity. Soon the Morehouse team was recognized for a level of sophistication in big data research not previously seen in a small minority institution. The synergies with Georgia Tech were essential, but no dependency had been created. No image of inferiority had been created. We each found benefit. But we needed a little white-splaining to set the stage.

Sometimes I've been given a seat at the table of decision-makers, where being quiet would mean being complicit. In 2023, I was in a meeting of Florida's State Health Improvement Plan steering committee, chaired by our ideology-driven State Surgeon General. He was surrounded by public health professionals but new to the field himself. He had begun making a series of decisions with little input from stakeholders or actual experts. In this case, he had personally scrubbed the State Health Improvement Plan of any mention of health equity, which used to be one of the plan's pillars. Health equity has been a core value of public health for decades, so I called him on it. Said I noticed. I asked him to explain, because I knew that no one else in the room could afford to call him out.

In that moment, I knew I would not win the day. But I put him on the record. The *Tampa Bay Times* picked up on it and pushed him to explain. If I'm a true ally and advocate, then I have to speak up when there are racial inequities being swept under the rug. If you see something, say something. Try to say it in a way that they can hear it, but say something. To be silent is to be complicit.

Throughout my career, I've had to be intentional about this question: What is the proper role for a white guy in the battle for health justice and health equity? My answer is, *"It depends."* There are times when an institution is so white and so male in its culture and norms that it just can't see itself. A white guy like me may need to lean in and speak up. Just like when I help a patient and their family to say the word "cancer" in front of each other, I may have to be the guy to say the word "racism" out loud. I may have to present data on unequal care and outcomes or question gender pay inequities. I may have to be open and transparent about my own straight cisgender white male biases to help others to see theirs.

Sometimes we need to be a voice for the voiceless, until we can shift the power so that their authentic voices can be heard without us. I have worked in a non-white world long enough to see (and occasionally feel) their realities. I have at moments experienced the powerlessness of the poor. I take those perspectives into white-world as an ally and as a voice that can sometimes be heard.

At times I have been the white guy who could say things in a hospital board meeting. I helped get Black physicians onto the previously all-white medical staff of two small southern hospitals. I have spoken up for racial diversity in NIH grant peer-review sessions when the lone African American scholar in the room didn't want to have to be "that guy" again. In our College of Medicine, I may speak up and ask for concrete action on minority faculty promotion and retention because my colleagues of color shouldn't have to be the only ones raising the issue.

In an interview with Alex Haley, Dr. Martin Luther King Jr. focused on this very question: "Where are the white voices speaking against injustice?"[20] In various settings, I have been able to walk into the C-suite of a hospital or the executive suite of a state Medicaid program. When they weren't ready to talk about racial justice, I could instead talk about six-sigma approaches to eliminating variation in clinical outcomes. They love to talk about one-year return on investment (ROI). And sometimes, when they genuinely wanted to do better but didn't know how, I could begin to help them.

We can't sit this one out. We can't be silent. On Transgender Day of Visibility, Allison Hope wrote an opinion piece and quoted their trans friend J. D. Melendez: "I need my loved ones to be bold. Show the courage I show by just existing," they said. "I feel more hurt by the silence of my loved ones and the people who claim to support us than I am about them coming for us. I expect that of them. . . . Y'all broke my heart."[21]

In other settings, I may need to play a supporting role, to hear and amplify and applaud voices of color who are speaking courageously of their own lived experience and the challenges of being in a majority institution. In those moments, I have no need to control or to "white-splain." In those settings, I can coach and mentor or just encourage. I can begin intentionally working myself out of a job, to give away power and privilege. At some point, I can step away, to make available another chair at the boardroom table or on the senior leadership team.

Working in a majority-minority setting, such as a community-governed migrant health center or a historically Black medical school, I could afford to listen more than I spoke. I could learn more than I taught. I could serve more than I led. To have any chance of relational healing, though, we have to get out of our comfort zones. We have to build relationships in settings where we are not in the majority, do not set the norms, and do not have the power. We have to be comfortable in our own skin. For me, that means being a white guy in a non-white, multigendered world.

FOR FURTHER READING

Johnson SK. *Inclusify—The Power of Uniqueness and Belonging to Build Innovative Teams.*

Morukian M. *Diversity Equity and Inclusion for Trainers: Fostering DEI in the Workplace.*

Obama M. *Becoming.*

Tannen D. *That's Not What I Meant! How Conversational Style Makes or Breaks Relationships.*

Tutu D. *No Future Without Forgiveness.*

Tutu D, Tutu M. *The Book of Forgiving: The Fourfold Path for Healing Ourselves and Our World.*

WK Kellogg Foundation. *Restoring to Wholeness: Racial Healing for Ourselves, Our Relationships and Our Communities.*

15.

Structural Healing
Toward Equity and Justice

A code blue is never a welcome event. It means that somebody has stopped breathing, and their heart has stopped beating. In a big institution, a code team responds. When I was a medical student on-call, I would run to a code. Up the stairwells from the on-call room, I might be the first to arrive, usually out of breath and clueless. Then I would just wait for the senior resident to arrive. They knew how to walk in a hurry but not run, keeping their adrenaline in check.

Codes in a university hospital were common and well organized. They had a system. The crash cart came to the bedside quickly. Nurses and techs had well-defined roles. Start CPR, one pressing on the chest and one doing bag-and-mask ventilation. Establish an IV line. Intubate. One person gets the clipboard, recording every medicine and every defibrillator shock. *"CLEAR!!!"* Take a step back so the shock doesn't get you through the metal bed rails. Sometimes the patient would regain rhythm and pulse. They went to the ICU. Often, the patient died. Their body went down to the morgue. We all went back to work.

Codes rarely happened in our little migrant clinic in small-town Groveland. We did outpatient primary care. High blood pressure and diabetes, flu and sore throats. The first code I experienced there was a disaster. It was a few months after I had arrived. A man came to the clinic with chest pain that had begun hours earlier at home. Instead of taking his heart attack to the emergency room (where he had past-due hospital bills), he came to our little community clinic. He was brought straight back to a room and placed on an exam table for an EKG. Almost immediately he flatlined. Cardiac arrest.

"CODE BLUE!!!" the nurse shouted down the hallway through the open door. Everyone outside the room froze. Panic broke out. *"Where's the crash cart? Get Dr. Rust! Has anybody called 9-1-1???"* I came rushing in to see all at once an unconscious patient, a flatline EKG rhythm, and a nurse standing frozen like a deer in the headlights.

"Let's get an IV," I said to the nurse as I started chest compressions. I saw our front desk receptionist standing in the hallway. *"Go call 9-1-1. Tell them to come to the back and wait for them with the door open. Go!!!"*

"This patient needs to breathe. You," I said to the nurse's aide. *"Can you use an Ambu-Bag?"* She looked at me like she knew she was supposed to say yes but just shook her head from side-to-side. *"Can you do CPR, chest compressions?"* She nodded meekly. *"Do it,"* I said. I grabbed the Ambu-Bag to squeeze breaths into the patient with my left hand, right hand clamping the mask to his face and jaw.

I looked back at the nurse. She had a bag of IV fluid with one tube hanging from the bag. There was another tube in her hand with a connector for an IV needle. She seemed flummoxed. There was no connector between the two tubes, but she just kept trying to put them together anyway. *"These don't fit,"* she said. Another nurse was scrambling through the drawers of the crash cart, look-ing for connectors and a needle.

She opened another drawer. *"Oh, here's an ET tube. Oooh, and here's the laryngoscope,"* she said as if she were on an Easter egg hunt. I grabbed them both and moved around to the head of the table to put the breathing tube down the man's throat. I snapped open the heavy metal-hinged laryngoscope as I had done dozens of times before, but this was the first time the little light didn't come on. The tiny bright light is essential for seeing the vocal cords and putting the tube in the trachea. Without the light, you're shooting blind. *"Battery's dead,"* an aide observed unhelpfully.

I went back to squeezing the Ambu-Bag. *"How're we doing with the IV line?"* I asked.

"Got it," the nurse said proudly, holding up a jury-rigged IV bag. The tubing had way too much tape at the connectors. A 20-gauge Jelco IV needle hung limply from the end. I handed her the Ambu-Bag with quick instructions to squeeze. I found a vein and started the IV, just as I had done hundreds of times at Cook County.

"Defibrillator?" I asked with little hope. We should have already shocked the patient by now. The nurses looked around at each other, deciding who was going to tell me that we didn't actually have one. I was ready to call it. This man might already be dead.

At that moment, the EMTs from the rural ambulance crew came striding down the hall, equipment in hand. *"Here's the defi-brillator,"* the tall, strong-voiced man said. His partner was a bit younger but just as confident. *"We've got this,"* she said, applying goop to the chest and placing the pads in just the right spot. *"CLEAR!!!"* she called. Instinctively, I took my step back and made sure my team did the same. The patient's body heaved with the shock. *"Hold CPR,"* the EMT called. *"We've got a rhythm."*

"Okay if we give lidocaine, doc?" she asked. I made a sweeping go-ahead gesture with my arms. They pushed meds through the

IV. *"We've got a pulse and a blood pressure. 90 over 70. Let's get him on the stretcher and go."*

I watched as they wheeled him down the hall out to the ambulance, a little chagrined but grateful and impressed. *"Nice work,"* I said sincerely.

"No worries," she said. *"We do this all the time."* And like the small-town EMTs and paramedics in rural areas all across America, they were the lifesavers. In that moment, to me they were like gods.

I vowed, though, that this would never happen to us again. I was a Cook County doc. We damned sure knew how to run codes. When I became medical director, I saw to it that all our clinics had up-to-date crash carts. We had *systems* for checking the med list and for changing batteries in the laryngoscopes, and by God we had tubing and connectors that fit together. We ran a mock-code drill in every clinic at least twice a year. Resusci-Annie would have a heart attack in the lab or in a dental chair. We practiced it all until it was routine. When it happened, we were ready.

It takes systems and practice and procedures and a well-trained team to get good outcomes. If you're waiting for heroes, it means your systems have failed. Racial disparities, unequal outcomes, and preventable suffering all mean that America's systems are failing. We need to be intentional. Better systems produce better outcomes.

There are systems we could change as organizations, as communities, and as a nation that would dramatically move the needle toward health justice. We need structural healing to achieve permanent change. We need far more radical change than the superficial stuff we have been doing if we're going to eliminate preventable suffering and death.

But what can I do? What can *we* do? What if we got organized? What if we all tried really hard, all at the same time?

Individual/Family Level

Think of all the decisions we make in the course of life that have health equity and social justice implications. What's my career focus? Do I hold a formal position, or do I have informal authority? Where do I choose to work? Do I work in a for-profit hospital system or a nonprofit, mission-driven community health center? A large, well-endowed elite university or a small community-based medical school? Big Pharma or an HBCU?

What school do we send our kids to? What neighborhood do we live in? In community, with whom are we connected? Is our faith community segregated by race? Is it welcoming to LGBTQ persons? How diverse is my network of friends and social support?

We can also choose to engage as citizens in core functions of our communities. One of my colleagues was medical director of a migrant health center in Texas in the 1980s. He decided to run for his local school board because of the corruption he saw. This led to a lifelong career of leaning into leadership roles in public health and academics.

When we vote, we can either vote out of self-interest or we can spend our votes on behalf of the poor and marginalized. Daniel Dawes reminds us that health justice is really just a downstream consequence of the *Political Determinants of Health*.[1] I may not have the luxury of remaining above politics.

What do we do with our money? Do we preferentially buy stuff from minority-owned businesses? Hire minority contractors? We can choose to support community-owned organizations that build power and resiliency among the poor and marginalized, instead of supporting charity that only helps the poor in a pitying "least-of-these" model. The goal is to support real structural change and empowerment and justice.

Many of us no longer have retirement pensions. Instead, we will rely on the money we save in 401(k) or other retirement accounts. What happens to all that money if we haven't spent it before we die? The default seems to be to let our kids inherit it, and I do love my kids. But we might also think of opportunities for at least some of that money to go to community-led organizations or minority-serving schools that don't have big endowments. Can our wealth be a force for good?

Department/Team/Organization/Agency Level

If you lead an agency or an organization, your responsibilities in the JEDI space (Justice, Equity, Diversity, and Inclusion) are even greater. If you have any authority over programs or budgets or people, then it's your job to create structural healing. Stefanie Johnson coined the word "inclusify" to emphasize the balance between inclusion and diversity.[2] Diversity means that everyone can be fully themselves, adding value to the team through their uniqueness. Inclusion means that every one of those diverse people fits into a cohesive team.

A third of my county's population is Black or African American. One in four Floridians is Hispanic or Latine. The proportion of adults who are openly LGBTQ is approaching 10 percent. If our teams don't match that, then we have to play catch up. Think about when your bath water has gotten cold. You add hot water (not warm) to bring it back to the desired temperature. In hiring and promotions, we need to far *exceed* the diversity of our community to get to a truly representative steady state. Other than historically Black or tribal institutions, where are the organizations that have committed to that?

Having done this, you may find yourself managing internal dynamics and conflicts that feel more like three-dimensional chess. Have the difficult conversations. As the team is *forming,* don't skip the *storming*. The critical guardrail is that people may not use their own identity or religion or ideology to demean or diminish the uniqueness of others.

Once hired, minoritized individuals must be supported to achieve career growth and purposeful accomplishments. Doesn't everybody need support? Sure. But marginalized and minoritized individuals need different kinds of support. If they are leaving or failing at different rates than white guys, then you are not there yet. Do equity.

Dana Brownlee tells the story of her aunt who was an elementary school educator. She was sitting at a student desk struggling to cut some construction paper for a bulletin board project. Finally, she exploded with frustration, "Why is everything designed for righties?"[3] To right-handed people, the chair and desk and scissors all seemed "normal." But to a left-handed person, they were made for someone else. That's how straight white-guy privilege works. How do we undo that?

First, our organizations must reflect vertically proportionate diversity up and down the org chart. It's not enough to have people of color as nurse's aides or at the reception desk. People of color should be in the board room and the C-suite and health professions in *at least* the same proportion as they are represented in your community. I say at least, because we need to oversample minority voices to hear the diversity within diversities.

There is power in our diversity, but equity requires diversity in power. Who approves the budget? Who hires? Who has the power to fire the president/dean/CEO? Typically, it's the white guys in charge. But there is a discipline of giving away control. Sometimes that means stepping away from leadership in order to create a seat at the table for others.

In an HBCU, I was very conscious that every leadership position I held could have been a launch pad for a minority scholar to rise from. Dr. David Satcher came to Morehouse School of

Medicine as chair of an academic department. From there, he became CDC director, then president of Meharry Medical College, and then the 16th Surgeon General of the United States. A white guy like me accepting a leadership position at an HBCU might be blocking someone else's next career step. I had to constantly reevaluate. *"Am I creating more opportunities than I'm taking up?"*

It's all about spending my privilege and giving away power. Stepping into leadership and knowing when to step away. White guys love to talk about being servant-leaders until someone actually treats us like servants. In a non-white world, we need to assume that *my job is to work myself out of a job.* It's hard to give up power and security. Nixon-era Watergate figure Charles Colson once said, "Power is like saltwater; the more you drink, the thirstier you get." Let it go.

Cultivating leaders of color is part of the job, especially for white men working in a non-white world. Dr. Dominic Mack had begun an academic career path when he joined the charter class of our Morehouse faculty development program more than three decades ago. At that time, he was providing primary care to low-income patients. He became medical director of one of the South's largest community health centers. When I taught workshops in the first year of our faculty development program, he was the person everyone loved. He was always smiling, always relaxed. I worried that maybe he wasn't taking the program seriously, until they did their projects. Dr. Mack made it look easy. Giving a talk? No sweat. Facilitating a small group? Easy-peasy. Writing papers? Best in class.

Over time, what started as a mentoring relationship grew into friendship and brotherly love. I have one brother by birth and another brother by choice. Dominic and I were there for each other in our work and in our family concerns. I drove to Augusta to attend his father's funeral, and he flew to Florida to attend my father's funeral. I love him dearly.

When Dr. Satcher asked me to once again step into the role of directing the National Center for Primary Care, I asked Dr. Mack to be my deputy director. He had amazing executive skills at a scale that I didn't have. He led an initiative to get thousands of physician practices across Georgia to adopt electronic health records. He had an MBA. He really deserved to be the executive leader of our center.

Our bosses weren't ready for it, so we became co-directors. We modeled collaborative leadership in a way that the institution had not seen before. Dr. Mack did executive leadership, and I did the scholarly stuff. He went to the budget meetings. He had the hire/fire authority. Symbols are important, so I moved out of the big office with floor-to-ceiling glass windows. I gave up the desk and chair from which Dr. Satcher had led our Center. Dr. Mack got the good parking space next to where the president and dean parked, while I went back to my old spot in the parking garage.

The messaging was clear. Dr. Mack was the executive leader of our National Center. It worked. It showed our institution a model of collaborative leadership, two strong men leading as brothers, with no jealousy or competition. I'm still proud of that.

At that time, it was African American men who held the medical school's top leadership positions. Our center managers and program managers, our executive assistants, and our project leaders were almost all women. They were (and are) super-competent. They really ran the place. We made sure that we helped women get the academic degrees or certificates they needed to move into executive-level positions. Sometimes they just needed us to visibly recognize their talents and accomplishments. Sometimes we just had to stop holding them back.

For white guys in leadership who feel threatened by affirmative action, I wish I could help you see how you can thrive in a non-white world. If you constantly have the goal of working yourself out of a job and nurturing diverse leaders to replace you, then all kinds of people will want you to join their team. Create more opportunities than you are sucking up. And when you leave that job, you will look back and find that you have created a more complete team, more effective precisely because it is equitable and diverse. It will have staying power—the kind of thing that lasts. And maybe you will have also found a new brother and a new family.

Expect pushback. Texas A&M University is now facing a class-action lawsuit over its efforts to increase recruitment of underrepresented minority faculty. A police chief in Fort Lauderdale, Florida, was fired for promoting six minority candidates (along with nine nonminority candidates) to leadership positions in his department. He was cited for commenting on photos of their current command team saying, "That wall is too white. I'm gonna change that." After his firing, he said this: "If promoting diversity is the hill I'm going to die on, I will sleep well tonight."[4]

As you build your team, build your objectives through an equity lens. What gets measured gets done. Are there services or outcomes that are subject to racial-ethnic or gender disparities? Make explicit your goals for eliminating those disparities. Designate people whose very job description is to achieve those objectives. Sometimes we can change structures and systems to make equity the default choice. Sometimes we don't have authority, but we all have influence. Moving toward equity should not always require heroic, disruptive action to overcome the status quo. Make it systemic. Make it automatic.

The starting point for each of us in leadership is to be honest with ourselves. Own the problem. Own our responsibility. I am (and my institution is) part of the problem. I (and my institution) can choose to be part of the solution. Take my current academic institution. Aside from state agencies, FSU is the largest employer in Leon County. Over 13,000 people work here. We have a $2.17 *billion* budget. Meanwhile, one in five Leon County residents lives below the poverty level. Black unemployment rate is twice the white rate. Huge inequalities in housing, education, income, and wealth are connected to a long arc of our history.

What if FSU decided that a $2 billion budget could make a dramatic difference in improving the social determinants of health in our small city of Tallahassee, Florida? What if our university spent every construction dollar, every contract for services, and every salary line with an *intention* to undo historic inequities? What could we accomplish for equity? It's not a zero-sum game. White people and white institutions don't lose, we gain! FSU and Tallahassee could become a model of equity for our entire nation.

Community Level

Equity requires balancing personal autonomy with community responsibility. We need a "we-all" rather than a "me-all" culture. In medicine, the phrase is "do no harm." In many faith traditions, it's "love your neighbor." If my neighbor is vulnerable to COVID, I get vaccinated even if I hate getting shots. I wear a mask even if the mask makes my face itch. Whether my neighbors are African American or indigenous or White or Latine or Asian or Republican or Muslim or gay or trans or straight, I choose to love them as my neighbors.

Health equity is all about sharing power with the community. When Dr. Jorge Prieto moved to Chicago, he started clinics in immigrant neighborhoods. He insisted on really listening to community leaders and people. The South Lawndale Health Center he founded was governed by a community board. We worked with and for the Latine residents of Pilsen-Little Village. Outsiders see La Villita as a neighborhood enmeshed in poverty and crime. My teachers and my patients saw *communidad* and *familismo*. They knew a community of strength and resiliency and hope.

Funding for the clinic came from the community health center program, born out of the 1960s war on poverty. Community development and health care were intentionally woven together. It was built on community strengths and assets, not needs and deficits. One of the first community health centers in the nation was co-founded in 1965 by Dr. Jack Geiger. He was an extraordinary white guy who taught many of us. He and Dr. John Hatch built the Delta Health Center in Mound Bayou, Mississippi.

Together, they had the vision to see health care beyond the clinic walls. They cultivated community gardens and community leadership. They created paths to health careers for young people. When Dr. Geiger saw extreme malnutrition, he wrote prescriptions for the clinic to pay for food at the grocery store. Challenged by his funding agency, Dr. Geiger had an answer. *"The textbooks all say that the medical treatment for malnutrition is food."*

Community health centers are designed to get the power dynamics right. Four Catholic nuns began working to address health issues in the 1970s in Apopka and Groveland, Florida. Asked in a community meeting to start a clinic, they demurred. *"We can't do this, we're just four white sisters."* An African American man stepped forward and proclaimed, *"Four white sisters and one Black brother."* And so it began, even though the KKK was still threatening these community organizers.

After starting in Apopka, one farmworker insisted for years that *"we need a clinic in Groveland too."* His name was Mr. Everardo Cortez. When I came to Groveland in the 1980s, he was chairman of the board of the entire community health organization. This board oversaw three clinics, a dozen physicians, and nearly a hundred staff, with licensed pharmacies and a birthing center. He led a nonprofit corporate board that was managing a $10 million budget in a highly regulated health care environment.

The farmworkers and low-income patients on our board had a majority that could hire or fire our CEO. They could hold us accountable and rattle my cage if I didn't hire enough fluently bilingual physicians. African American residents of Deep South small towns were also on our board. They insisted on a racially diverse staff that showed respect and dignity to every patient. They had the power. As it should be.

John McKnight is the thought leader behind Asset-Based Community Development (ABCD). He asks one specific question about any initiative: "Does the proposed activity have a timetable for training and transferring ownership to indigenous leadership?"[5] If not, why not? Every community-serving program should have this plan.

Here's a Chinese poem that someone showed me early in my learning about community health development. A tattered copy has been taped to my computer monitor for the past 30 years.

Go to the people.
> Live among them.
>> Learn from them.
>> Love them.

Build on what they have.
> Grow from what they know.

But of the very best leaders,
> The people will say,
>> We have done it ourselves.

Community ownership is key. Southcentral Foundation provides health care to a large area surrounding Anchorage, Alaska. Some years ago, the Indian Health Service finally transferred ownership to the Alaska Native community. They quickly began transforming themselves into a culturally relevant system of care they call "Nuka." It means "strong, giant structures and living things." Patients became "Customer-Owners."

Their primary care teams have doctors and nurses, but also mental health specialists and native healers, who are together responsible for actual health outcomes. And while all this may sound like soft fuzzy stuff, they decreased emergency department visits and hospital admissions by over a third. They decreased dollar costs and decreased human suffering. They got objectively better outcomes by being culturally relevant and getting the community power dynamics right.

The other day, some of our school's research leaders were meeting with community stakeholders. The FSU folks were mostly white professionals with high salaries. Community stakeholders were African American individuals, some with lower-wage jobs. Expressing their frustration, a community member said this: *"Why do you keep asking us to give our input? Why don't you just hire us to run the program???"*

Why not indeed?

Even more important than having a variety of programs is to have them work in harmony together in a common direction. Collective action can achieve collective impact.[6] We need collective action to build cohesive, comprehensive systems of health care. We need collective impact to eliminate the Black–white infant mortality gap, to save a baby's life every day here in Florida. We also need collective action to improve the social determinants of health. We must act in partnership *with* communities, rather than paternalistically doing *for* communities. As disability advocates say, *"Nothing about us without us."*

Too often, our organizations act as if we are the only ones working for good in our communities. We limit our collaborations with other agencies because we compete for grants or for clients. Frankly, I've had enough of this "stay in your lanes" bullshit that separates medicine from mental health from addiction treatment. For that matter, why do we separate health needs from housing and education? Only together will we solve the complex syndemic of health inequities. Let's build more health equity coalitions.[7] Says Don Lemon, "Imagine the life-changing, world-shifting power of solidarity between people of color and people of conscience."[8]

We talk of upstream and downstream factors that drive health outcomes. Caring for sick people is the downstream activity. Social determinants are midstream. Policy and politics flow from upstream. But this river of equity is a magical river that flows in both directions. Social determinants may drive health outcomes, but health care systems can provide an operational base for improving socioeconomics. A migrant clinic in Groveland, Florida, was the community's largest year-round employer. It was a hub for training our diabetic *promotoras*. It was a leadership development program for our community board. But we had to be *intentional*.

If your organization engages in community partnerships, you have an incredible opportunity to demonstrate or to undermine your own trustworthiness. Too many universities think they're being progressive when they invest resources in community "engagement." But that continues to treat the community as "other."

In my own community work, my mantra is this—don't say "partnership" unless you really mean it.

- Real partners share the money.
- Real partners share the power.
- Real partners share the vision.
- Real partners share the work.
- Real partners share the future.

State and Federal Levels

Look at the root causes of inequities. Consider the kinds of community-level change that would be required to fix them. It all starts with the simple, powerful right to vote.

Voting Rights

The ongoing effort to suppress voters of color has echoes of Jim Crow. Republican state legislatures continue to gerrymander

districts to make sure that African Americans are not propor-
tionately represented. It's anathema to democracy. Let's at least
pass the John Lewis Voting Rights Act. But why stop there?
Countries from Australia to Uruguay have 90 percent voter turnout in their national elections. Why not in America? Why not
have universal voter registration? Why not designate national
elections as national holidays? Why not mandate online voting
and mail-in ballot options in all federal elections? If we really believe in democracy, don't we believe in everyone voting?

Civil Rights

We need our laws to bind and protect us all equally, not just the
in-groups. The Equal Rights Amendment to the Constitution was
first passed by Congress over 50 years ago. It has now been rati-
fied by 38 states. How long is this going to take? In 1873, Susan B.
Anthony reminded us, "It is 'we the people', not 'we the white male
citizens', . . . , who formed the Union."[9] We the people, the whole
people, includes all racial/ethnic and language groups. It includes
straight and lesbian and gay Americans, cis and trans Americans,
queer and questioning Americans—all of us. Yet anti-LGBTQ laws
are being enacted across many states.[10] They cruelly target trans
youth. They are bizarrely obsessed with drag shows. The Equality Act would protect all of us from discrimination in jobs and
housing and health and education.[11] Why is this so hard?

Immigration

Frederick Douglass is known for his passionate advocacy for racial justice, but not just for Black people. In his 1869 Composite
Nation speech, he also argued against restrictions on Chinese immigration, proclaiming, "There are such things in the world as
human rights."[12] In a nation of immigrants, advancing civil rights

has to include immigration reform. Protect the Dreamers. Turn the Deferred Action for Childhood Arrivals (DACA) program into law. Pass the Fairness for Farm Workers Act. Ultimately, we need comprehensive immigration reform. Immigrants refresh our nation and build our future.

Environmental Injustice

In caring for refugees, I often see high lead levels in children. It's easy to explain if they were exposed to burn pits in Afghanistan or if their families use traditional pottery or certain cosmetics. But I shouldn't see it in US children. In Flint, Michigan, children had lead poisoning for years before physicians' voices were heard and city water pipes examined. In Jackson, Mississippi, residents have had to rely on bottled water for months. Instead of fixing the water system, a white-dominated state legislature is trying to take control of a majority-Black city from its African American elected officials.

None of this is new. The placement of landfills in communities of color impacts air and water quality. Routing highways through poor neighborhoods is linked to childhood asthma. Think of where Black neighborhoods are situated in so many communities, from small towns to big cities, North and South. White people in nice houses are on the high ground. Black housing is relegated to "the bottoms," those areas of swampy, poorly drained land, often on the other side of the tracks. Imagine how such neighborhoods will be affected by increasing sea levels, floods, and hurricanes related to climate change.

Educational Inequities

Educational inequalities are a national embarrassment, an American shame. We raised our own kids inside Atlanta's perimeter in

Decatur, Georgia. Progress there has been complicated. Decatur made the decision to desegregate their schools in 1967, over a dozen years after the Supreme Court's *Brown v. Board of Education* decision. It took pressure from the courts and federal agencies as well as from local advocates.

While many other schools in Georgia were still resisting desegregation, Decatur City Schools finally decided to move ahead. By the early 1970s, there was only one middle school and one high school, where Black and white kids all attended together.

Mr. Clifford Chandler had been first a student, then a teacher, in Decatur's all-Black Trinity High School. He lived the years of segregation and then desegregation. Asked if Decatur integrated before they were forced to, he answered, "No." But in 1972, he was asked by the same superintendent who had initially resisted desegregation to become the first principal of a newly opened and racially integrated middle school.

Our kids finished their elementary years at a Quaker school and then moved on to attend Decatur's Middle School and High School, where Black and white and immigrant kids all went to school together.

But still there were educational inequities. Elementary schools on the majority-Black side of the city south of the tracks were underperforming relative to schools in whiter neighborhoods. Decatur paid attention, and in one of many efforts to achieve educational equity, they reengineered their schools. They moved away from the wealth-driven neighborhood school model.

Seven early elementary schools were consolidated into three. For fourth and fifth grades, all the kids would move together into an academy, which adopted an International Baccalaureate curriculum. All our kids would learn together and form one community together.

But progress takes persistence. It's complicated. Now there are again five early elementary schools and two upper elementary schools before kids finally come together at the middle school.

The school board has adopted an educational equity plan. They continue to innovate and try new things. The current school superintendent, Dr. Gyimah Whitaker, insists that "equity is the vehicle to excellence." They're trying. They're working. They're persisting. They're progressing.

In so doing, Decatur City Schools remains one of the most excellent school systems in the Atlanta metro area. They lost a few families but gained many more, because of the clarity of their vision.

Income Inequality

In global health, we talk of extreme poverty, not having enough income to even sustain life. Poverty in the United States is not often so extreme, but it is still demeaning and still life-threatening. It's certainly not fair. Income inequality could first be addressed with a livable minimum wage indexed to keep up with inflation. A more radical yet evidence-based approach would be to provide a floor of minimum income for all Americans.

Here's an interesting thought experiment. What if the Social Security retirement age were set at *either* 68 years old *or* at 85 percent of the average life expectancy of your racial-ethnic group, whichever came first? African American people could retire at 64, while white people would have to wait until age 68. "*It isn't fair,*" we white people would wail. And we'd be right, but in the wrong direction. If we waited until 85 percent of our life expectancy, we should have to retire at 70. Think about all the African American men and women who have died before they ever got a dime of Social Security or a single doctor visit paid by Medicare because they died prematurely. Is that fair?

Residential Segregation/Wealth Inequality

America continues to have neighborhoods largely segregated by race, despite fair housing laws. In the 1980s, Oak Park, Illinois, decided to fight "white flight" by actively steering renters to mixed neighborhoods. They worked intentionally to maintain racial balance across their community, even as Chicago was becoming increasingly segregated. Across the city line in Chicago's Austin neighborhood, increasing racial isolation and concentrated poverty created conditions ripe for crime and social decline. Cultivating racial integration helped Oak Park preserve property values and quality of life for all.

White families have a net worth on average 7 to 10 times greater than that of Black families in America. Much of this wealth gap is due to our history of residential segregation, institutionally enforced by redlining neighborhoods and devaluing Black property by law or by practice.[13] In 2019, Evanston, Illinois, began acknowledging these historic inequities. They are now seeking to make amends, through a program of financial reparations to Black homeowners directly impacted by this history.

California's Commission on Reparations is struggling with how to redress broader historic inequities such as health disparities, housing discrimination, and mass incarceration. At a national level, it's hard to imagine what reparations might look like. That's why we need a Reparations Study Commission. The devil would be in the details. Should dollars go to individuals or to services in marginalized communities? Either way, we must explicitly tie our repentance to some form of recompense and justice. In America, that means money.

Policing and Public Safety

Many communities are trying to move from policing to public safety. Less than a third of 911 calls involve life-threatening situations. Why call the police if a person with mental illness is acting out in front of a local store? De-escalate the situation. Eugene, Oregon, sends a medic and a mental health crisis worker on calls for people with mental health issues or intoxication. Rarely is police intervention needed.

The National League of Cities seeks to reduce use of jails while focusing on reentry. They recommend violence interruption strategies and civilian oversight for accountability of law enforcement. Police departments employing four or more of Campaign Zero's "Eight Can't Wait" strategies have not only the lowest rates of killings by police but also the lowest rates of officer deaths.[14] Safer for everyone.

Guns are now the leading cause of death for children.[15] We live in an era (and nation) of mass shootings. Most Americans support common-sense gun laws. The 1994 federal ban on assault rifles saved lives before it expired. The law also limited high-capacity magazines, which should have no effect on hunters. If you need more than 10 bullets to shoot a deer, you're doing it wrong.

Background checks should be universal. No loopholes. For those who should not have guns, 19 states have passed red flag laws. With all the warning signs of the recent mass shooting in Maine, a red flag law could have impounded the guns of the shooter and prevented 18 tragic deaths. Under these laws, thousands of extreme risk protection orders have temporarily removed weapons, preventing hundreds of shootings and suicides in those states.

Criminal Justice System

The disproportionate jailing of Black men is wrong. This pattern has persisted in America ever since the Black codes were used to provide a post-slavery plantation workforce. Our country incarcerates humans at a rate far exceeding that of other industrialized nations. We have developed an entire industry of privatized prisons, in part to create jobs in poor rural communities.

Another injustice is the schools-to-prison pipeline, by which minoritized students are disciplined and detained at far greater rates than are white students. The Black Lives Matter at School Movement advocates four principles of school reform—more teachers of color, more teaching of Black history and sociology, more racial trauma–informed counselors, and more social support systems. They seek to replace suspensions and expulsions with "mediation and restorative justice."

The jailing of individuals who cannot afford cash bail or fines or court fees further drives inequities. Poor people wait for trial in jail, while rich people live free. Criminal justice reform could start with bail reform and sentencing reform. We also need aggressive civil rights enforcement against jurisdictions with unequal arrest rates, unequal charging decisions, and unequal sentencing.[16] Let's make justice just.

Health Equity

The quickest step toward health equity would be for our nation to enact universal health care coverage. Every other Western industrialized nation has been able to do it but us. They have very different models, but at their core, they try very hard not to leave anyone out. Look at Britain or Canada or Germany or Sweden or Japan or New Zealand or any one of a dozen other countries.[17] Let's do one of these models, or let's create our own. But let's stop leaving people out. Let's put an end to preventable suffering.

Until then, 12 states could choose at last to embrace Medicaid expansion. That would improve access to health care and decrease preventable suffering for at least 3.7 million people. It would also lower medical debt, bankruptcies, and poverty in the very states that have the highest poverty rates and the worst health outcomes.[18] Medicaid expansion has even been associated with lower high school dropout rates, home evictions, and crime rates.[19]

The Mental Health Parity Act was a step forward but needs to be more consistently enforced. To achieve real parity, we need a dramatic increase in public funding for mental health and substance use treatment. We need a tenfold increase in funding for supportive housing for those with chronic and persistent mental illness. Wouldn't this be better than spending our tax dollars on prisons? Why couldn't we be intentional about building recovery-nurturing, resiliency-building, healthy, and therapeutic communities across America?

In the 1960s, segregation of hospital wards was eliminated in just a few years through bold government action. Here's a simple idea—if a hospital or managed care organization (MCO) wants to get Medicare payments, they have to deliver equitable care to achieve *equality of outcomes*. Do the same for state Medicaid programs. Spend the dollars however you wish, and deliver care and social support in whatever ways meet each patient's unique needs. But in the end, we'll pay you for equitable care that achieves equal outcomes. We could decrease costs and decrease human suffering at the same time—why wouldn't we?

One of the great strengths of public health is our day-to-day surveillance of communicable diseases. We track COVID and flu, leprosy and malaria, and even brain-eating amoebas. If there's a meningitis case or a whooping cough outbreak, I get a phone call. We have dashboards and data systems to monitor outbreaks that drive interventions in real time. Our surveillance systems tell us very quickly whether our interventions are working or not.

So why don't we use actionable data to eliminate health disparities in premature deaths and preventable suffering? How many kids had emergency department visits for asthma this week? How many adults had uncontrolled high blood pressure or diabetes, or preventable strokes? On current trend lines, when will we eliminate the Black–white gap in infant mortality?

We need rapid-cycle feedback loops and dynamic interventions to reduce preventable death and suffering. We need to know when we are moving the needle toward equity. And when we are not, we must change the interventions.

International/Global Level

Going global is beyond the scope of this book and beyond my level of competence. Read Paul Farmer's book *To Repair the World*.[20] Perhaps with intentionality, read from authors who are African[21,22,23] and Latine.[24] Read works by Indigenous native peoples.[25,26] Hear them speaking their truth. See the world through the eyes of the two-thirds world, the Brown and Black world, the colonized and nonnuclear nations. Embrace the notion of "de-colonizing global health," but notice the irony in how many authors seeking to define this are from the Global North. Remember how shocked the white-guy CIA agent is in the *Black Panther* movie, when the tech-savvy Shuri casually calls him "colonizer"? He ends up being a good guy but not the hero of the story. He's an ally, not a savior. If you're a white guy like me, try doing that.

Bottom Line

What will it take to achieve such structural change? What will it take to achieve optimal and equitable outcomes for all? Equal outcomes will require "unequal" (but equitable) interventions. In the face of old white guys like me clinging to power and privilege and leadership, what will it take to eliminate historical and ongoing inequities? What will it take to make social justice systemic?

Here's a laundry list of what it might take:

- More Money (and a redistribution of spending priorities)
- More People (a more diverse and better-trained workforce)

- Bigger Vision and Better Values (love our neighbor, build the beloved community)
- More Power to the People (community-owned and responsive leadership)
- More Votes (building political will and public support by building coalitions)
- More Collective Impact (cohesive, coordinated community action)
- More Focus (eyes on the prize—optimal and equitable outcomes for all)

But we cannot wait any longer. In the words of Dr. Martin Luther King Jr., "We have come to this hallowed spot to remind America of the fierce urgency of *now*. . . .

Now is the time to make real the promises of Democracy. . . .
Now is the time to open the doors of opportunity to all of God's children. . . .
Now is the time to lift our nation from the quicksands of racial injustice to the solid rock of brotherhood."[27]

Now . . . is the time.
Now!

FOR FURTHER READING

Brettschneider M, Burgess S, Keating C. *LGBTQ Politics: A Critical Reader.*

Dawes D. *The Political Determinants of Health.*

Farmer P. *To Repair the World.*

King ML Jr. *Where Do We Go From Here: Chaos or Community?*

Reid TR. *The Healing of America: A Global Quest for Better, Cheaper, and Fairer Health Care.*

16.

Healing and Hope in the Time of Exhaustion

The most common phrase I hear these days is, *"I'm just exhausted."* I hear it from teachers. I hear it from public health workers. I hear it from women. I hear it from LGBTQ friends, and I hear it most often from people of color. During the trial of the police who killed George Floyd, the video of his killing was replayed endlessly on cable news. New videos of more killings of Black men by police came forward almost every day. Keith Boykin called 2021 "our weary year."[1]

New York City Public Advocate Jumaane Williams was interviewed at a press conference after these killings and spoke with tears. "I am not okay today," he said. "I want to give the Black community permission to say I am not okay. I am tired. I am tired. . . . I have not watched the video of George Floyd. It is too much. Black people have to go to work the next day and be alright. I am not okay. I am tired. I am tired of racism."[2]

Of course, these killings were not a new phenomenon. They were merely a constellation of highly visible Black deaths in a world where such deaths occur frequently. And it's not just in the Black community. Similar patterns of brutality and hate crimes occur daily against American Indian women, Latine workers, Asian elders, trans people, queer people, Muslim people, and Jewish people all across our nation. To read the news and to care about the human race is exhausting in itself.

Here in Florida, we feel progress slipping backward. The "Stop-Woke Act" made it illegal to teach about racial inequities. The "Don't Say Gay" bill dehumanized LGBTQ teachers and parents. Teachers began self-censoring, because felony charges could be brought against any of us for discussing topics that made (straight, white) kids "uncomfortable." Books were pulled from shelves or stricken from reading lists.

A colleague of mine sadly remembered a time when *"it was illegal to be gay, illegal to be me."* He thought we were past all that, but not now. The polarizing anti-gay, anti-trans bullying is somehow okay, but social-emotional learning is not. Our legislature just made it legal to carry a concealed gun with no training or permit. Apparently, drag shows are the real danger.

Meanwhile, the COVID pandemic was killing jobs and small businesses, but mostly killing people. School closures were forcing people to juggle childcare and working from home. Hospital nurses found themselves burning out in caring week after week for people critically ill from a preventable illness. Ventilators and oxygen supplies ran short. Just when it seemed that COVID was dying down, the surge of a new variant would overwhelm the ICUs.

In public health, we experienced a similar sense of exhaustion. In mask and gown and double-gloves in a Tallahassee parking lot, I leaned into cars in the drive-through COVID testing line to stick a probe up people's noses. Reflexively, they coughed in my face. Dozens of my colleagues and students risked their own health to help with the testing.

At the same time, some political leaders actively undermined the rational and scientific public health response. Public health leaders were the targets of vitriol and even death threats across the nation. Our governor prohibited school boards from implementing mask mandates to protect our children. He bullied high school kids for wearing masks. School staff died. Teachers died. Children died.

The governor's response was to take down the COVID data dashboard and to stop releasing mortality statistics. Denial is his chosen defense. He prohibited county public health departments from sharing their local data. He chose as his State Surgeon General a California-based academic internist with no background or credentials in public health.

Dr. Ladapo sent out an official state health directive warning of the "dangers" of mRNA vaccines based on his personal (and flawed) analysis. In a rare action, the FDA and CDC wrote him a joint letter "to correct the associated misinterpretations and misinformation about the data."[3] A quote often misattributed to Einstein applies perfectly. "The only thing more dangerous than ignorance is arrogance."

Resources were shifted from vaccine outreach (preventing disease and its spread) to monoclonal antibody treatment centers (treating people once they got sick). Public health officials in my county were prohibited from sharing mask and vaccine messaging with local media. The governor wanted to be the sole voice speaking on COVID. His preferred message was that it was over. Nothing to see here. Let's move on to a more distracting and divisive issue, such as attacking woke folks or drag queens. Denial was the strategy for COVID and the strategy for racism.

Mary Frances-Winter wrote a book called *Black Fatigue*.[4] She describes "the fear, frustration, anguish, and yes, rage that is a regular part of many Black people's daily lives." She goes on to say this: "Black people have been marching, protesting, resisting, writing, orating, praying, legislating, and commentating for centuries for equity and justice, and—young and old—*we are fatigued*."[5]

Dr. Sam Rae describes how "it is so expensive to be marginalized. There are so many invisible taxes that marginalized folks pay." She cited a neurodiversity tax, a poverty tax, a Black and Brown tax, a woman tax, an LGBTQ+ tax, and a non-Christian religion tax, among many others, and then said this: "Now imagine if you fit into all of these categories. . . . It is a lot. The point is people are tired."[6]

One reason for the exhaustion is that white folks in general, and white men specifically, are too often willing to sit back and let minoritized colleagues fight the battle. We act as if we don't have a dog in this fight. Sometimes we stay silent because we are afraid that we might say the wrong thing. But that leaves our friends and colleagues fighting for equality and inclusion by themselves, with no allies or support. They can never be sure that we've got their backs. It's exhausting.

Chief Joseph of the Nez Perce said it this way: "I am tired of fighting. Our Chiefs are dead. . . . The old men are dead. . . . He who led the young men is dead . . . I am tired; my heart is sick and sad. From where the sun now stands, I will fight no more forever."[7]

In preparing for a discussion panel at the National Press Club, I suggested a question our moderator could ask me: *"How do we mobilize white men to get in the game?"* He shook his head and let out a long breath.

"Man, if you can say that, then say it. Because I am exhausted, tired of trying to get white men to step up and do the right thing. I'm tired of having to fight this battle alone."

To be honest, exhaustion is the reason I didn't want to write this book. Engaging on racial issues is in itself exhausting. Hearing feedback on what I get wrong is even tougher. Sometimes I just can't heal any faster. So I've learned enough about self-care to be able to say, *"I'm bone-dry, exhausted. I need to consolidate the gains*

I've already made. I'm going to circle back to this, but right now I just desperately need a nap."

There are days when I want to engage and days when I just want to go fishing. I'm okay with that. I've learned over a few decades that if I go fishing now, I'll have more energy to engage tomorrow. It's a marathon, not a sprint. But I also recognize it as a form of privilege. I can choose my moments to engage or not engage.

I first noticed this sense of cultural exhaustion doing community health among the farmworkers and low-income patient population we served in Groveland. In the exam room, I would struggle with my imperfect Spanish. In the hallways, we would sometimes shift back and forth in *Spanglish*. After seeing a Spanish-speaking migrant mother and her three children, I might go to an exam room with my favorite older couple. They always sat together. He would say in a Jamaican accent, *"How's your father? We're praying for him."* Then to a room with a grandmother raising grandchildren. Then to a young African American woman who owned her own home-based hairstyling business.

There was physical exhaustion running from exam room to exam room to care for too many patients. There was intellectual exhaustion trying to sort out all the medical and social and behavioral complexities of our patients. There was spiritual exhaustion, trying to give them the best care I could with such limited resources. And there was also a cultural exhaustion. I was trying to speak two languages, to relate to Black and white racial dynamics, and trying to be all things to all people. I've said earlier that I'm a chameleon. I am constantly and often unconsciously expending energy to be less white or less Anglo and sometimes working just as hard to fit in with white folks. It's exhausting.

I found myself craving a lunch break where I could just go and sit by myself to recharge. I would often go to places whose norms were firmly centered in white-world. If I had to do quick rounds at the hospital, lunch was at McDonald's. A plastic, commercial, mass-consumption bubble of white-world.

Years later at Morehouse, I would be perfectly comfortable at the mostly Black West End mall or at one of the storefront Caribbean food vendors. But at times of exhaustion, I would find myself driving out to one of the white suburban shopping mall food courts. Was it the introvert in me wanting to have some quiet time in the car? Or was it the white guy exhausted from shape-shifting to fit into other cultures? Maybe I just didn't want to stick out as the one white guy in the food court. Is that how my Black friends feel in white-world?

The work of embracing diversity in the workplace requires re-aligning our norms, our language, and our behavior. This too is exhausting. In the words of the researchers, it may result in "cognitive resource depletion."[8] I still struggle with burnout and exhaustion.

Times like these test our very souls.[9] We are working for health equity in a time of overt, aggressive opposition. There are forces actively fighting *against* health for all. We hear a dialectic in which the collective good is placed in opposition to individual freedoms. At times I have an aching desire to escape back into a white world of postracist denial. I need time to breathe and refresh and regain strength before turning back to fight the dragons of racial injustice. Sometimes hope is all that sustains me. We have to nurture that hope.

"Hope is a good thing, maybe the best of things." These words were spoken by a wrongly convicted prisoner in the movie *Shawshank Redemption*. What restores your hope? Figure out what recharges your batteries. Then have the discipline to do it, no matter what other urgencies intrude.

It would be easy to lose hope. Good people working to address poverty or public health are attacked. Ideologues fight to limit the role of government in addressing health equity. They work to roll back recent gains while offering no real alternatives. Across the Western world, the rekindled fires of anti-immigrant white nationalism have achieved new levels of influence.

Health disparities continue to be pervasive and persistent. The language of social "determinants" can be demoralizing as well. It can lead to despair if we believe that they "determine" our outcomes. Children born in a low-income census tract are on average destined to be poor adults, with poor health outcomes. Indeed, poverty can actually damage brain development from earliest infancy.

On the other hand, hope is found in our brain's neuroplasticity. We can reshape our brains. Early interventions matter. Long-term follow-up studies show that Head Start programs improve long-term educational outcomes. They permanently enhance social, emotional, and behavioral development.[10]

Hope is essential in forging a path toward health equity and social justice. We can't afford to just wring our hands and say, *"Ain't it awful!"* There is mounting evidence that disparities can be eliminated. Health equity can be achieved. Over 60 US counties have already achieved lower Black male mortality rates than the average US white male mortality rate.[11] Some states will achieve racial equality in infant survival within my lifetime if they can just maintain their current rate of progress.

Senator Cory Booker put it this way: "Hope confronts. It does not ignore pain, agony, or injustice. . . . You can't have hope without despair, because hope is a response. Hope is the active conviction that despair will never have the last word."[12]

Globally, too, there is reason for hope. The worldwide under-five child mortality rate was cut in half in the two decades from 1990 to 2010. It is on track to drop another 50 percent in the following decades. What once seemed to be an impossible vision was achieved through effective efforts to address extreme poverty. In the most underresourced two-thirds world settings, we see the combined impact of economic development, access to safe water and food, and vaccinations against deadly childhood illnesses.

Since then, the United Nations has established Sustainable Development Goals such as "no poverty," "zero hunger," and "good health and well-being." Specific targets include *eliminating* preventable deaths of infants and children under age five by 2030. Such hopeful, aspirational goals may seem naively optimistic. Yet consider the global eradication of smallpox—was that goal not naively ambitious? From 1960 to 1973, the world eliminated the deadly disfiguring disease of smallpox. Not just controlled it. Eradicated it. Worldwide. And we're on a path to doing the same with polio.

We must create an affirmative expectation that health equity is achievable. And we must hold each other accountable for measuring our progress, accelerating that progress, and ultimately achieving our goal. No more wringing of the hands and saying that the poor will always be with you. No more soul-sucking talks on the tragedies of health disparities. Dr. David Satcher once said that "living through the Civil Rights movement showed me that I could be a part of change. I realized then that you don't have to accept things the way they are."[13] And more than almost anyone on the planet, he has been the voice for eliminating health disparities and achieving health equity in our lifetime.

Migrant farmworkers have faced some of the greatest injustices of any group in America. Yet the Coalition of Immokalee Workers (CIW) has made incredible progress through unity and community organizing. Starting with the Taco Bell boycott, CIW effectively pressured the grocery stores and fast-food chains that purchase tomatoes. Since then, CIW has managed to get most tomato growers in their area to sign the fair food agreement. It guarantees safer fields and better pay for the workers who harvest our food. The *Washington Post* called CIW "one of the great human rights success stories of our day."[14]

History is on our side. "The arc of the moral universe is long, but it bends toward justice."[15] Martin Luther King Jr. paraphrased this from an abolitionist minister, who had said it a century before. Both sought to speak their vision of justice into being. History shows that this arc bends toward justice even more strongly when leaders articulate a clear vision. They provide the optimism and faith to build movements.

One could argue that there was no earthly cause for optimism or hope in Selma, Alabama, in 1965, or during the United Farmworkers' Delano march and grape boycott, or in South Africa during apartheid. But leaders acted as if the outcome of justice was already assured. In his American Dream speech, Dr. King called us to "rise . . . from the fatigue of darkness to the buoyancy of hope."[16]

Ta-Nehisi Coates cautions us against the naive assumption that we will inevitably have a happy redemptive ending. He says, "You must resist the common urge . . . toward fairy tales that imply some irrepressible justice."[17] We have to work for the future we hope for, not just sit back and wait for it to inevitably find us.

None of the visionaries who changed our world were naive about their realities, yet they voiced hope. In the same poem in which Langston Hughes said, "There's never been equality for me, nor freedom in this 'homeland of the free,'"[18] he went on to say this:

O, yes,
I say it plain,
America never was America to me,
And yet I swear this oath—
America will be!

We cannot act toward a just and equitable future without first imagining it. We need to have a vision. Desmond Tutu acknowledged that "apartheid did look invincible" but also said that "hope is being able to see that there is light despite all of the darkness."[19] Nelson Mandela said simply, "It seems impossible until it's done."[20]

Tutu and Mandela, Chavez and Huerta, Marsha Johnson and Harvey Milk, MLK and John Lewis all had a dream. They all voiced aspirational, wildly unrealistic, yet strangely specific expressions of hope. They articulated for us a clear vision of a just future.

The key is not to be overwhelmed or to underestimate the challenges. In the book *Good to Great*, Jim Collins summarized lessons learned by a prisoner of war during eight years of isolation and torture in Viet Nam.[21] He called it the Stockdale Paradox—honestly confront the brutal facts, but never lose faith.

Is it really achievable? Yes!

Our team at the National Center for Primary Care at Morehouse School of Medicine built a body of research around the mantra that *"disparities are not inevitable."* In a study of infant mortality, our team identified a specifically "resilient" stratum of counties. Each had moved from high racial disparities in infant mortality in 1979 to paradoxically low Black infant mortality rates by 2001. It was still true even after controlling for education, poverty, and income levels.[22]

For at least a decade now, our research in health disparities has shifted to focus on building an affirmative expectation of success. How do we move toward optimal and equitable outcomes for all? Our research articles have titles like these:

- What If We Were Equal?
- Disparities Are Not Inevitable
- Triangulating on Success
- Progress in Reducing the Black–White Infant Mortality Gap
- Paths to Cancer Health Equity

Realistic hope demands an affirmative vision of a positive outcome. In several studies on cancer mortality, we identified US counties that had moved from high levels of racial disparity to near equality over a 20-year period.[23] This work also reminded us that the cure is not always the inverse of the cause. Finding potential paths to health equity may push us to understand and learn from paradoxically successful, equality-achieving communities.

My former colleagues at Morehouse and Emory are now conducting a whole portfolio of research on what drives more positive health outcomes. How is one community able to swim upstream against the tide of adverse social determinants? What makes a person more resilient to ongoing stressors of race and poverty? What makes some impoverished neighborhoods more resilient than others?

Disparities are not inevitable. Health equity is achievable. In certain conditions and in certain communities, it is already happening. We must commit to achieving equality of outcomes. We must find the combinations of interventions that can drive the elimination of health disparities. We must use surveillance of real-time data to create rapid-cycle feedback loops. We have to know if and when we are moving the needle toward equity. When we are not, we must change the interventions to do more, do it better, and do it cohesively. We must have an affirmative expectation of a positive outcome. Finally, we must hold ourselves and each other accountable to achieve optimal and equitable outcomes for all.

And what about the larger vision of social justice? How do we make equal the social determinants that drive so many disparities in health outcomes? I choose not to look just at the massive challenge of poverty but at the huge opportunity to make it better. Take one example. Before the passage of Medicare and Social Security, roughly half of all elderly people in America lived below the poverty level. Even now, 37 percent of older adults would be living below the poverty level if they didn't have Social Security income. Instead, the number of elderly persons below the poverty level is now just 9.2 percent.[24] Amazing progress. More left to do. Challenge accepted.

There recently was an event in which the descendants of Robert E. Lee gathered at his National Memorial on a hill in Arlington National Cemetery with descendants of people whom Lee's family had enslaved. They talked of remembering hard history and remembering ancestors but also of finding new paths of reconciliation and healing. A park ranger who works at the site said, "Just seeing all of these people come together in this moment, at this site, it symbolizes hope for me; hope for our country because if they can do it, we all can do it."[25]

What gives me hope today, as exhausted and exasperated as I am with my beloved Florida and my beloved nation, are the people of hope, young and old:

- Students whose friends were killed at Marjorie Stoneman Douglass High School in Parkland, Florida, are organized and fighting for common-sense gun laws. One has been elected to Congress.
- Students and faculty of our state universities are speaking out against the bullying of trans and gay people and standing up for teaching our racial history. Black History Professor Ndiangui said, "We're going to stand for the truth. . . . Love will always prevail. Justice will always prevail."[26]
- In Florida, a 100-year-old woman, Grace Linn, testified before the Martin County school board against the banning of books.[27] She showed a quilt that she had made, each patch representing a book that was banned. She said, "I was born the year after women got the right to vote. My first husband was killed in action in World War II. He died for freedom. One of the freedoms that the Nazis crushed was the freedom to read the books that they banned."
- High school kids are organizing to elect supportive school board members. One student who experienced

anti-LGBTQ discrimination in Florida schools said, "The thing about Gen Z is that we are passionate about the injustices we witness and vocal against its perpetrators."[28]

- In Des Moines, a group of 11-year-olds started a basketball team for non-binary kids. Said a supportive parent, "I want for these kids to have more soft places in the world to land."
- Hennepin County, Minnesota, reduced homelessness by 80 percent in five years by investing heavily in transitional and long-term supportive housing for the chronically homeless. The county has committed to ending chronic homelessness by the end of 2025, saying not that no one will be homeless, but "that instances will be rare, brief and nonrecurring, and more people will exit homelessness than enter it."
- Across an increasingly conservative "anti-woke" Florida, eight Florida cities have earned a perfect score on the Human Rights Campaign's Municipal Equality Index of LGBTQ inclusiveness.[29]
- In 2023, Kentucky's Democratic governor issued an election-year veto of a Republican bill banning access to gender-affirming health care. While advocating for women's reproductive rights, he was reelected by a large majority in a very red state.[30]

I take hope from my colleagues, each in their own way seeking to become more open and healing in their relationships. They live the change they seek, through teaching and research and community involvement and advocacy, forging new paths to social justice and health equity.

And I take the greatest hope of all from my kids, and their friends, and their generation. I find hope in the ways that they actively engage with their diverse, multicultural, multigendered world. I take hope from how they are raising their kids (my grandkids) to be far better at all this than I could ever be.

Some describe our goal of achieving health equity as being a journey, a destination we never see until we get there. A current meme sums it up this way—*call me when you reach Nirvana*. Instead, Dr. Camara Jones has given us the parable of the Gardner's Tale, "an allegory about a gardener with 2 flower boxes, rich and poor soil, and red and pink flowers."[31] I love this imagery.

I choose to imagine health equity as a garden of beauty, bursting with rainbow colors and lush, lavish, resplendent life. Imagine an abundance of flowers and trees and ponds and streams. Now imagine that it's not some faraway place. Imagine instead that each of us can create these beautiful gardens of abundant life exactly where we are, right here and right now.

We must first cultivate and nurture the garden of our own healing, deep in our own heart and headspace. We must see our own vision for equity. We must cultivate the emerging passion for justice within ourselves. Nurture the garden within.

We can then begin to think about all of the spaces and relationships in which we have some influence. These are places we can begin. Wherever we are, in even the smallest spheres of influence, we can till the soil and plant the seeds and water the garden and nourish life. Each of us can build gardens of health equity and social justice, first in our own lives and in our families. Perhaps then we can nurture beauty and equity in our work setting. Maybe it's in a medical practice or in one unit of a hospital, or perhaps a social agency or a business or even one block of a neighborhood.

Many of us are not in charge of anything. We feel like we have no power to make gardens of equity or to make justice blossom. But where we do not have control, we often have influence. We can speak up when we see injustice. We can ask the naive question—*how could we make things better?* We can reflect bias or ugliness back to the speaker—*"What did you mean when you said that?"*

We can be an ally. We can stand with those who have authentic lived experience or who are effective advocates for their community. We can notice when hierarchy or systems of power or a culture of denial are making it too risky for them to speak up. In those moments, we can step into that danger and speak as an ally.

Perhaps we will be near enough to others to find connections. We begin to see our gardens merge and blend and fill spaces that once were barren with death and injustice. Imagine thousands of us across this country and millions across the world committed to nurturing gardens of equity in all the spaces we touch. Imagine those vibrant, colorful gardens becoming the ecosystem of our nation and injustice merely the weeds that we must occasionally dig out.

Wouldn't that be worth doing? Wouldn't that be cool? Wouldn't you want to play your part? We don't have to be perfect. We just have to do our best to grow and tend the garden. But we have to be intentional.

In the words of the Hebrew prophet Amos, "Let justice roll down like the living waters, and goodness as an ever-flowing stream." In the end, hope is not a strategy. It is far more important than that! Like President Obama, we need to embrace "the audacity of hope" in a brutally honest but stubbornly optimistic commitment to optimal and equitable health for all. Sixteen years before apartheid ended, then-bishop Desmond Tutu spoke at the funeral of murdered activist Stephen Biko. He declared that "the powers of injustice, of oppression, of exploitation, have done their worst, and they have lost."[32]

I recently attended a concert presented by the Florida A&M University (FAMU) Concert Choir and the Tallahassee Symphony Orchestra at Lee Hall on the historically Black FAMU campus. I chose this venue intentionally instead of going to the large concert hall on my comfortable turf at FSU. Make these conscious choices. If you've never watched *Black Panther* at a downtown movie theater with a mostly Black audience, you've never really experienced *Black Panther*.

Powerful Voices was a newly commissioned piece, celebrating the two FAMU students who refused to move to the back of the bus in 1956. They were arrested for "causing a riot." That was two months before I was born and six months after Rosa Parks had been arrested in Montgomery.

The piece also celebrated the FAMU students who rallied around them in the very building in which I was listening to the concert. And it celebrated C. K. Steele and other civil rights leaders who joined the moment to organize the Tallahassee bus boycott and withstand the white backlash. Crosses were burned in front of houses, but people stood strong. The choir sang of moving from terror to indignation.

In a county whose population was 73 percent enslaved people in 1860, in a state that seems to be racing backward on racial justice, for one night I was part of a broadly multiracial audience melding our hearts together with a mostly Black choir and a mostly white orchestra. We were all together as one community celebrating our local civil rights heroes and the spirit that seeks justice.

When we heard the first notes of "Lift Every Voice and Sing," people of all races stood out of respect and sang as one. And when every soul in the room joined with the choir and the symphony to sing "We Shall Overcome," I began again to believe it.

It gave me hope for our nation. Even for Florida.

C. K. Steele was the faith leader and civil rights champion who was so central to the success of the Tallahassee bus boycott in 1956. He spoke nearly a quarter-century later to students here at FSU. He saw in these protests "the great opportunity to fulfill the purpose of this great nation . . . , where there would be a real brotherhood and economic fairness and justice for all." He went on to say, "Somehow," he said, "in spite of hell and high water, I believe that the great day will come."[33]

I too hope for that great day to come. I hope for health equity and social justice. I hope we build the diverse, multicultural, multigendered human family in which we all have a place. I hope I live to see Dr. King's beloved community. I hope to walk in the beautiful gardens of equity and justice we must all work to cultivate. I hope with the robust, complex hope of the clear-eyed realist who sees the hell and the high water but also the beautiful gardens beyond.

One physician recently wrote a personal essay about the importance of hope in a time of her own grief. She said, "Hope is not delusion, and hope is not denial. . . . Hope was the steady whisper that goodness was still possible."[34]

May we all hear that whisper of hope. Goodness is still possible!

Cling to the hope. Build out the goodness.

Care for ourselves. Embrace one another.

Be the beloved community.

Tend our gardens.

Hope.

Love.

Heal.

FOR FURTHER READING

Goodall J, Abrams D, Hudson G. *The Book of Hope: A Survival Guide for Trying Times.*

Jackson JL, Kim GJ-S, ed. *Keeping Hope Alive: Sermons and Speeches of Rev. Jesse L. Jackson, Sr.*

Meacham J. *His Truth Is Marching On: John Lewis and the Power of Hope.*

Obama B. *The Audacity of Hope.*

Obama B. *A Promised Land.*

NOTES

Chapter 1. Leaving White-World

1. Wilkerson I. *Caste: The Origins of Our Discontents*. Random House; 2020:118–120.

2. Chozick A. How Hillary Clinton went undercover to examine race in education. *New York Times*. December 27, 2015. https://www.nytimes.com/2015/12/28/us/politics/how-hillary-clinton-went-undercover-to-examine-race-in-education.html.

3. Quarshie M, Slack D. Census: US sees unprecedented multiracial growth, decline in the white population for first time in history. *USA TODAY*. August 12, 2021. https://www.usatoday.com/story/news/politics/2021/08/12/how-2020-census-change-how-we-look-america-what-expect/5493043001/.

4. Krogstad JM. Reflecting a demographic shift, 109 U.S. counties have become majority nonwhite since 2000. Pew Research Center. August 21, 2019. https://www.pewresearch.org/fact-tank/2019/08/21/u-s-counties-majority-nonwhite/.

5. James Baldwin, *Notes of a Native Son*, 1955, as quoted in Boykin K. *Race Against Time: The Politics of a Darkening America*. Bold Type Books; 2021:5.

6. Tatum BD. *Why Are All the Black Kids Sitting Together in the Cafeteria? And Other Conversations About Race*. Basic Books; 2017.

7. Martin R, Lakins L. *White Fear: How the Browning of America Is Making White Folks Lose Their Minds*. Benbella Books; 2022.

8. Gonyea D. Majority of white Americans say they believe whites face discrimination. *NPR*. October 24, 2017. https://www.npr.org/2017/10/24/559604836/majority-of-white-americans-think-theyre-discriminated-against.

9. Gonella C. Survey: 20 percent of Millennials identify as LGBTQ. *NBC News*. March 31, 2017. https://www.nbcnews.com/feature/nbc-out/survey-20-percent-millennials-identify-lgbtq-n740791.

10. Frank Wilhoit (classical music composer, not the political scientist of the same name) blogpost on crookedtimber, March 22, 2018, https://

crookedtimber.org/2018/03/21/liberals-against-progressives
/#comment-729288, as quoted in *Slate*, https://slate.com/business
/2022/06/wilhoits-law-conservatives-frank-wilhoit.html.

11. Silliman D. Decline of Christianity shows no signs of stopping. *Christianity Today*. September 13, 2022, https://www.christianitytoday
.com/news/2022/september/christian-decline-inexorable-nones-rise
-pew-study.html.

12. Booker C. United: *Thoughts on Finding Common Ground and Advancing the Common Good*. Ballantine Books; 2016.

13. Will GF. Opinion: How America became a nation of the woke and the wary, walking on eggshells. *Washington Post*. March 11, 2022. https://
www.washingtonpost.com/opinions/2022/03/11/how-america
-became-woke-and-wary/.

Chapter 2. Unnecessary Suffering

1. Egan BM, Li J, Sutherland SE, Rakotz MK, Wozniak GD. Hypertension control in the United States 2009 to 2018: factors underlying falling control rates during 2015 to 2018 across age- and race-ethnicity groups. *Hypertension*. 2021;78(3):578-587. doi:10.1161/HYPERTENSIONAHA.120.16418.

2. Muntner P, Hardy ST, Fine LJ, Jaeger BC, Wozniak G, Levitan EB, Colantonio LD. Trends in blood pressure control among US adults with hypertension, 1999-2000 to 2017-2018. *JAMA*. 2020; 324(12): 1190-1200. doi:10.1001/jama.2020.14545.

3. Brown TM, Fee E. Rudolf Carl Virchow: medical scientist, social reformer, role model. *Am J Public Health*. 2006;96(12):2104-2105. doi:10.2105/AJPH.2005.078436.

4. Satcher D, Fryer GE Jr, McCann J, Troutman A, Woolf SH, Rust G. What if we were equal? A comparison of the Black-white mortality gap in 1960 and 2000. *Health Aff (Millwood)*. 2005;24(2):459-464. doi:10.1377/hlthaff.24.2.459.

5. Murray CJL, Kulkarni SC, Michaud C, et al. Eight Americas: investigating mortality disparities across races, counties, and race-counties in the United States. *PLoS Med*. 2006;3(9):e260. doi:10.1371/journal.pmed.0030260.

6. McCord C, Freeman HP. Excess mortality in Harlem. *N Engl J Med*. 1990;322:173-177. doi:10.1056/NEJM199001183220306.

7. Davis MA, Guo C, Sol K, Langa KM, Nallamothu BK. Trends and disparities in the number of self-reported healthy older adults in the United States, 2000 to 2014. *JAMA Intern Med*. 2017;177(11):1683-1684. doi:10.1001/jamainternmed.2017.4357.

8. Agency for Healthcare Research and Quality (AHRQ). *2021 National Healthcare Quality and Disparities Report Executive Summary Agency for Healthcare Research and Quality (AHRQ)*. https://www.ahrq.gov /sites/default/files/wysiwyg/research/findings/nhqrdr/2021qdr-final -es.pdf.

9. Caraballo C, Massey DS, Ndumele CD, et al. Excess mortality and years of potential life lost among the Black population in the US, 1999-2020. *JAMA*. 2023;329(19):1662-1670. doi:10.1001/jama.2023 .7022.

10. Agency for Healthcare Research and Quality (AHRQ). Executive summary. 2021 National Healthcare Quality and Disparities report. https://www.ahrq.gov/sites/default/files/wysiwyg/research/findings /nhqrdr/2021qdr-final-es.pdf.

11. 250,000 dumped from Medicaid rolls in Florida alone. *Washington Post*. https://www.washingtonpost.com/politics/2023/06/06/states -find-there-more-than-one-way-unwind-medicaid/.

12. Phelan JC, Link BG, Diez-Roux A, Kawachi I, Levin B. "Fundamental causes" of social inequalities in mortality: a test of the theory [published correction appears in *J Health Soc Behav*. 2005;46(1):v]. *J Health Soc Behav*. 2004;45(3):265-285. doi:10.1177/002214650404500303.

13. King WD, Minor P, Ramirez Kitchen C, et al. Racial, gender and geographic disparities of antiretroviral treatment among US Medicaid enrolees in 1998. *J Epidemiol Community Health*. 2008;62(9):798-803. doi:10.1136/jech.2005.045567.

14. US DHEW. Report of the Secretary's Task Force on Black and Minority Health. 1985. https://collections.nlm.nih.gov/catalog/nlm:nlmuid -8602912-mvset.

15. US DHEW. Report of the Secretary's Task Force on Black and Minority Health. 1985. https://minorityhealth.hhs.gov/assets/pdf/checked/1 /ANDERSON.pdf.

16. Giles Bruce, quoting William D. Leading Harvard expert on disparities urges journalists to be a "tiny ripple of hope." July 21, 2020. USC Annenburg Center for Health Journalism. https://centerforhealthjour nalism.org/2020/07/21/leading-harvard-researcher-disparities-urges -journalists-be-tiny-ripple-hope.

17. Dyson ME. *The Tears We Cannot Stop*. St. Martin's Griffin Edition; 2021.

18. Moon M. White feminism won't cut it. *Reporter*. Rochester Institute of Technology; November 30, 2016. https://reporter.rit.edu/views/white -feminism-wont-cut-it.

19. National LGBTQ Task Force. Injustice at every turn: a report of the National Transgender Discrimination Survey, as cited in *Analysis*

Shows Startling Levels of Discrimination Against Black Transgender People. September 16, 2011. https://www.thetaskforce.org/news /analysis-shows-startling-levels-of-discrimination-against-black -transgender-people/.

20. Centers for Disease Control and Prevention. Drug overdose: death rate maps & graphs. https://www.cdc.gov/drugoverdose/deaths/index.html.

21. Brown Speights JS, Goldfarb SS, Wells BA, Beitsch L, Levine RS, Rust G. State-level progress in reducing the Black-white infant mortality gap, United States, 1999–2013 [published correction appears in *Am J Public Health.* 2018;108(4):e14–e16]. *Am J Public Health.* 2017;107(5): 775–782. doi:10.2105/AJPH.2017.303689.

22. Dr. Martin Luther King Jr. in 1966, while addressing the second convention of the Medical Committee for Human Rights. PNHP. MLK's vision and the right to healthcare. https://pnhp.org/news/mlks-vision -and-the-right-to-healthcare/.

23. Lockhart PR. What Serena Williams's scary childbirth story says about medical treatment of Black women. *Vox.com.* January 11, 2018. https:// www.vox.com/identities/2018/1/11/16879984/serena-williams-child birth-scare-Black-women.

24. Patterson E, Becker A, Baluran D. Gendered racism on the body: an intersectional approach to maternal mortality in the United States. *Popul Res Policy Rev.* 2022;41:1–34. doi:10.1007/s11113-021-09691-2.

25. CNN. 4 out of 5 pregnancy-related deaths in the US are preventable, CDC finds. https://www.cnn.com/2022/09/19/health/maternal -mortality-preventable-cdc/index.html.

26. Martin N, Montagne R. Lost mothers: nothing protects Black women from dying in pregnancy and childbirth. ProPublic. NPR News. December 7, 2017. https://www.propublica.org/article/nothing-protects-Black -women-from-dying-in-pregnancy-and-childbirth.

27. Mullan F. Tin-cup medicine. *Health Aff (Millwood).* 2001;20(6):216–221. doi:10.1377/hlthaff.20.6.216.

28. LaVeist TA, Pérez-Stable EJ, Richard P, et al. The economic burden of racial, ethnic, and educational health inequities in the US. *JAMA.* 2023;329(19):1682–1692. doi:10.1001/jama.2023.5965.

29. National Center for Health Statistics. *Healthy People 2010 Final Review.* National Center for Health Statistics; 2012. file:///C:/Users/georu/ Downloads/cdc_12360_DS1.pdf.

30. Byrd WM, Clayton LA. An American health dilemma: a history of Blacks in the health system. *J Natl Med Assoc.* 1992;84(2):189–200.

31. King ML Jr. Where do we go from here: chaos or community? *Newsweek.* https://www.newsweek.com/martin-luther-king-inspiring -quotes-mlk-day-2022-1668511.

32. Swietek K, Gianattasio KZ, Henderson S, et al. Association between racial segregation and COVID-19 vaccination rates. *J Public Health Manag Pract.* 2023;29(4):572–579. doi:10.1097/PHH.0000000000 001738.

33. Institute of Medicine (US) Division of Health Care Services. *Community Oriented Primary Care: A Practical Assessment: Volume I: The Committee Report.* National Academies Press; 1984. https://www.ncbi .nlm.nih.gov/books/NBK217635/.

Chapter 3. Unmentionable History

1. Holland B. The father of modern gynecology performed shocking experiments on slaves. History.com. August 29, 2017. https://www .history.com/news/the-father-of-modern-gynecology-performed -shocking-experiments-on-slaves.

2. Gamble VN. Under the shadow of Tuskegee: African Americans and health care. *Am J Public Health.* 1997;87(11):1773–1778. doi:10.2105/ ajph.87.11.1773.

3. Holland B. The father of modern gynecology performed shocking experiments on slaves. History.com. August 29, 2017. https://www .history.com/news/the-father-of-modern-gynecology-performed -shocking-experiments-on-slaves.

4. Sims JM. *The Story of My Life.* D. Appleton and Company; 1884. https://ia800303.us.archive.org/1/items/storyofmylifoosims /storyofmylifoosims.pdf.

5. Smith ND. Virginia Republicans vote against apology for misusing Black bodies for medical research, citing "no-end" to number of amends needed. *Atlanta Black Star.* February 26, 2023. https://atlantaBlackstar .com/2023/02/26/virginia-republican-politicians-vote-down-an -official-apology-for-misusing-Black-bodies-for-medical-research/.

6. Kenney JA. Second Annual Oration on Surgery: the Negro's contribution to surgery. *J Natl Med Assoc.* 1941;33(5):203–214.

7. AAMC. Diversity facts & figures. https://www.aamc.org/data-reports /workforce/report/diversity-facts-figures.

8. AAMC News. At a glance: Black and African American physicians in the workforce. February 20, 2017. https://www.aamc.org/news-insights /glance-Black-and-african-american-physicians-workforce.

9. Wilson DE, Kaczmarek JM. The history of African-American physicians and medicine in the United States. *J Assoc Acad Minor Phys.* 1993;4(3):93–98.

10. Tweedy D. *Black Man in a White Coat.* Picador; 2015:121.

11. Downey M. Morehouse held a crown over his head. Harvard held a question mark. *Philadelphia Tribune.* September 24, 2019. https://www

.phillytrib.com/news/across_america/morehouse-held-a-crown-over
-his-head-harvard-held-a-question-mark/article_cca8224e-d599-58a7
-a12f-48dd91fcbf43.html.

12. Russell T. Mortality rate for Black babies is cut dramatically when Black doctors care for them after birth, researchers say. *Washington Post.* January 13, 2021. https://www.washingtonpost.com/health /Black-baby-death-rate-cut-by-Black-doctors/2021/01/08/e9f0f850 -238a-11eb-952e-0c475972cfc0_story.html, citing Greenwood BN, Hardeman RR, Huang L, Sojourner A. Physician-patient racial concordance and disparities in birthing mortality for newborns. *Proc Natl Acad Sci U S A.* 2020;117(35):21194–21200. doi:10.1073/ pnas.1913405117.

13. Satcher D. *My Quest for Health Equity: Notes on Learning While Leading.* Johns Hopkins University Press; 2020.

14. Call J. FSU faculty say it's "rubbish" as Christopher Rufo targets FSU "radical" diversity programs. *Tallahassee Democrat.* February 23, 2023. https://www.tallahassee.com/story/news/politics/2023/02/03/new -college-trustee-christopher-rufo-blasts-fsu-diversity-programs -florida-state-says-its-rubbish/69869875007/.

15. "The American Dream," July 4th Speech Transcript—Martin Luther King Jr. July 1965. Transcribed on rev.com. https://www.rev.com/blog /transcripts/the-american-dream-july-4th-speech-transcript-martin -luther-king-jr

16. Frederick Douglass gave a speech he titled, "What to the Slave Is the Fourth of July?" https://nmaahc.si.edu/explore/stories/nations-story -what-slave-fourth-july.

17. Robinson J. *I Never Had it Made.* HarperCollins; 1995.

18. Meacham J. *His Truth Is Marching On: John Lewis and the Power of Hope.* Random House; 2020:241.

19. Ellison R. What America would be like without Blacks. *Time* magazine, 1970, as quoted by Jones J. Black history, uncensored: Ralph Ellison envisioned an American nightmare. MSNBC. February 15, 2023. https://www.msnbc.com/the-reidout/reidout-blog/ralph-ellison -Black-history-uncensored-rcna70849.

20. Hughes L. Let America be America again. In: *The Collected Poems of Langston Hughes.* Alfred A. Knopf; 1994. Copyright © 1994 the Estate of Langston Hughes. https://poets.org/poem/let-america-be-america -again.

21. Cane C. Not just Tulsa: Race massacres that devastated Black communities in Rosewood, Atlanta, and other American cities. BET.com. May 31, 2021. https://www.bet.com/article/fqn5oc/five-other-race -massacres-that-devastated-Black-america.

22. Brockell G. The long, ugly history of anti-Asian racism and violence in the U.S. *Washington Post*. March 18, 2021. https://www.washing tonpost.com/history/2021/03/18/history-anti-asian-violence -racism/.

23. Ledette J. Racism worsening for BIPOC children across US—study shows Black, Indigenous children increasingly experiencing racism. Black Information Network. November 14, 2022. https://www .binnews.com/content/2022-11-14-study-shows-Black-indigenous -children-increasingly-experiencing-racism/.

24. Tutu D, Tutu M. *The Book of Forgiving: The Fourfold Path for Healing Ourselves and Our World*. Edited by Douglas C. Abrams. Harper Collins; 2014:72–74.

25. Bump P. What does "woke" mean? Whatever Ron DeSantis wants. *Washington Post*. December 5, 2022. https://www.washingtonpost.com /politics/2022/12/05/desantis-florida-woke-critical-race-theory/.

26. Stripling J. Channeling Orwell, judge blasts Florida's "dystopian" ban on "woke" instruction. *Chronicle Higher Educ*. November 17, 2022. https://www.chronicle.com/article/conjuring-orwell-florida-judge -blasts-dystopian-ban-on-woke-instruction

27. Kendi IX. *How to Be an Anti-Racist*. One World; 2019:14–15.

28. Gilbreath E. A prophet out of Harlem. *Christianity Today*. September 16, 1996. https://www.christianitytoday.com/ct/1996/september 16/6ta036.html.

29. Milbank D, Glenn Youngkin's no-guilt history of Virginia for fragile white people. *Washington Post*. February 1, 2022. https://www.wash ingtonpost.com/opinions/2022/02/01/racist-virginia-textbooks -history-youngkin/.

30. Pornoy J. Glenn Youngkin's health chief doubts racial disparities in health care. *Washington Post*. June 15, 2022. https://www.washington post.com/dc-md-va/2022/06/15/racial-disparities-health-care -youngkin/.

31. Rothstein R. *The Color of Law: A Forgotten History of How Our Govern- ment Segregated America*. Liveright Publishing (Norton); 2018.

32. Nehisi-Coates T. *Between the World and Me*. One World (Penguin Random House); 2005:8.

33. Perkins J. *Let Justice Roll Down*, quoted in: *The Beloved Community: How Faith Shapes Social Justice from the Civil Rights Movement to Today*. Basic Books; 2005:246.

34. Mastrovita M. Architectural records documenting segregated health care facilities in Baldwin, Richmond, Treutlen, Ware, and Wayne counties in Georgia now available online. *Galileo*. February 3, 2021. https://blog.dlg.galileo.usg.edu/?p=7709.

35. "Diagram of Fourth Floor of Detroit Memorial Hospital Where Negro Patients Are Concentrated." Detroit Urban League Collection, Bentley Historical Library; University of Michigan. Image posted by Charlene Galarneau in blog titled King's Words on Health Injustice: what did he actually say? *International Journal of Feminist Approaches to Bioethics*. April 19, 2018. https://www.ijfab.org/blog/2018/04/kings-words-on -health-injustice-what-did-he-actually-say/.

36. Largent EA. Public health, racism, and the lasting impact of hospital segregation. *Public Health Rep.* 2018;133(6):715-720. doi:10.1177/003 3354918795891.

37. Brooks DD, Smith DR, Anderson RJ. Medical apartheid: an American perspective. *JAMA*. 1991;266(19):2746-2749. doi:10.1001/jama.1991 .03470190094036.

38. Vinekar K. Pathology of racism: a call to desegregate teaching hospitals. *N Engl J Med*. 2021;385(13):e40. doi:10.1056/NEJMpv2113508.

39. Byrd WM, Clayton LA. An American health dilemma: a history of Blacks in the health system. *J Natl Med Assoc*. 1992;84(2):189-200.

40. Tutu D. *No Future Without Forgiveness*. Random House; 1999:31.

41. Grossman R. 50 years ago: MLK's march in Marquette Park turned violent, exposed hate. *Chicago Tribune*. July 28, 2016. https://www .chicagotribune.com/opinion/commentary/ct-mlk-king-marquette -park-1966-flashback-perspec-0731-md-20160726-story.html.

42. The Martin Luther King, Jr. Research and Education Institute, Stanford University. Chicago Campaign. https://kinginstitute .stanford.edu/encyclopedia/chicago-campaign.

43. Kozol J. *Savage Inequalities: Children in America's Schools*. Broadway Books; 1991:51.

44. Kozol J. *Savage Inequalities: Children in America's Schools*. Broadway Books; 1991.

45. Gianaros PJ, Horenstein JA, Cohen S, et al. Perigenual anterior cingulate morphology covaries with perceived social standing. *Soc Cogn Affect Neurosci*. 2007;2(3):161-173. doi:10.1093/scan/nsm013.

46. Betancourt LM, Avants B, Farah MJ, et al. Effect of socioeconomic status (SES) disparity on neural development in female African-American infants at age 1 month. *Dev Sci*. 2016;19(6):947-956. https://doi.org/10.1111/desc.12344.

47. Schilbach F, Schofield H, Mullainathan S. The psychological lives of the poor. *Am Econ Rev*. 2016;106(5):435-440. doi:10.1257/aer.p20161101.

48. Muñoz E, Robins RW, Sutin AR. Perceived ethnic discrimination and cognitive function: a 12-year longitudinal study of Mexican-origin adults. *Soc Sci Med*. 2022;311:115296. doi:10.1016/j.socscimed .2022.115296.

49. McCloskey E. The deadly consequences of inequality. March 22, 2023. https://patrioticmillionaires.org/2023/03/22/the-deadly-conseq uences-of-inequality/

50. Pickett K, Wilkinson R. *The Spirit Level: Why More Equal Societies Almost Always Do Better.* Allen Lane; 2009.

51. Brown M. "Our history is like a compass": seven Tallahassee seniors reflect during Black *History Month Tallahassee Democrat.* February 13, 2021. https://www.tallahassee.com/story/life/2021/02/13/seven -tallahassee-seniors-think-back-during-black-history-month /6731237002/.

52. Sandra Mattar, as quoted by Zimmerman R. How does trauma spill from one generation to the next? *Washington Post.* June 12, 2023. https://www.washingtonpost.com/wellness/2023/06/12/generational -trauma-passed-healing/.

Chapter 4. The Unspeakable R-Word: Racism

1. Omowale Akintunde, as quoted by DiAngelo R. *White Fragility: Why It's So Hard for White People to Talk About Racism.* Beacon Press; 2018:72.

2. DiAngelo R. *White Fragility: Why It's So Hard for White People to Talk About Racism.* Beacon Press; 2018:7.

3. Kendi IX. *How to Be an AntiRacist.* Random House; 2019:47.

4. Rust G, Levine RS, Fry-Johnson Y, Baltrus P, Ye J, Mack D. Paths to success: optimal and equitable health outcomes for all. *J Health Care Poor Underserved.* 2012;23(2)(suppl):7-19. doi:10.1353/hpu.2012.0084.

5. Rust G, Zhang S, Malhotra K, et al. Paths to health equity: local area variation in progress toward eliminating breast cancer mortality disparities, 1990–2009. *Cancer.* 2015;121(16):2765-2774. doi:10.1002/ cncr.29405.

6. Brown Speights JS, Goldfarb SS, Levine RS, Rust G. Racial equality in infant outcomes: a call to action. *Am J Public Health.* 2019;109(5):666-668. doi:10.2105/AJPH.2019.305028.

7. Quarles C. New study indicates that invoking "white privilege" often backfires. *PsyPost.* May 21, 2022. https://www.psypost.org/2022/05 /new-study-indicates-that-invoking-white-privilege-often-backfires -63189.

8. Campbell J. Why this predominantly white county in Southern California is declaring racism a public health crisis. *CNN.* December 9, 2022. https://www.cnn.com/2022/12/08/us/orange-county-racism -public-health-crisis-reaj/.

9. Agarwal P. Neuroimaging our unconscious biases. *Sci Am.* Special edition. Summer 2021:34-35.

10. Gee GC, Ro A. Racism and discrimination. In: Trinh-Shevrin C, Islam NS, Rey MJ, eds. *Asian American Communities and Health: Context, Research, Policy, and Action.* Jossey Bass; 2009.

11. Bonilla-Silva E. Rethinking racism: toward a structural interpretation. *Am Sociol Rev.* 1997;62(3):465–80.

12. Hurston ZN. *You Don't Know Us Negroes.* HarperCollins; 2022:186–187.

13. Farah B. *America Made Me a Black Man.* HarperCollins; 2022.

14. Hughes L. Mother and child. In: *The Ways of White Folks.* Vintage Books; 1933/1990:190.

15. King ML Jr. Letter from a Birmingham Jail. https://www.africa.upenn .edu/Articles_Gen/Letter_Birmingham.html.

16. Kessler G. Stephen Miller's disingenuous ad charging "anti-White" racism. *Washington Post.* November 4, 2022. https://www.washington post.com/politics/2022/11/04/stephen-millers-disingenuous-ad -charging-anti-white-racism/.

17. Brownlee D. Dear white people: when you say you "don't see color," this is what we really hear. *Forbes.* June 19, 2022. https://www.forbes .com/sites/danabrownlee/2022/06/19/dear-white-people-when-you -say-you-dont-see-color-this-is-what-we-really-hear/?sh=50005d 2a26d6.

18. Myhre KGT. How to explain white supremacy to a white supremacist. March 7, 2016. https://guante.info/2016/03/17/how-to-explain-white -supremacy-to-a-white-supremacist-new-video/.

19. Lemon D. *This Is the Fire: What I Say to My Friends About Racism.* Little, Brown; 2021:22.

20. Ledet J. "Get me a real doctor": Black physician left in tears by racist remarks. Black Information Network. August 4, 2022. https://www .binnews.com/content/2022-08-04-get-me-a-real-doctor-Black -physician-left-in-tears-by-racist-remarks/.

21. Saini A. The racist history of race science. Union of Concerned Scientists. October 6, 2020. https://www.ucsusa.org/resources/racist -history-race-science.

22. Linnaeus C. Systema Naturae, 10th edition, 1758. In: Encyclopedia .com. https://www.encyclopedia.com/social-sciences/encyclopedias -almanacs-transcripts-and-maps/scientific-racism-history.

23. Jardina A, Piston S. 2021. Hiding in plain sight: dehumanization as a foundation of white racial prejudice. *Sociol Compass.* 2021;15(9): e12913. https://compass.onlinelibrary.wiley.com/doi/10.1111/soc4 .12913.

24. Michelle Obama "ape in heels" post causes outrage. BBC. November 17, 2016. https://www.bbc.com/news/election-us-2016-37985967.

25. Wilkerson I. *Caste: The Origins of Our Discontents*. Random House; 2020:141–164.

26. Institute of Medicine (US) Committee on Understanding and Eliminating Racial and Ethnic Disparities in Health Care; Smedley BD, Stith AY, Nelson AR, eds. *Unequal Treatment: Confronting Racial and Ethnic Disparities in Health Care*. National Academies Press; 2003. https://www.ncbi.nlm.nih.gov/books/NBK220355/.

27. Schulman KA, Berlin JA, Harless W, et al. The effect of race and sex on physicians' recommendations for cardiac catheterization [published correction appears in *N Engl J Med*. 1999;340(14):1130]. *N Engl J Med*. 1999;340(8):618–626. doi:10.1056/NEJM199902253400806.

28. Weisse CS, Sorum PC, Sanders KN, Syat BL. Do gender and race affect decisions about pain management? *J Gen Intern Med*. 2001;16(4):211–217. doi:10.1046/j.1525-1497.2001.016004211.x.

29. Smith J, Spodak C. Black or "Other"? Doctors may be relying on race to make decisions about your health. CNN Health. July 6, 2023. https://www.cnn.com/2021/04/25/health/race-correction-in-medicine-history-refocused/index.html.

30. Rivas C. *Brown Enough*. Row House Publishing; 2022.

31. Keveney B. LA City Council racism scandal shows ugly side of creating political maps. Can redistricting reform help? *USA TODAY*. October 18, 2022. https://news.yahoo.com/la-city-council-racism-scandal-091203838.html.

32. Pereira KM, Telles EE. The color of health: skin color, ethnoracial classification and discrimination in the health of Latin Americans. *Soc Sci Med*. 2014;116:241–250.

33. Telles E. *Pigmentocracies: Ethnicity, Race, and Color in Latin America*. University of North Carolina Press; 2014. https://www.jstor.org/stable/10.5149/9781469617848_telles.

34. Flores RD, Telles E. Social stratification in Mexico: disentangling color, ethnicity and class. *Am Sociol Rev*. 2012;77(3):486–494.

35. Gross B. Education Justice Research and Organizing Collaborative (New York City) as quoted by Gail Cornwall in "Diverse schools are taking a new approach to anti-racism: training white parents." *USA TODAY*. April 12, 2022. https://www.usatoday.com/story/news/education/2022/04/12/diverse-schools-anti-racism-training-white-parents/9461020002/?gnt-cfr=1.

36. Michelle Obama, as quoted by Asmelash L. Michelle Obama: it's up to everyone to root out racism. *CNN*. May 30, 2020. https://www.cnn.com/2020/05/30/politics/michelle-obama-george-floyd-statement-trnd/index.html.

Chapter 5. Fear and Oppression

1. Petersen AH. Running while Black: a conversation with Alison Désir. November 2, 2022. https://annehelen.substack.com/p/running-while -Black.

2. Willingham AJ. Study of 100 million police stops finds Black motorists are more likely to be pulled over. *CNN.* March 21, 2019. https://www .cnn.com/2019/03/21/us/police-stops-race-stanford-study-trnd/index .html.

3. NAACP. Criminal Justice Fact Sheet. https://naacp.org/resources /criminal-justice-fact-sheet.

4. Cavna M. A Black father wrote a book about "the talk"—to show why it's necessary. *Washington Post.* June 6, 2023. https://www.washing tonpost.com/comics/2023/06/06/darrin-bell-the-talk/.

5. Karimi F. What Black drivers are doing to protect themselves during traffic stops. *CNN.* April 14, 2021. https://www.cnn.com/2021/04/14 /us/driving-while-Black-precautions-trnd/index.html.

6. Fara B. *America Made Me a Black Man.* HarperCollins; 2022:2.

7. Lemon D. *This Is the Fire: What I Say to My Friends About Racism.* Little, Brown; 2021:128-129.

8. Fatal Force: 1,128 people have been shot and killed by police in the past 12 months (as of Jan 31, 2024). *Washington Post.* https://www .washingtonpost.com/graphics/investigations/police-shootings -database/.

9. Bor J, Venkataramani AS, Williams DR, Tsai AC. Police killings and their spillover effects on the mental health of Black Americans: a population-based, quasi-experimental study. *Lancet.* 2018;392(10144):302-310. doi:10.1016/S0140-6736(18)31130-9.

10. Coates T. *Between the World and Me.* Spiegel and Grau; 2015.

11. John Lewis, speech at the March on Washington for Jobs and Freedom, 1963, as quoted in Martin R, Lakins L. *White Fear: How the Browning of America Is Making White Folks Lose Their Minds.* BenBella Books; 2022.

12. Novak S. Half of the 250 kids expelled from preschool each day are Black boys. *Sci Am.* January 12, 2023. https://www.scientificamerican .com/article/half-of-the-250-kids-expelled-from-preschool-each-day -are-Black-boys/.

13. Cooper B. *Eloquent Rage.* Picador Paperback; 2019:13.

14. UCLA School of Law. Discrimination and harassment by law enforce- ment officers in the LGBT community. March 2015. https://williams institute.law.ucla.edu/publications/lgbt-discrim-law-enforcement/.

15. Anti-Violence Project. Hate violence against transgender communities fact sheet. https://avp.org/wp-content/uploads/2017/04/ncavp _transhvfactsheet.pdf, as cited by the Innocence Project. https://

innocenceproject.org/lbgtq-pride-month-san-antonio-four-police
-violence/.

16. Dyson ME. *The Tears We Cannot Stop*. St. Martin's Press; 2021:177.

17. Dyson ME. *The Tears We Cannot Stop*. St. Martin's Press; 2021:174, 193.

18. Scoon V. FSU Film school faculty to present new documentary on history of plantations and the enslaved in North Florida. May 6, 2021. FSU College of Motion Picture Arts, https://film.fsu.edu/2021/05/06 /fsu-film-school-faculty-to-present-new-documentary-on-history-of -plantations-and-the-enslaved-in-north-florida/.

19. American History, Race, and Prison. Vera: Reimagining Prison Web Report. https://www.vera.org/reimagining-prison-web-report /american-history-race-and-prison.

20. Duke Sanford World Food Policy Center. Sharecropping, Black land acquisition, and white supremacy (1868–1900). https://wfpc.sanford .duke.edu/north-carolina/durham-food-history/sharecropping-Black -land-acquisition-and-white-supremacy-1868-1900/.

21. Bresin M. Betton Hills neighborhood president: offensive covenants matter, action needed. *Tallahassee Democrat.* July 2, 2019. https://www .tallahassee.com/story/opinion/2019/07/02/betton-hills-neighbor hood-president-offensive-covenants-matter-action-needed/16286 04001/.

22. Dunn M. Lynching incidents, 1916–1923. In: *A History of Florida Through Black Eyes*. CreateSpace Independent Publishing Platform; 2016:94–123.

23. The Story of Lynching in America: A Classified Listing (Tuskegee Lynching List). As shown by Dunn M. *A History of Florida Through Black Eyes*. CreateSpace Independent Publishing Platform; 2016: 259–273.

24. Nellis A. The color of justice: racial and ethnic disparity in state prisons. The Sentencing Project. October 13, 2021. https://www .sentencingproject.org/reports/the-color-of-justice-racial-and-ethnic -disparity-in-state-prisons-the-sentencing-project/.

25. Michelle Alexander, as quoted by hooks b. *Writing Beyond Race: Living Theory and Practice*. Routledge; 2013:127.

26. Patrice J. Prosecutor's typed rulebook demands harsher plea deals if defendant has criminal history "and/or Hispanic" . . . wait, what?!? *AboveTheLaw.* April 20, 2023. https://abovethelaw.com/2023/04 /prosecutors-typed-rulebook-demands-harsher-plea-deals-if -defendant-has-criminal-history-and-or-hispanic-wait-what/.

27. Miller K, Murphy S. Oklahoma sheriff says recording of killing talk was illegal. *APNews.* April 18, 2023. https://apnews.com/article/mccurtain

-oklahoma-racist-killing-journalists-recording-196ab0bf32fe8a5c0b4
8ef25c0af3c9f.

28. Lai KKR, Lee JC. Why 10% of Florida adults can't vote: how felony convictions affect access to the ballot. *New York Times*. October 6, 2016. https://www.nytimes.com/interactive/2016/10/06/us/unequal -effect-of-laws-that-block-felons-from-voting.html.

29. Boyd LM. Murder of James Byrd, Jr.: United States history. *Brittanica*, updated February 2, 2024. https://www.britannica.com/event/murder -of-James-Byrd-Jr.

30. Explained: COVID-19 and the rise in anti-Asian hate. An OCA-Asian Pacific American Advocates project. https://www.aapihatecrimes.org /facts.

31. Cramer RJ, Kaniuka AR, Yada FN, et al. An analysis of suicidal thoughts and behaviors among transgender and gender diverse adults. *Soc Psychiatry Psychiatr Epidemiol*. 2022;57(1):195–205. doi:10.1007/ s00127-021-02115-8.

32. National Crime Victimization Survey: LGBTQ Americans are 9 times more likely to be victimized by a hate crime. *Conversation*. December 21, 2022. https://theconversation.com/lgbtq-americans-are-9-times-more -likely-to-be-victimized-by-a-hate-crime-196717.

33. Matthew Shepard Foundation. Matthew's story. https://www.matthew shepard.org/about-us/our-story/.

34. Movement Advancement Project. *Policy Spotlight: Hate Crime Laws*. July 2021. www.lgbtmap.org/2021-report-hate-crimes.

35. Moore R. Man who killed 23 at El Paso Walmart pleads guilty to hate crimes. *Texas Tribune*. February 8, 2023. https://www.texastribune.org /2023/02/08/el-paso-walmart-shooting-pleads-guilty/.

36. Tanno S. A third of young men in Germany think violence against women is "acceptable," study finds. *CNN*. June 11, 2023. https://www .cnn.com/2023/06/11/europe/germany-violence-against-women -study-intl/index.html.

37. Ray M. Orlando shooting of 2016: United States history. *Brittanica*. December 28, 2023. https://www.britannica.com/event/Orlando -shooting-of-2016.

38. Driggers C. What it's like to be an LGBTQ+ high schooler in DeSantis's Florida. *Advocate*. March 21, 2023. https://www.advocate.com/voices /school-desantis-florida.

39. Ali W. Wajahat Ali's helpful guide to becoming an American. *The Daily Beast*. January 23, 2022. https://www.thedailybeast.com/wajahat-alis -helpful-guide-to-becoming-an-american.

40. Jefferson M. *Negroland: A Memoir*. Pantheon Books/Penguin Random House; 2015:163–164, 173.

41. Parker HW, Abreu AM, Sullivan MC, Vadiveloo MK. Allostatic load and mortality: a systematic review and meta-analysis. *Am J Prev Med.* 2022;63(1):131–140. doi:10.1016/j.amepre.2022.02.003.

42. Blake J. There's one epidemic we may never find a vaccine for: fear of Black men in public spaces. *CNN.* May 27, 2020. https://www.cnn.com /2020/05/26/us/fear-Black-men-blake/index.html.

43. Metzl JM. *Dying of Whiteness.* Basic Books; 2019:71.

44. Kuhn C, Mixon G. Atlanta Race Massacre of 1906. In: *New Georgia Encyclopedia.* September 3, 2005. https://www.georgiaencyclopedia .org/articles/history-archaeology/atlanta-race-massacre-of-1906/.

45. W. E. B. Du Bois, "A Litany at Atlanta," as quoted by Cone JH. *God of the Oppressed.* Orbis Books; 1997/2002:171.

46. Timsit A, McDaniel J. White neighbor shoots Black mother of four through door in Ocala. *Washington Post.* June 6, 2023. https://www .washingtonpost.com/nation/2023/06/06/ajike-aj-owens-shooting -ocala-florida/.

Chapter 6. Anger and Rage

1. Gray J. Watts Riots of 1965 | Factors & Aftermath. Study.com. https:// study.com/learn/lesson/watts-riots-1965-causes-aftermath-los -angeles.html#:~:text=The%20riots%20began%20due%20to,National %20Guard%20instated%20a%20curfew.

2. Villarosa L. *Under the Skin: Racism, Inequality, and the Health of a Nation.* Scribe Publications; 2022:116.

3. Grier WH, Cobbs PM. *Black Rage: Two Black Psychiatrists Reveal the Full Dimensions of the Inner Conflicts and the Desperation of Black Life in the United States.* Basic Books; 1968/1980:205.

4. Grier WH, Cobbs PM. *Black Rage: Two Black Psychiatrists Reveal the Full Dimensions of the Inner Conflicts and the Desperation of Black Life in the United States.* Basic Books; 1968/1980:181–199.

5. Haley A. Alex Haley's 1965 Playboy Interview with Rev. Martin Luther King Jr. *Daily Beast.* January 19, 2014. https://www.thedailybeast.com /alex-haleys-1965-playboy-interview-with-rev-martin-luther-king-jr.

6. Cornel West, "Malcolm X and Black Rage," as quoted by hooks b. *Writing Beyond Race: Living Theory and Practice.* Routledge; 2013: 18–19.

7. Tutu D, Tutu M. *The Book of Forgiving: The Fourfold Path for Healing Ourselves and Our World.* Edited by Douglas C. Abrams. Harper Collins; 2014:178–179.

8. Tutu D, Tutu M. *The Book of Forgiving: The Fourfold Path for Healing Ourselves and Our World.* Edited by Douglas C. Abrams. Harper Collins; 2014:108.

9. Cooper B. *Eloquent Rage*. Picador Paperback; 2019:273–275.

10. Yael Danieli, *International Handbook of Multigenerational Legacies of Trauma*, as quoted by DeGruy J. *Post-Traumatic Slave Syndrome: America's Legacy of Enduring Injury and Healing*. Uptone Press; 2005/2017:104.

11. Chemaly S. *Rage Becomes Her: The Power of Women's Anger*. Atria Books; 2018.

12. Tutu D, Tutu M. *The Book of Forgiving: The Fourfold Path for Healing Ourselves and Our World*. Edited by Douglas C. Abrams. Harper Collins; 2014:179.

13. Blake, J. Why Obama doesn't dare become the "angry black man." *CNN*. June 9, 2010. https://www.cnn.com/2010/POLITICS/06/08/rage.obama/index.html.

14. Morgan T. The NRA supported gun control when the Black Panthers had the weapons. March 22, 2018. https://www.history.com/news/Black-panthers-gun-control-nra-support-mulford-act.

15. Burrough B. *Days of Rage: America's Radical Underground, the FBI, and the Forgotten Age of Revolutionary Violence*. Penguin Books; 2016.

16. Brownlee D. If America is "beyond racism," why does Ketanji Brown Jackson's Supreme Court nomination seem like a miracle? *Forbes.com*. March 2021. https://www.forbes.com/sites/danabrownlee/2022/03/21/if-america-is-beyond-racism-why-does-ketanji-brown-jacksons-supreme-court-nomination-seem-like-a-miracle/?sh=d139ded3fcbf.

17. Reinhard B, Dawsey J. How a Trump-allied group fighting "anti-white bigotry" beats Biden in court. *Washington Post*. December 12, 2022. https://www.washingtonpost.com/politics/2022/12/12/stephen-miller-america-first-legal-biden-race-policies/.

18. Kessler G. Stephen Miller's disingenuous ad charging "anti-White" racism. *Washington Post*. November 4, 2022. https://www.washingtonpost.com/politics/2022/11/04/stephen-millers-disingenuous-ad-charging-anti-white-racism/.

19. Anderson C. *White Rage: The Unspoken Truth of Our Racial Divide*. Bloomsbury; 2017.

20. Cineas F. White rage won't just go away. *Vox*. January 27, 2021. https://www.vox.com/22243875/white-rage-white-nationalism.

21. Michael Kimmel, as interviewed by Simons S. The one thing all angry men have in common. *Fatherly.com*. May 4, 2023. https://www.fatherly.com/life/anger-management-expert-why-men.

22. Conroy JO. "Angry white men": the sociologist who studied Trump's base before Trump. *Guardian*. February 27, 2017. https://www.theguardian.com/world/2017/feb/27/michael-kimmel-masculinity-far-right-angry-white-men.

23. Collins O. *Speeches That Changed the World*. Westminster John Knox Press; 1998:208.
24. LeVine M. Trump calls political enemies "vermin," echoing dictators Hitler, Mussolini. *Washington Post*. November 13, 2023. https://www .washingtonpost.com/politics/2023/11/12/trump-rally-vermin -political-opponents/.

Chapter 7. Trust and Mistrust

1. Cooper B. *Eloquent Rage*. Picador Paperback; 2019:262.
2. Bates KG. Is it genocide? *Essence*. 1990;76–78(116):118. Quoted by Gamble VN. Under the shadow of Tuskegee: African Americans and healthcare. *Am J Public Health*. 1997;87(11):1773-1778.
3. Heller J. Rumors and realities: making sense of HIV/AIDS conspiracy narratives and contemporary legends. *Am J Public Health*. 2015;105(1):e43-e50. doi:10.2105/AJPH.2014.302284.
4. McClay C. The story of historically black colleges in the US. *BBC*. February 15, 2019. https://www.bbc.com/news/world-us-canada -47234239.
5. Beard KV, Julion WA. Does race still matter in nursing? The narratives of African-American nursing faculty members. *Nurs Outlook*. 2016;64(6):583–596. doi:10.1016/j.outlook.2016.06.005.
6. Hudson B, Campbell KM. Does criticism of minority faculty result from a lack of senior leadership training and accountability? *Acad Med*. 2020;95(12):1792. doi:10.1097/ACM.0000000000003735.
7. SD Gould. Trust, distrust, and trustworthiness. *J Gen Intern Med*. 2002;17(1):79-81.
8. Hall MA, Dugan E, Zheng B, Mishra AK. Trust in physicians and medical institutions: what is it, can it be measured, and does it matter. *Milbank Q*. 2001;79(4):613-639.
9. Pearson D, Raeke LH. Patients' trust in physicians: many theories, few measures, and little data. *J Gen Intern Med*. 2000;15(7):509-513.
10. Egede LE, Ellis C. Development and testing of the multidimensional trust in HealthCare Systems Scale. *J Gen Intern Med*. 2008;23(6):808-815.
11. Mosely KL, Freed GL, Bullard CM, Goold SD. Measuring African-American parents' cultural mistrust while in a healthcare setting: a pilot study. *J Natl Med Assoc*. 2007;99(1):15-21.
12. LaVeist TA, Nickerson KJ, Bowie JV. Attitudes about racism, medical mistrust, and satisfaction with care among African American and White cardiac patients. *Med Care Res Rev*. 2000;57(1)(suppl): 146-161.
13. Obama M. *Becoming*. Crown Books; 2018.

14. Adams LB, Richmond J, Corbie-Smith G, Powell W. Medical mistrust and colorectal cancer screening among African Americans. *J Community Health*. 2017;42(5):1044–1061. doi:10.1007/s10900-017-0339-2.

15. Mullins MA, Peres LC, Alberg AJ, et al. Perceived discrimination, trust in physicians, and prolonged symptom duration before ovarian cancer diagnosis in the African American Cancer Epidemiology Study. *Cancer*. 2019;125(24):4442–4451. doi:10.1002/cncr.32451.

16. Birkhäuer J, Gaab J, Kossowsky J, et al. Trust in the health care professional and health outcome: a meta-analysis. *PLoS One*. February 7, 2017. https://doi.org/10.1371/journal.pone.0170988. As mentioned in https://www.modernhealthcare.com/opinion-editorial/commentary-erosion-trust-threatens-essential-element-practicing-medicine.

17. Losin EAR, Woo CW, Medina NA, Andrews-Hanna JR, Eisenbarth H, Wager TD. Neural and sociocultural mediators of ethnic differences in pain [published correction appears in *Nat Hum Behav*. 2020;4(6): 656–658]. *Nat Hum Behav*. 2020;4(5):517–530. doi:10.1038/s41562-020-0819-8.

18. Hoffman KM, Trawalter S, Axt JR, Oliver MN. Racial bias in pain assessment and treatment recommendations, and false beliefs about biological differences between Blacks and whites. *Proc Natl Acad Sci U S A*. 2016;113(16):4296–4301. doi:10.1073/pnas.1516047113.

19. Wiltshire JC, Person SD, Allison J. Exploring differences in trust in doctors among African American men and women. *J Natl Med Assoc*. 2011;103(9–10):845–851. doi:10.1016/s0027-9684(15)30439-9.

20. Lynn B, Yoo GJ, Levine EG. "Trust in the Lord": religious and spiritual practices of African American breast cancer survivors. *J Relig Health*. 2014;53(6):1706–1716. doi:10.1007/s10943-013-9750-x.

21. Benkert R, Hollie B, Nordstrom CK, Wickson B, Bins-Emerick L. Trust, mistrust, racial identity and patient satisfaction in urban African American primary care patients of nurse practitioners. *J Nurs Scholarsh*. 2009;41(2):211–219. doi:10.1111/j.1547-5069.2009.01273.x.

22. Nazione S, Perrault EK, Keating DM. Finding common ground: can provider-patient race concordance and self-disclosure bolster patient trust, perceptions, and intentions? *J Racial Ethn Health Disparities*. 2019;6(5):962–972. doi:10.1007/s40615-019-00597-6.

23. Lynn B, Yoo GJ, Levine EG. "Trust in the Lord": religious and spiritual practices of African American breast cancer survivors. *J Relig Health*. 2014;53(6):1706–1716. doi:10.1007/s10943-013-9750-x.

24. Sullivan LS. Trust, risk, and race in American medicine. *Hastings Center Rep*. 2020;50(1):18–26. doi:10.1002/hast.1080.

25. Sullivan LS. Trust, risk, and race in American medicine. *Hastings Center Rep.* 2020;50(1):18–26. doi:10.1002/hast.1080.

26. Commonwealth Fund. Understanding and ameliorating medical mistrust among Black Americans. January 14, 2021. https://www .commonwealthfund.org/publications/newsletter-article/2021/jan /medical-mistrust-among-black-americans.

27. AAMC. Principles of trustworthiness. https://www.aamc.org/trust worthiness#principles.

28. Sullivan LS. Trust, risk, and race in American medicine. *Hastings Center Rep.* 2020;50(1):18–26. doi:10.1002/hast.1080.

29. Graham JL, Giordano TP, Grimes RM, Slomka J, Ross M, Hwang LY. Influence of trust on HIV diagnosis and care practices: a literature review. *J Int Assoc Physicians AIDS Care.* 2010;9(6):346–352. doi:10.1177 /1545109710380461.

30. Jamison AM, Quinn SC, Freimuth VS. "You don't trust a government vaccine": narratives of institutional trust and influenza vaccination among African American and white adults. *Soc Sci Med.* 2019;221: 87–94. doi:10.1016/j.socscimed.2018.12.020.

31. Bogart LM, Ojikutu BO, Tyagi K, et al. COVID-19 related medical mistrust, health impacts, and potential vaccine hesitancy among Black Americans living with HIV. *J Acquir Immune Defic Syndr.* 2021;86(2):200–207. doi:10.1097/QAI.0000000000002570.

32. Corbie-Smith G, Thomas SB, St George DM. Distrust, race, and research. *Arch Intern Med.* 2002;162(21):2458–2463. doi:10.1001/ archinte.162.21.2458.

33. Cunningham A. Medical racism didn't begin or end with the syphilis study at Tuskegee. *ScienceNews.* December 20, 2022. https://www .sciencenews.org/article/tuskegee-syphilis-study-medical-racism.

34. Gamble VN. Under the shadow of Tuskegee: African Americans and health care. *Am J Public Health.* 1997;87(11):1773–1778. doi:10.2105/ ajph.87.11.1773.

35. Corbie-Smith G, Thomas SB, Williams MV, Moody-Ayers S. Attitudes and beliefs of African Americans toward participation in medical research. *J Gen Intern Med.* 1999;14(9):537–546.

36. AAMC. Principles of trustworthiness. https://www.aamc.org/trust worthiness#principles.

37. Prevention Research Center at Morehouse School of Medicine. Community values. https://www.msm.edu/Research/research _centersandinstitutes/PRC/communityPartnerships/community values.php.

38. MacDonald G. https://www.brainyquote.com/topics/trust-quotes.

Chapter 8. Respect and Disrespect

1. Ellison R. *Invisible Man*. Random House; 1952/1995:1.
2. Ellison R. *Invisible Man*. Random House; 1952/1995:1.
3. Lena Williams. *It's the Little Things: Everyday Interactions That Anger, Annoy, and Divide the Races*. Harcourt, Inc.; 2000.
4. African Studies Center, University of Pennsylvania. Letter from a Birmingham Jail [King, Jr.]. https://www.africa.upenn.edu/Articles _Gen/Letter_Birmingham.html.
5. Dr. Carrie Rosario asked a Greensboro, N.C. official to call her 'doctor.' He refused. *Lily*. https://www.thelily.com/a-white-city-official-refused -to-address-this-Black-professor-as-doctor-he-got-fired/.
6. Ritterhouse J. *Growing Up Jim Crow: How Black and White Southern Children Learned Race*. University of North Carolina Press; 2006.
7. Davis RLF. *Racial Etiquette: The Racial Customs and Rules of Racial Behaviour in Jim Crow America*. California State University, Northridge. https://files.nc.gov/dncr-moh/jim%20crow%20etiquette.pdf.
8. Glasgow J. Racism as disrespect. *Ethics*. 2009;120(1):64–93. https:// www.journals.uchicago.edu/doi/full/10.1086/648588#xref_fn8.
9. Jagsi R, Griffith K, Krenz C, et al. Workplace harassment, cyber incivility, and climate in academic medicine. *JAMA*. 2023;329(21): 1848–1858. doi:10.1001/jama.2023.7232.
10. Douglas PS. Disrespectful conduct in the medical profession: we have met the enemy and they are us. *JAMA*. 2023;329(21):1829–1831. doi:10.1001/jama.2023.3694.
11. Thomas KL, Mehta LS, Rzeszut AK, Lewis SJ, Duvernoy CS, Douglas PS; ACC Diversity and Inclusion Task Force and ACC Women in Cardiology Section. Perspectives of racially and ethnically diverse US cardiologists: insights from the ACC professional life survey. *J Am Coll Cardiol*. 2021;78(17):1746–1750. doi:10.1016/j.jacc.2021.09.002.
12. Thomson J. BigThink.com. September 2022. https://bigthink.com /thinking/epistemic-injustice-prejudice/.
13. Briggs H, Kothari B, Briggs AC, Bank L, DeGruy J. Initial testing of the Racial Respect Scale for Adult African Americans. *J Soc Soc Work Res*. 2015;6(2):269–302. doi:10.1086/681625.

Chapter 9. Consider Culture and Show Respect

1. Portions of this chapter were originally published in *Ethnicity and Disease*: Rust G, Kondwani K, Martinez R, et al. A crash-course in cultural competence. *Ethn Dis*. 2006;16(2)(suppl 3):29–36.
2. The Core Collaborative Learning Lab. Beyond the Surface: Exploring the Iceberg of Culture, 2024. https://thecorecollaborative.com /beyond-the-surface-exploring-the-iceberg-of-culture/.

3. Berlin EA, Fowkes WC Jr. A teaching framework for cross-cultural health care. Application in family practice. *West J Med.* 1983;139(6):934–938.

4. Steele D, Harrison J. Challenging Physician-Patient Interactions (Self-Study Guide). American Academy of Family Physicians; 2002.

5. Kleinman A. *Patients and Healers in the Context of Culture: An Exploration of the Borderland Between Anthropology, Medicine, and Psychiatry.* University of California Press; 1980.

6. Kendi IX. Introduction. In: Kendi IX, Blain KN, eds. *Four Hundred Souls.* One World; 2022:xiv.

7. Morukian M. *Diversity Equity and Inclusion for Trainers: Fostering DEI in the Workplace.* ATD Press; 2022:215–216.

8. Edwards J. Michelle Obama says Americans weren't ready for her natural Black hair. *Washington Post.* November 17, 2022. https://www.washingtonpost.com/nation/2022/11/17/michelle-obama-Black-hair-braids/.

9. ACLU. My son's hair is part of a thousand-year-old tribal culture. His school called it a "fad." https://www.aclu.org/news/racial-justice/my-sons-hair-is-part-of-a-thousand-year-old-tribal-culture-his-school-called-it-a-fad.

10. Johnson RL, Saha S, Arbelaez JJ, Beach MC, Cooper LA. Racial and ethnic differences in patient perceptions of bias and cultural competence in health care. *J Gen Intern Med.* 2004;19(2):101–110.

11. Kennedy BP, Kawachi I, Lochner K, Jones C, Prothrow-Stith D. (Dis)respect and black mortality. *Ethn Dis.* 1997 Autumn;7(3):207–214.

12. Morrison T, Conaway WA. *Kiss, Bow, or Shake Hands, 2nd Edition: The Bestselling Guide to Doing Business in More Than 60 Countries Paperback—Illustrated.* Adams Media; 2006.

13. Deborah Tannen, as quoted by Xu N. In real life, not all interruptions are rude. *New York Times.* September 25, 2021. https://www.nytimes.com/2021/09/25/opinion/interrupting-cooperative-overlapping.html.

Chapter 10. Assess and Affirm Differences

1. McLaren BD. *A Generous Orthodoxy.* Zondervan; 2004:28.

2. Madaras L, Stonington S, Seda CH, Garcia D, Zuroweste E. Social distance and mobility—a 39-year-old pregnant migrant farmworker. *N Engl J Med.* 2019;380(12):1093–1096. doi:10.1056/NEJMp1811501.

3. Rosado J. *After the Harvest: A Story About Saying Goodbye.* http://www.fsustress.org/separation.html

4. Alvarez J. *How the Garcia Girls Lost Their Accents.* Algonquin Books; 1991:293.

5. Fadiman A. *The Spirit Catches You and You Fall Down: A Hmong Child, Her American Doctors, and the Collision of Two Cultures.* Farrar, Straus and Giroux; 2012.

6. Dr. Seuss. *Oh the Places You'll Go.* Random House Books for Young Readers; 1990.

7. Niebuhr R. The original Serenity Prayer as cited in Proactive 12 Steps. https://proactive12steps.com/serenity-prayer/.

Chapter 11. Show Sensitivity

1. Short-Handled Hoe. Behind the Scenes with the curators of the National Museum of American History. https://objectofhistory.org/objects/brieftour/shorthandledhoe/index.html.

2. Centers for Medicare & Medicaid Services. Accountable Health Communities (AHC) model evaluation: first evaluation report. https://innovation.cms.gov/data-and-reports/2020/ahc-first-eval-rpt.

3. Resnicow K, Baranowski T, Ahluwalia JS, Braithwaite RL. Cultural sensitivity in public health: defined and demystified. *Ethn Dis.* 1999;9(1):10–21.

4. Williams L. *It's the Little Things: Everyday Interactions That Anger, Annoy, and Divide the Races.* Harcourt, Inc.; 2000.

5. CROWN Coalition. The official campaign of The CROWN Act led by the CROWN Coalition. https://www.thecrownact.com/.

6. Senate Republicans Block Passage of CROWN Act. December 14, 2022. https://watsoncoleman.house.gov/newsroom/press-releases/senate-republicans-block-passage-of-crown-act.

7. Katsha H. Microaggressions are the "norm" for Black people at work. Here's proof. *HuffPost.* July 14, 2022. https://www.huffingtonpost.co.uk/entry/microaggressions-the-norm-for-Black-people-at-work_uk_62cfca25e4b007c97c86f9b0.

8. Sue DW, Capodilupo CM, Torino GC, et al. Racial microaggressions in everyday life: implications for clinical practice. *Am Psychol.* 2007;62(4):271–286. doi:10.1037/0003-066X.62.4.271.

9. Pierce C, Carew J, Pierce-Gonzalez D, Willis D. An experiment in racism: TV commercials. In: Pierce C, ed. *Television and Education.* Sage; 1978:62–88.

10. Sue DW, Spanierman LB. *Microaggressions in Everyday Life.* 2nd ed. John Wiley; 2020, chap. 1, p. 3.

11. Sue DW. Microaggressions: "Death by a thousand cuts." *Sci Am.* Special edition. Summer 2021;30(3s):48–49.

12. Sloss M. Latine people are sharing the "unwritten rules" they follow that other people are clueless about. *Buzzfeed.* https://www.buzzfeed.com/morgansloss1/latine-people-unwritten-rules.

13. Black patients dress up and modify speech to reduce bias, California Health Care Foundation Survey. March 2023. https://sacobserver.com /2023/03/Black-patients-dress-up-and-modify-speech-to-reduce-bias -california-survey-shows/.

14. Torres-Harding SR, Andrade AL, Romero Diaz CE. The Racial Microaggressions Scale (RMAS): a new scale to measure experiences of racial microaggressions in people of color. *Cultur Divers Ethnic Minor Psychol.* 2012;18(2):153–164. doi:10.1037/a0027658.

15. Grant G. What is racial battle fatigue? A school psychologist explains. *The Conversation; Triad City Beat.* January 14, 2023. https://triad-city -beat.com/what-is-racial-battle-fatigue-a-school-psychologist -explains/.

16. Rude comments and bottom slaps: the things female doctors put up with. *The Washington Post.* May 23, 2023. https://www.washingtonpost .com/wellness/2023/05/23/women-doctors-mistreatment-obuobi/.

17. Lighthouse. 7 Microaggressions trans people face in health and mental healthcare settings. https://blog.lighthouse.lgbt/transgender-health care-microaggressions/.

18. University of Edinburgh. Common trans and/or non-binary based microaggressions. February 8, 2021. https://www.ed.ac.uk/equality -diversity/students/microaggressions/lgbtq-microaggressions/trans -and-or-non-binary-microaggressions/commontrans-and-non-binary -based-microaggression.

19. Borresen K. 14 Microaggressions LGBTQ people deal with all the time. *HuffPost.* 2021. https://www.huffpost.com/entry/microaggressions -lgbtq-people-deal-with_l_60c12080e4b059c73bd556e2.

20. Guthrie J. Rosalynn Carter—advocate for the mentally ill. *San Francisco Chronicle.* August 11, 2010. https://www.sfgate.com/entertain ment/article/Rosalynn-Carter-Advocate-for-the-mentally-ill-31782 70.php.

21. Barber S, Gronholm PC, Ahuja S, Rüsch N, Thornicroft G. Microaggressions towards people affected by mental health problems: a scoping review. *Epidemiol Psychiatr Sci.* 2019;29:e82. doi:10.1017/ S2045796019000763.

Chapter 12. Nurture Self-Awareness and Humility

1. Tangermann V. GPT-4 was deeply racist before OpenAI muzzled it. *Futurism.* March 30, 2023. https://futurism.com/gpt-4-deeply-racist -before-openai-muzzled-it.

2. Braswell P. Code-switching may be a survival strategy but "culture coding" can be a superpower. *FastCompany.com.* June 21, 2022. https://www.fastcompany.com/90761872/code-switching-may-be-a

-survival-strategy-but-culture-coding-can-be-a-superpower
?partner=rss.

3. Dyson ME. *The Tears We Cannot Stop*. St. Martin's Griffin Edition, St. Martin's Press; 2021:65–66.

4. Hughes L. *The Ways of White Folks*. Vintage Books; 1933/1990.

5. Dyson ME. *The Tears We Cannot Stop*. St. Martin's Griffin Edition, St. Martin's Press; 2021:135.

6. Waxman SR. Racial awareness and bias begin early: developmental entry points, challenges, and a call to action. *Perspect Psychol Sci*. 2021;16(5):893–902. doi:10.1177/17456916211026968.

7. DiAngelo R. *White Fragility: Why It's So Hard for White People to Talk About Racism*. Beacon Press; 2018.

8. Ellison R. *Invisible Man*. Random House; 1952/1995:1.

9. Love S. White people who got placebo from white doctors felt better, study says. *Vice.com*. August 9, 2022. https://www.vice.com/en/article /g5vyxb/white-people-who-got-placebo-from-white-doctors-felt -better-study-says.

10. Dyson ME. *The Tears We Cannot Stop*. St. Martin's Griffin Edition, St. Martin's Press; 2021:67.

11. Nordell J. *The End of Bias: A Beginning: The Science and Practice of Overcoming Unconscious Bias*. Metropolitan; 2021.

12. Tervalon M, Murray-García J. Cultural humility versus cultural competence: a critical distinction in defining physician training outcomes in multicultural education. *J Health Care Poor Underserved*. 1998 May;9(2):117–125.

Chapter 13. Inner Healing

1. Hemfelt R, Minirth F, Meier P. *We Are Driven: The Compulsive Behaviors America Applauds*. Thomas Nelson; 1991.

2. Brin D. Self-addiction and self-righteousness. In: Oakley B, Knafo A, Madhavan G, Wilson DS, eds. *Pathologic Altruism*. Oxford University Press; 2012:77.

3. McGrath M, Oakley B. Codependency and pathological altruism. In: Oakley B, Knafo A, Madhavan G, Wilson DS, eds. *Pathologic Altruism*. Oxford University Press; 2012:58.

4. Widiger TA, Crego C. The Five Factor Model of personality structure: an update. *World Psychiatry*. September 9, 2019. https://doi.org/10 .1002/wps.20658.

5. Farmer P. *To Repair the World: Paul Farmer Speaks to the Next Generation*. University of California Press; 2013.

6. Kidder T. *Mountains Beyond Mountains*. Random House; 2004.

7. King R. *Mindful of Race: Transforming Racism from the Inside Out.* SoundsTrue; 2018.

8. Menakem R. *My Grandmother's Hands: Racialized Trauma and the Pathway to Mending Our Hearts and Bodies.* Central Recovery Press; 2017.

9. Magee R. *The Inner Work of Racial Justice.* TarcherPerigree; 2019:100.

10. Attributed to Michele McDonald, as cited by King R. *Mindful of Race: Transforming Racism from the Inside Out.* Sounds True; 2018:109.

11. King R. *Mindful of Race: Transforming Racism from the Inside Out.* Sounds True; 2018:93.

Chapter 14. Relational Healing

1. Coates T-N. *We Were Eight Years in Power: An American Tragedy.* One World; 2017.

2. Malcolm X, as quoted by Boykin K. *Race Against Time: The Politics of a Darkening America.* Bold Type Books; 2021:11.

3. bell hooks, *All About Love,* as quoted by Asare JG. Five bell hooks quotes to carry with you while trying to create a more equitable world. *Forbes.* December 15, 2021. https://www.forbes.com/sites/janice gassam/2021/12/15/five-bell-hooks-quotes-to-carry-with-you-while -trying-to-create-a-more-equitable-world/?sh=71c4ca246f29.

4. Tutu D. Ubuntu: on the nature of human community. In: *God Is Not a Christian.* Rider; 2011. E-book. As quoted in https://www.lookingfor wisdom.com/ubuntu/.

5. Tutu D, Tutu M. *The Book of Forgiving: The Fourfold Path for Healing Ourselves and Our World.* Edited by Douglas C. Abrams. HarperCollins Publishers; 2014:198.

6. Tutu D, Tutu M. *The Book of Forgiving: The Fourfold Path for Healing Ourselves and Our World.* Edited by Douglas C. Abrams. HarperCollins Publishers; 2014:5.

7. Tutu D, Tutu M. *The Book of Forgiving: The Fourfold Path for Healing Ourselves and Our World.* Edited by Douglas C. Abrams. HarperCollins Publishers; 2014:190.

8. Dyson ME. *The Tears We Cannot Stop.* St. Martin's Griffin Edition, St. Martin's Press; 2021:46, 67.

9. James Cone, *God of the Oppressed,* as quoted by Wallis J. Why James Cone was the most important theologian of his time. *Sojourners.* May 2, 2018. https://sojo.net/articles/why-james-cone-was-most-important -theologian-his-time.

10. DiAngelo R. *White Fragility: Why It's So Hard for White People to Talk About Racism.* Beacon Press; 2018:150.

11. Dyson ME. *The Tears We Cannot Stop*. St. Martin's Griffin Edition, St. Martin's Press; 2021:78.

12. Harris JF, Fletcher MA. Six decades later, an apology. *Washington Post*. May 17, 1997. https://www.washingtonpost.com/archive/politics/1997/05/17/six-decades-later-an-apology/2e196b6a-87af-434a-b151-0a50202fb215/. As quoted by Tuskegee University at https://www.tuskegee.edu/about-us/centers-of-excellence/bioethics-center/coverage-of-the-apology.

13. Tutu D. *No Future Without Forgiveness*. Random House; 1999:218.

14. Tutu D. *No Future Without Forgiveness*. Random House; 1999:125.

15. Meacham J. *His Truth Is Marching On: John Lewis and the Power of Hope*. Random House; 2020:243, 247.

16. Wiesel E. The Nobel Acceptance Speech delivered by Elie Wiesel in Oslo on December 10, 1986. The Elie Wiesel Foundation for Humanity; https://eliewieselfoundation.org/about-elie-wiesel/nobel-prize-speech/.

17. Jerome F. Einstein and racism in America. *Physics Today*. 2005;58(9):54–55. https://doi.org/10.1063/1.2117824.

18. Breen K. What to know about the "Tennessee Three": why were two of the Democratic lawmakers expelled, and what happens now? *CBS News*. April 12, 2023. https://www.cbsnews.com/news/tennessee-expulsion-house-democrats-expelled-what-happens-now/.

19. Lemon D. *This Is the Fire: What I Say to My Friends About Racism*. Little, Brown; 2021:116.

20. Alex Haley's 1965 Playboy interview with Rev. Martin Luther King Jr. *The Daily Beast*. January 19, 2014. https://www.thedailybeast.com/alex-haleys-1965-playboy-interview-with-rev-martin-luther-king-jr.

21. Hope, A. Opinion: if you say you're a trans ally, this is what you have to do. CNN.com, March 31, 2023. https://edition.cnn.com/2023/03/31/opinions/transgender-day-visibility-wellness.

Chapter 15. Structural Healing

1. Dawes D. *The Political Determinants of Health*. Johns Hopkins University Press; 2020.

2. Johnson SK. *Inclusify—The Power of Uniqueness and Belonging to Build Innovative Teams*. HarperCollins; 2020:xiii.

3. Brownlee D. Anti-Racism 101: let's clarify "white privilege" once and for all. *Forbes*. August 16, 2022. https://www.forbes.com/sites/danabrownlee/2022/08/16/dear-white-people-lets-clarify-white-privilege-once-and-for-all/?sh=4bb6f0a156ea.

4. Afshar P, Dominguez C. Fort Lauderdale police chief fired over minority-first practices in hiring and promotions, report says. *CNN*.

March 5, 2022. https://www.cnn.com/2022/03/05/us/fort-lauderdale -police-chief/index.html.

5. Lupton RD. *Toxic Charity: How Churches & Charities Hurt Those They Help.* HarperCollins; 2011:145.

6. Collective Impact Forum. What is collective impact? https:// collectiveimpactforum.org/what-is-collective-impact/.

7. Culture of Health Leaders. National Collaborative for Health Equity. https://cultureofhealth-leaders.org/.

8. Lemon D. *This Is the Fire: What I Say to My Friends About Racism.* Little, Brown; 2021:179.

9. Collins O. *Speeches That Changed the World.* Westminster John Knox Press; 1998:340–341.

10. ACLU. Past legislation affecting LGBTQ rights across the country 2022. January 14, 2022. https://www.aclu.org/documents/legislation -affecting-lgbtq-rights-across-country-2022.

11. Equality Act, H.R. 5, 117th Congress., 1st sess. (March 2, 2021). https://www.congress.gov/bill/117th-congress/house-bill/5.

12. Douglass F. 1869 Composite Nation speech. https://reason.com/volokh /2023/02/04/the-continuing-relevance-of-frederick-douglass/.

13. Rothstein R. *The Color of Law: A Forgotten History of How Our Government Segregated America.* Liveright Publishing (Norton); 2018.

14. https://8cantwait.org/as cited by McKenna S. Beyond de-escalation training. *Sci Am.* Special edition. Summer 2021;30(3s):94–97.

15. Goldstick JE, Cunningham RM, Carter PM. Current causes of death in children and adolescents in the United States. *N Engl J Med.* 2022;386(20):1955–1956. doi:10.1056/NEJMc2201761. Cited by National Institutes of Health. Preventing gun violence, the leading cause of childhood death. https://www.nichd.nih.gov/about/org/od/directors _corner/prev_updates/gun-violence-July2022.

16. Benjamin R. *Viral Justice.* Princeton University Press; 2022:136.

17. Reid TR. *The Healing of America: A Global Quest for Better, Cheaper, and Fairer Health Care.* Penguin Books; 2010.

18. Donohue JM, Cole ES, James CV, Jarlenski M, Michener JD, Roberts ET. The US Medicaid program: coverage, financing, reforms, and implications for health equity. *JAMA.* 2022;328(11):1085–1099. doi:10.1001/jama.2022.14791.

19. Chen AH, Ghaly MA. Medicaid as a driver of health equity. *JAMA.* 2022;328(11):1051–1052. doi:10.1001/jama.2022.14911.

20. Farmer P. *To Repair the World: Paul Farmer Speaks to the Next Generation.* University of California Press; 2013.

21. Ujewe SJ, van Staden WC. Inequitable access to healthcare in Africa: reconceptualising the "accountability for reasonableness framework"

to reflect indigenous principles. *Int J Equity Health*. 2021;20:139. https://doi.org/10.1186/s12939-021-01482-7.

22. Mbali M, Rucell J. African voices in global health: knowledge, creativity, accountability. *Glob Public Health*. 2022;17(12):3993-4001. doi:10.1080/17441692.2022.2139853.
23. Oti SO, Ncayiyana J. Decolonising global health: where are the Southern voices? *BMJ Glob Health*. 2021;6(7):e006576. doi:10.1136/bmjgh-2021-006576.
24. Córdoba-Flores C. Instituciones y políticas de salud pública en la Ciudad de México, de la Colonia al Porfiriato (Institutions and Politics of Mexico's City Public Health, from the Colony to the Porfiriato). *HiSTOReLo. Revista de Historia Regional y Local*. October 2019. https://revistas.unal.edu.co/index.php/historelo/article/view/80770/74886 or https://doi.org/10.15446/historelo.v12n24.80770.
25. Pan American Health Organization. Indigenous and Afro-descendant voices must be front and center of COVID-19 response in the Americas, says PAHO. October 30, 2020. https://www.paho.org/en/news/30-10-2020-indigenous-and-afro-descendant-voices-must-be-front-and-center-covid-19-response.
26. Natarajan M. Moving from cultural competency to decolonizing health care. *Mad in America*. June 28, 2021. https://www.madinamerica.com/2021/06/moving-cultural-competency-decolonizing-health-care/.
27. National Public Radio. Read Martin Luther King Jr.'s "I Have a Dream" speech in its entirety. NPR.org. Updated January 16, 2023. https://www.npr.org/2010/01/18/122701268/i-have-a-dream-speech-in-its-entirety.

Chapter 16. Healing and Hope in the Time of Exhaustion

1. Boykin K. *Race Against Time: The Politics of a Darkening America*. Bold Type Books; 2021:1.
2. Frances-Winter M. *Black Fatigue: How Racism Erodes the Mind, Body, and Spirit*. Berrett-Koehler Publishers; 2020:1-2.
3. Centers for Disease Control and Prevention. FDA and CDC response to the Florida surgeon general. March 10, 2023. https://www.cdc.gov/media/releases/2023/p0313-letter.html.
4. Frances-Winter M. *Black Fatigue: How Racism Erodes the Mind, Body, and Spirit*. Berrett-Koehler Publishers; 2020:ix-x.
5. Frances-Winter M. *Black Fatigue: How Racism Erodes the Mind, Body, and Spirit*. Berrett-Koehler Publishers; 2020:1-2.
6. LinkedIn post by Dr. Sam Rae, E., 2nd CEO & Founder, DSRD Consulting. December 13, 2022.

7. Chief Joseph of the Nez Perce. Collins O. *Speeches That Changed the World*. Westminster John Knox Press; 1998:350.

8. Koopman J, Lanaj K, Lee YE, Alterman V, Bradley C, Stoverink AC. Walking on eggshells: a self-control perspective on workplace political correctness. *J Appl Psychol*. 2023;108(3):425-445. doi:10.1037/apl0001025.

9. Some material adapted from a previously published article: Rust G. Perspective: hope for health equity. *Ethn Dis*. 2017;27(2):117-120. doi:10.18865/ed.27.2.117.

10. Schanzenbach DW, Bauer L. The long-term impact of the Head Start program. Brookings Institute. August 19, 2016. https://www.brookings.edu/articles/the-long-term-impact-of-the-head-start-program/.

11. Levine RS, Rust G, Aliyu M, et al. United States counties with low Black male mortality rates. *Am J Med*. 2013;126(1):76-80. doi:10.1016/j.amjmed.2012.06.019.

12. Booker C. *United: Thoughts on Finding Common Ground and Advancing the Common Good*. Ballantine Books; 2016.

13. The Community Foundation for Greater Atlanta. http://www.cfgreateratlanta.org/Giving/Donor-Stories/The-David-Satcher-Fund1.aspx.

14. Burkhalter H. Fair Food Program helps end the use of slavery in the tomato fields. *Washington Post*. September 2, 2012. https://www.washingtonpost.com/opinions/fair-food-program-helps-end-the-use-of-slavery-in-the-tomato-fields/2012/09/02/788f1a1a-f39c-11e1-892d-bc92fee603a7_story.html.

15. Martin Luther King Jr. (paraphrased from abolitionist minister Theodore Parker's sermon "Of Justice and the Conscience" [in an 1853 compilation of sermons]). http://quoteinvestigator.com/2012/11/15/arc-of-universe/.

16. "The American Dream" July 4th Speech Transcript—Martin Luther King Jr. https://www.rev.com/blog/transcripts/the-american-dream-july-4th-speech-transcript-martin-luther-king-jr.

17. Nehisi-Coates T. *Between the World and Me*. One World (Penguin Random House); 2005.

18. Hughes L. Let America be America again. In: *The Collected Poems of Langston Hughes*. Alfred A. Knopf; 1994. Copyright © 1994 the Estate of Langston Hughes. https://poets.org/poem/let-america-be-america-again.

19. Solomon D. The priest. *New York Times Magazine*. March 4, 2010. http://www.nytimes.com/2010/03/07/magazine/07fob-q4-t.html.

20. Durando J. 15 of Nelson Mandela's best quotes. *USA TODAY.* December 5, 2013. https://www.usatoday.com/story/news/nation-now/2013 /12/05/nelson-mandela-quotes/3775255/.

21. Collins J. Confront the brutal facts (but never lose faith). In: *Good to Great: Why Some Companies Make the Leap . . . and Others Don't.* Harper Collins Publishers; 2001.

22. Fry-Johnson YW, Levine R, Rowley D, Agboto V, Rust G. United States Black:white infant mortality disparities are not inevitable: identification of community resilience independent of socioeconomic status. *Ethn Dis.* 2010;20(1)(suppl 1):131–135.

23. Rust G, Zhang S, Malhotra K, et al. Paths to health equity: local area variation in progress toward eliminating breast cancer mortality disparities, 1990–2009. *Cancer.* 2015;121(16):2765–2774. doi:10.1002/ cncr.29405.

24. Share of adults 65 and over in poverty before and after the effects of Social Security benefits from 2019 to 2021, by state. *Statista.* November 23, 2023. https://www.statista.com/statistics/1318055/share-adults -poverty-before-after-social-security-us/.

25. Elliott D. They're strangers with a painful shared bond: Robert E. Lee enslaved their ancestors. *Morning Edition, NPR.* April 24, 2023. https://www.npr.org/2023/04/24/1171498241/arlington-house-robert -e-lee-reconciliation.

26. Fleischer P, Pellegrino J. Future of education uncertain as DeSantis targets DEI. *WINK News.* April 28, 2023. https://winknews.com/2023 /04/28/future-of-education-uncertain-as-desantis-targets-dei/.

27. Seat D. 100-year-old Martin County woman criticizes Florida's book ban, creates quilt to show opposition. *WPTV.* March 22, 2023. https:// www.wptv.com/news/treasure-coast/region-martin-county/100-year -old-martin-county-woman-criticizes-floridas-book-ban-creates-quilt -to-show-opposition.

28. McMenamin L. Organizers are fighting Ron DeSantis's educational bans with free books. *Teen Vogue.* February 17, 2023. https://www .teenvogue.com/story/fighting-desantis-bans-free-books.

29. City of St. Petersburg receives perfect score on human rights campaign's municipal equality index for ninth consecutive year. St. Petersburg. November 30, 2022. https://www.stpete.org/news_detail_T30 _R578.php.

30. Kentucky governor vetoes sweeping GOP transgender care ban. *PBS NewsHour.* March 24, 2023. https://www.pbs.org/newshour/politics /kentucky-governor-vetoes-sweeping-gop-transgender-care-ban.

31. Jones CP. Levels of racism: a theoretic framework and a gardener's tale. *Am J Public Health*. 2000;90(8):1212–1215. doi:10.2105/ajph .90.8.1212.

32. Perry A. The laughing bishop. *Time*. October 11, 2010. http://content .time.com/time/magazine/article/0,9171,2022647,00.html?iid=sr -link6.

33. C. K. Steele, "Non-Violent Resistance: The Pain and the Promise," as quoted by Alice-Rabby G. *The Pain and the Promise: The Struggle for Civil Rights in Tallahassee, Florida*. University of Georgia Press; 1999/2016:266.

34. Olson RM. Cradling hope. *JAMA*. 2023;329(10):795-796.

INDEX

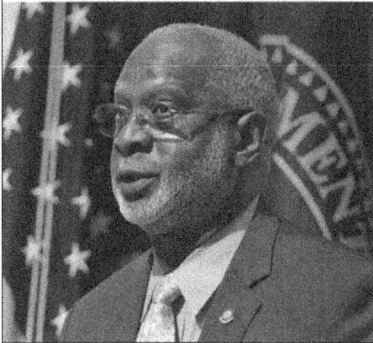